Diagnostic Ultrasound

PRINCIPLES AND INSTRUMENTS

Diagnostic Ultrasound

PRINCIPLES AND INSTRUMENTS

Fourth Edition

Frederick W. Kremkau, Ph.D.

Professor and Director
Center for Medical Ultrasound
Bowman Gray School of Medicine
Wake Forest University
Medical Center Boulevard
Winston-Salem, North Carolina

W.B. SAUNDERS COMPANY
A Division of
Harcourt Brace & Company

Philadelphia   London   Toronto
Montreal   Sydney   Tokyo

W.B. SAUNDERS COMPANY
A Division of
Harcourt Brace & Company

The Curtis Center
Independence Square West
Philadelphia, PA 19106

Library of Congress Cataloging-in-Publication Data

Kremkau, Frederick W.
  Diagnostic ultrasound : principles and instruments /
Frederick W. Kremkau.—4th ed.
    p. cm.
  Includes bibliographical references and index.
  ISBN 0–7216–4308–6
  1. Diagnosis, Ultrasonic. 2. Diagnosis, Ultrasonic—Problems,
exercises, etc. I. Title.
  [DNLM: 1. Ultrasonography. WB 289 K92d]
  RC78.7.U4K745 1993
  616.07′543—dc20
  DNLM/DLC   92–48829

The cover photograph was provided by Advanced Technology Laboratories.

Diagnostic Ultrasound: Principles and Instruments   ISBN   0–7216–4308–6

Printed in the United States of America

Last digit is the print number: 9   8   7   6   5   4   3   2

To Lil

PREFACE

Diagnostic ultrasound includes diagnostic sonography and Doppler ultrasound. Sonography is medical cross-sectional anatomic and flow imaging using pulse-echo ultrasound. This book is written for sonographers, vascular technologists, and sonologists who need a basic knowledge of the physical principles and instrumentation of diagnostic sonography. Its purpose is to explain how diagnostic sonography works. It does not describe how to perform diagnostic examinations or how to interpret the results, except in the consideration of artifacts in Chapter 6. Little background in mathematics and physics is assumed. For the sake of brevity and comprehension, many of the statements made in this book are simplifications of the actual situation.

This book and that listed in Reference 1 are complementary in that this book contains an expansion of Chapter 2 in Reference 1 and Reference 1 contains an expansion of Chapter 5 in this book (Fig. P.1). They are, therefore, companion texts that together cover in detail the principles of both diagnostic sonography and Doppler ultrasound.

Several hundred exercises are provided to check the reader's progress, strengthen concepts, and provide practice for registry and specialty board examinations. Answers are given beginning on page 341. Exercises at the end of each chapter may be used as pretests or posttests to determine knowledge in specific subject areas. A comprehensive multiple-choice examination, with explanatory referenced answers, is presented in Appendix B.

Many of the equations included in previous editions of this text have been eliminated from this edition to make the book less mathematical. The qualitative messages from some of these equations (represented in the previous edition by up and down arrows) have been retained. Only the most basic and important equations have been included in the text of this edition. A more complete set of equations is contained in Appendix A for those desiring more precise mathematical relationships.

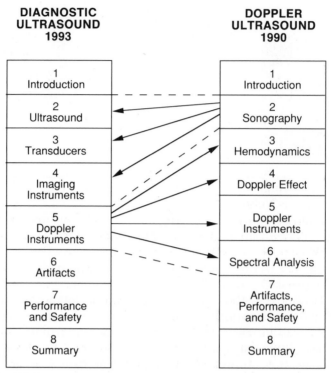

Figure P.1. This book contains an expansion of Chapter 2 in Reference 1, whereas Reference 1 contains an expansion of Chapter 5 in this book.

Superscript numbers refer to citations in the reference list, which begins on page 393.

This fourth edition contains new and expanded material, particularly in the areas of transducer arrays (Chapter 3), temporal and contrast resolution (Chapter 4), Doppler ultrasound (Chapter 5), and safety (Chapter 7). More than 100 new sonographic images are included to enhance the explanation and understanding of principles and concepts. Sections 7.3 and 7.4 are a revision of an earlier chapter on the subject (Reference 35), which was used as a basis for these sections with permission from Mosby–Year Book.

The author gratefully acknowledges helpful comments and suggestions from instructors and students who have used previous editions of the book. These have resulted in clarifications and improvements in the text and exercises. For assistance with figure acquisition, he thanks Gene Adamowski, Pam Burgess, Jackie Carlson, Jackie Challender, George Cook, Larry Crum, Jean Ellison, Tracey Heriot, Sharon Hughes, Teresa

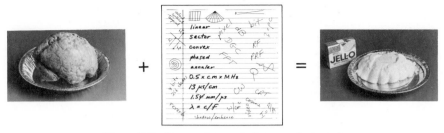

Figure P.2. Your opinion of ultrasound physics?

Jones, Marie King, Dana Meads, Chris Merritt, Mort Miller, Terry Needham, Lewis Nelson, Mohsen Nomeir, Roy Preston, Joe Roselli, Ken Taylor, Paul Tesh, Barbara Weinstein, Neil Wolfman, and the following companies: Acuson, Advanced Technology Laboratories, ATS Laboratories, Bruel and Kjaer, Diasonics, General Electric, Hewlett-Packard, JJ&A Instruments, Medisonics, Nuclear Associates, Nuclear Enterprises, Philips, Radiation Measurements, Inc., Shimadzu, and Siemens/Quantum. He thanks Louise Nixon for typing the manuscript and Marie King and Jo Patterson for proofreading.

Your view of physics might be described by Figure P.2. This book is offered in the hope that, as you read it, you will not only understand the physics of ultrasound but will actually enjoy it (maybe just a little bit)! Best wishes for your professional ultrasound future!

CONTENTS

Diagnostic Ultrasound

PRINCIPLES AND INSTRUMENTS

COLOR
PLATES

PLATE I

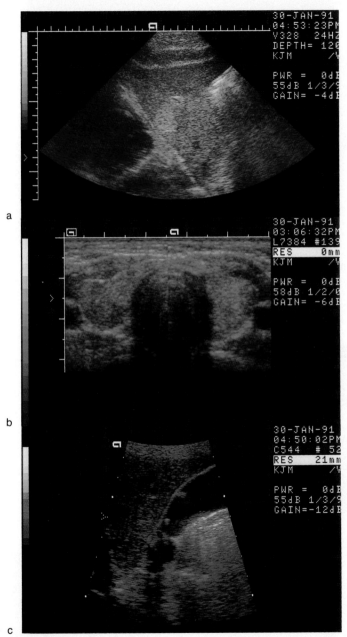

Figure 4.28. Color displays of a hemangioma (*a*) (compare with Fig. 4.27), thyroid (*b*), and gall bladder (*c*). Color assignments, shown in the color bars on the left, are designated as follows: (*a*) temperature (increasing intensity assigned dark orange through yellow to white), (*b*) magenta (dark magenta through light magenta to white), and (*c*) rainbow (dark violet through various colors to white).

PLATE II

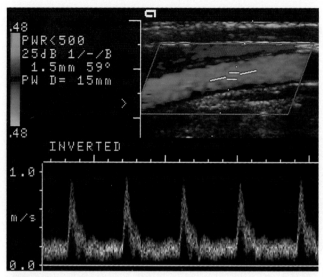

Figure 5.10. Color-flow display of a common carotid artery, including a color-coded pulsed-Doppler spectrum. Colors are assigned to the spectrum according to Doppler shift amplitudes. (Reproduced from Kremkau, F. W.: Doppler principles. Sem. Roentg. *27*: 6–16, 1992, with permission.)

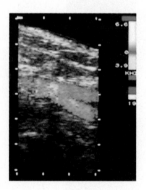

Figure 5.11. Superficial femoral artery and profunda branch flow are shown in color; a wedge was used to avoid 90-degree Doppler angle.

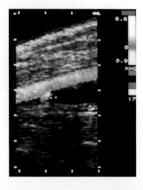

Figure 5.13. The profunda branch off the femoral artery appears to have no flow (no color within it) because of the 90-degree Doppler angle between the scan lines and the flow. Compare this with Figure 5.11, in which the wedge has been reversed.

PLATE III

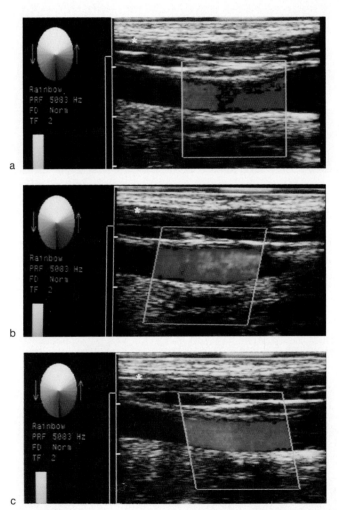

Figure 5.12. Color scan lines are directed (*a*) vertically, (*b*) to the left of vertical, and (*c*) to the right of vertical. Flow is from left to right, producing positive and negative Doppler shifts depending on the relationship between scan lines and flow. (Reproduced from Kremkau, F. W.: Doppler principles. Sem. Roentg. *27*: 6–16, 1992, with permission.)

PLATE IV

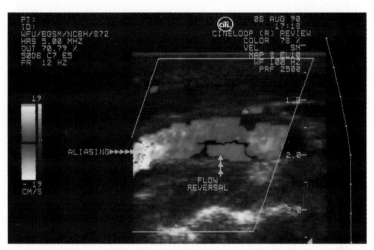

Figure 6.28. Color-flow presentation of common carotid artery flow, including flow reversal and aliasing. The two can be distinguished because the boundary between the different directions with flow reversal passes through the baseline (*black*), whereas the aliasing boundary passes through the upper and lower extremes of the color bar (*white*). In this particular color bar assignment, the maximum positive Doppler shifts are assigned the color green so that there is a thin green region showing the exact boundary where aliasing occurs. The aliasing occurs in the distal portion of the vessel because it is curving down, reducing the Doppler angle between the flow and the scan lines. (Reproduced from Kremkau, F. W.: Doppler principles. Sem. Roentg. *27*: 6–16, 1992, with permission.)

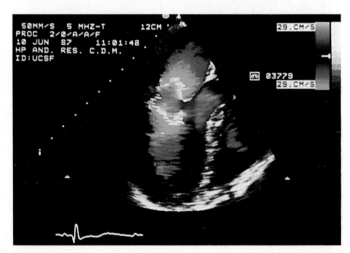

Figure 6.29. Transesophageal cardiac color-flow image of the long axis in diastole. The blue colors between the left atrium and left ventricle represent blood traveling away from the transducer. However, because of high flow speeds through the mitral valve, aliasing has occurred and the yellow and orange colors have replaced the blue colors.

PLATE V

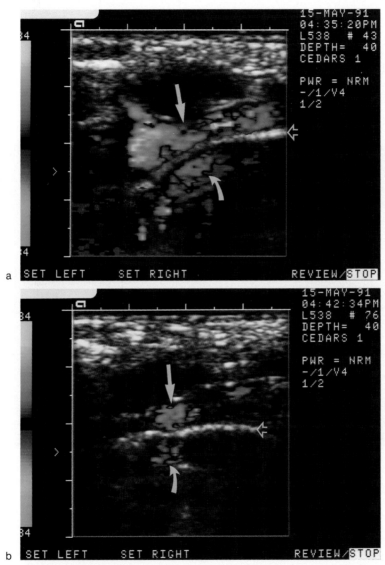

Figure 6.30. Color-flow imaging of the subclavian artery (*straight arrow*) in longitudinal (*a*) and cross-sectional (*b*) views. The pleura (*open arrow*) causes the mirror image (*curved arrow*).

PLATE VI

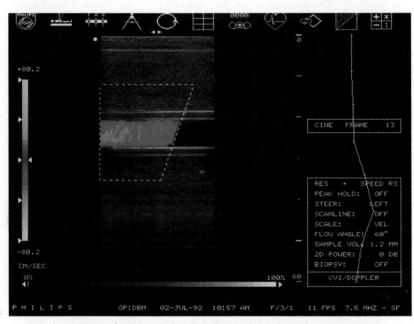

Figure 7.10. (*c*) Color-flow image from flow phantom.

CHAPTER 1

Introduction

This book is intended to help readers understand how diagnostic sonography works, what causes artifacts, and how to scan safely and prudently, conduct instrument performance measurements, and prepare for registry and board examinations.

The word *sonography* comes from the Latin *sonus* (sound) and the Greek *graphein* (to write). Sonography, or more precisely, ultrasonography, means imaging with ultrasound. Diagnostic sonography is medical cross-sectional anatomic and flow imaging using pulse-echo ultrasound.

Ultrasound imaging is not a passive push-button activity. Rather, it is an interactive process involving the sonographer, patient, transducer, instrument, and sonologist. Understanding the physical principles involved contributes to the quality of medical care involving diagnostic sonography.

An image (from the Latin term for "imitate") is a reproduction or imitation of the form of a person or thing. In the ultrasound field, it is the visible counterpart of an object produced by an electronic instrument. In this chapter, we consider the question: How does ultrasound look inside the human body (Fig. 1.1) to image anatomy? Anatomic imaging with ultrasound is accomplished with a pulse-echo technique. Pulses of ultrasound (see Chapter 2) are generated by a transducer (see Chapter 3) and sent into the patient (Fig. 1.2), where they produce echoes at organ boundaries and within tissues. These echoes return to the transducer, where they are detected and then imaged on an instrument (see Chapter 4). The transducer (Fig. 1.3) both generates the ultrasound pulses and detects the returning echoes. Sonography requires knowledge of the location of origin and the strength of the echoes returning from the patient. The ultrasound instrument (Fig. 1.4) processes the echo information and generates appropriate dots, which form the ultrasound image on the display. The brightness of each dot corre-

1

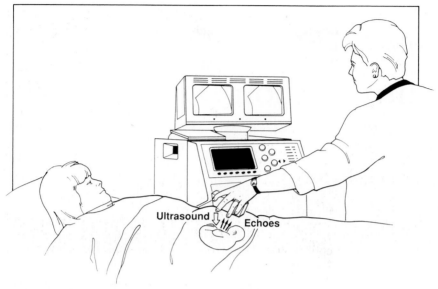

Figure 1.1. Ultrasound provides a window into the human body. (Courtesy of American Institute of Ultrasound in Medicine.)

sponds to the echo strength, producing what is known as a gray-scale image. The location of each dot corresponds to the anatomic location of the echo-generating structure. The positional information is determined by knowing the direction of the pulse when it enters the patient and

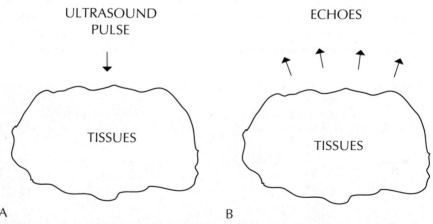

Figure 1.2. (*a*) In diagnostic ultrasound, ultrasound pulses are sent into the tissues to interact with them and obtain information about them. (*b*) Echoes return from the tissues, providing information useful for imaging, flow measurement, and diagnosis.

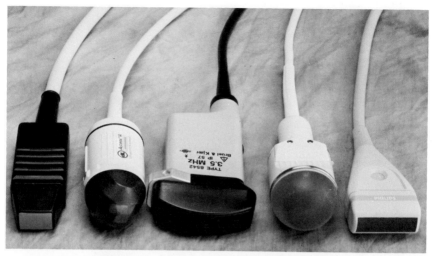

Figure 1.3. Several transducers of various types.

measuring the time for its echo to return to the transducer. From an assumed starting point on the display (usually at the top), the proper location for presenting the echo can then be derived, provided the direction in which to travel from that starting point to the appropriate distance is known. With knowledge of the sound propagation speed, the echo arrival time can be converted to the distance to the structure that produced the echo.

Figure 1.5 shows an image of nylon lines located at two depths in an ultrasound test object (see Chapter 7). Ultrasound instruments use the arrival times of the echoes to locate such objects properly in depth. If one pulse of ultrasound is emitted, one series of dots (one line of information or one scan line) is displayed (Fig. 1.6). Therefore, not all of the

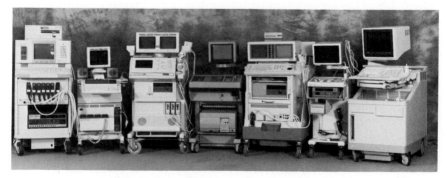

Figure 1.4. Several sonographic instruments.

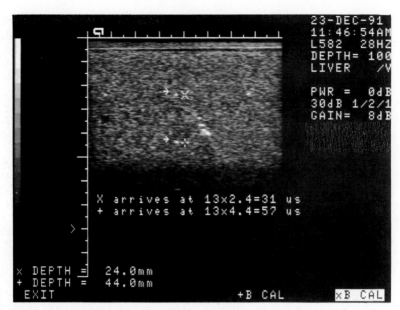

Figure 1.5. An image of nylon lines located at depths of 24 and 44 mm from the transducer in an ultrasound test object. The ultrasound instrument uses the arrival times of the echoes to locate these lines properly in terms of depth. The transducer location is at the top of the image.

ultrasound pulse is reflected back from any interface. Rather, a portion of the original pulse will continue on and be reflected back from deeper interfaces. This is demonstrated in Figure 1.6e, which shows a scan line for a tissue-equivalent ultrasound phantom. If the process is repeated, but with different starting points for each subsequent pulse, a cross-sectional image of the phantom begins to build up (Fig. 1.7). In this case, each pulse travels in the same direction but starts from a different point. This yields parallel scan lines and a rectangular display, as shown in Figure 1.8. This cross-sectional image has been produced with vertical parallel scan lines that are so close together that they cannot be identified individually. The rectangular display resulting from this procedure is often called a linear scan. A second approach to sending ultrasound pulses through the object to be imaged is shown in Figure 1.9. Using this method, each pulse originates from the same starting point, but subsequent pulses go out in slightly different directions from the previous ones. This results in a sector scan, which is shaped like a slice of pie (Fig. 1.10).

Scan formats are commonly limited to two types: linear and sector. Other formats are sometimes used, but in all cases what is required is that ultrasound pulses be sent through all portions of the cross section

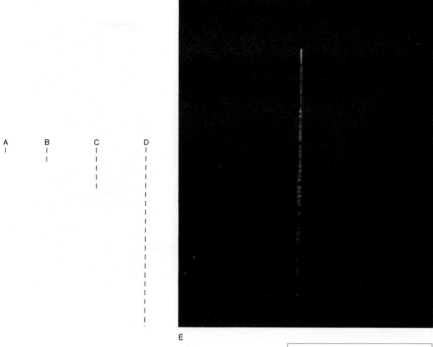

A B C D

E

Figure 1.6. One pulse of ultrasound generates a single scan line (series of echoes) as it travels through tissue. Echoes are presented in sequence on a scan line as they return from tissue as a pulse travels. (*a*) The first echo is displayed. (*b*) The second echo is added. (*c*) Three more echoes are added. (*d*) All the echoes from a single pulse have been received and displayed as a completed scan line. (*e*) A scan line resulting from a pulse traveling into a tissue-equivalent phantom. (*f*) The pulse-echo imaging principle: one pulse traveling through tissues produces a series of echoes that becomes a scan line on the display.

Pulse

↓

Echoes

↓

Scan Line

F

that is to be imaged. Each pulse generates a series of echoes, which results in a series of dots (a scan line) on the display. The resulting cross-sectional image is made up of many (typically around 200) of these scan lines. The scan format determines the starting points and paths for the individual scan lines according to the starting point and path for each pulse used in generating each scan line. Figures 1.8 and 1.10 are examples of clinical cross-sectional gray-scale ultrasound images of the linear and sector types, respectively. These are sometimes called B scans, reflecting the fact that the images are produced by scanning the ultrasound through the imaged cross section (i.e., sending pulses through all

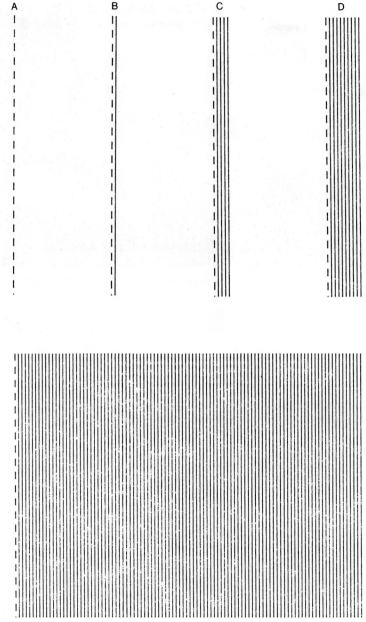

Figure 1.7. A single linear image or scan (frame) is made up of many parallel scan lines; each represents a series of echoes returning from a pulse traveling through the tissues. (*a*) One scan line from one pulse as generated in Figure 1.6. (*b*) A second scan line is added. (*c* and *d*) Five and 10 scan lines, respectively. (*e*) A complete linear frame consisting of (in this example) 100 scan lines.

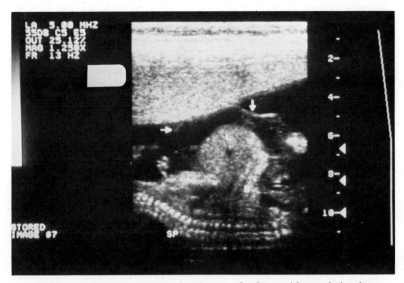

Figure 1.8. Linear (rectangular) image of a fetus with omphalocele.

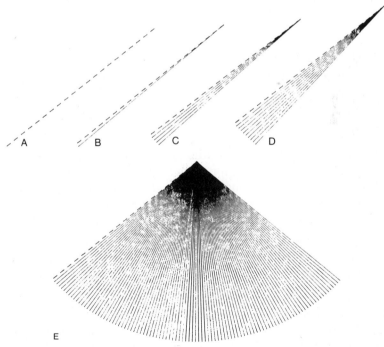

Figure 1.9. A single sector frame is built up by (*a*) 1, (*b*) 2, (*c*) 5, (*d*) 10, and (*e*) 100 scan lines in sequence. These all originate from the same location and travel out in different directions.

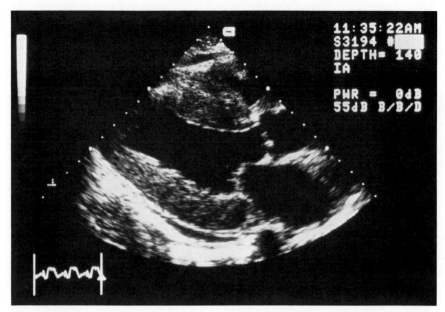

Figure 1.10. Sector image (shaped like a pie slice) of a heart showing left ventricular hypertrophy.

regions of the cross section) and converting echo strength into brightness of each represented echo on the display (hence, B scan, or brightness scan).

If an echo-generating structure is moving, the echo will have a different frequency than that of the pulse emitted from the transducer. This is the Doppler effect, which is put to use in blood flow detection and measurement. The Doppler instrument determines the change in frequency resulting from the motion, converting it to an audible sound and presentation on a display that represents the flow. This topic is covered briefly in Chapter 5 and more extensively in Reference 1. References 2 through 10 are other appropriate sources for the study of the physical principles underlying diagnostic ultrasound.

EXERCISES

1.1 The diagnostic ultrasound imaging (sonography) method has two parts:
  1. Sending _____ of _____ into the body.
  2. Using _____ received from the tissues to produce an _____ of internal structures.

1.2 Ultrasound gray-scale scans are _____-_____ images of tissue cross sections.

1.3 The brightness of an echo, as presented on the display, represents its _____.

1.4 A linear scan is made up of many _____ scan lines.

1.5 A sector scan is made up of many scan lines with a common _____.

1.6 A linear scan has a _____ shape.

1.7 A sector scan is shaped like a _____ of _____.

1.8 Sonography is accomplished by using a _____-_____ technique. The information of importance in doing this is the _____ from which the echo originated and the _____ of the echo. From these, the echo _____ and _____ on the display are determined.

CHAPTER 2

Ultrasound

Ultrasound is like the ordinary sound that we hear except that it has a frequency (discussed in the next section) higher than that to which the human hearing system responds. In this chapter, we consider the following questions: What is ultrasound and how does it behave? How are continuous and pulsed ultrasound described? How is ultrasound weakened as it travels through tissue? How are echoes generated? In addition, the following terms are discussed in this chapter:*

absorption	echo
acoustic	energy
acoustic propagation properties	force
acoustic variables	frequency
amplitude	hertz (Hz)
anechoic	impedance
attenuation	incidence angle
attenuation coefficient	intensity
backscatter	intensity reflection coefficient
compressibility	intensity transmission coefficient
continuous wave (cw)	interference
continuous-wave mode	longitudinal wave
coupling medium	kilohertz (kHz)
cycle	logarithm (log)
decibel (dB)	medium
density	megahertz (MHz)
displacement	oblique incidence
duty factor	particle

---

*Terms listed at the beginning of each chapter are defined in the glossary starting on page 327. Definitions are also given in the review section of each chapter in which the terms are discussed.

particle motion
penetration
period
perpendicular
perpendicular incidence
power
pressure
propagation
propagation speed
pulse
pulse duration
pulse repetition frequency (PRF)
pulse repetition period
pulsed ultrasound
range equation
rarefaction
rayl
reflection
reflection angle

reflector
refraction
scatterer
scattering
sound
spatial pulse length
specular reflection
speed
stiffness
strength
temperature
transmission angle
ultrasound
velocity
wave
wavelength
wave variables
work

2.1
Sound

Sound is a wave. A wave is a propagating (traveling) variation in quantities called wave variables. For example, a water wave is a traveling variation in water surface height (the wave variable in this case). Waves carry energy, not matter, from one place to another. Energy is the capability of doing work. They can also carry information from one place to another, as in radio, television, radiography, and diagnostic ultrasound. Sound is one particular type of wave. It is a propagating variation in quantities called acoustic variables. These acoustic variables include pressure, density, temperature, and particle motion. A particle is a small portion of the medium through which the sound is traveling. Particles oscillate back and forth as a sound wave travels. At any point in the medium, pressure, density, and temperature increase and decrease in repetitive cycles as the sound wave travels. Regions of low pressure and density (rarefactions) and regions of high pressure and density (compressions) travel through the medium in such a wave. Unlike light waves and radio waves, sound requires a medium through which to travel; that is, it cannot pass through a vacuum. Sound is a mechanical longitudinal (compressional) wave in which back-and-forth particle motion is parallel to the direction of wave travel.

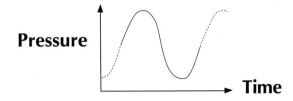

Figure 2.1. One complete variation (cycle) of an acoustic variable (pressure). This variation may repeat as time passes, as indicated by the dashed lines.

Sound is described by a few terms common to all waves. These include frequency, period, wavelength, propagation speed, amplitude, and intensity. Frequency, period, amplitude, and intensity are determined by the sound source. Propagation speed is determined by the medium, and wavelength is determined by both the source and the medium.

Recall that sound is a traveling variation in acoustic variables. Frequency describes how many complete variations (cycles) an acoustic variable goes through in 1 second of time—that is, how many cycles occur in 1 second. Take pressure as an example of an acoustic variable. Pressure may start at its normal (undisturbed) value, increase to a maximum value, return to normal, decrease to a minimum value, and return to normal (Fig. 2.1). This describes a complete cycle of variation of pressure as an acoustic variable. The positive and negative half-cycles are compression and rarefaction, respectively. As a sound wave travels past some point, this cycle is repeated over and over. The number of times that it occurs in 1 second is called the frequency (Fig. 2.2). Thus, frequency is the number of cycles that occur per second.

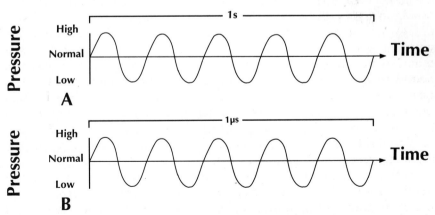

Figure 2.2. Frequency is the number of complete variations (cycles) that an acoustic variable (pressure, in this case) goes through in 1 second. (*a*) Here, five cycles occur in a second; thus, the frequency is five cycles per second, or 5 Hz. (*b*) If five cycles occur within one millionth of a second, also known as a microsecond (1 μs) (i.e., 5 million cycles occurring within a second), the frequency is 5 MHz.

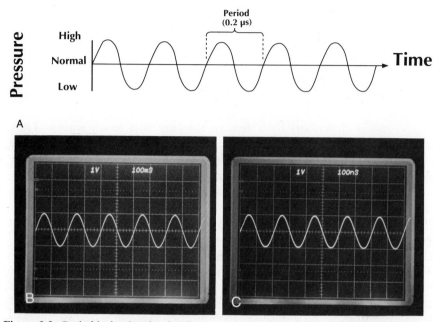

Figure 2.3. Period is the time it takes for one cycle to occur. (*a*) Here, each cycle occurs in 0.2 *μ*s, so the period is 0.2 *μ*s. If one cycle takes 0.2 (one fifth) millionths of a second to occur, then five million cycles occur in a second, so the frequency is 5 MHz. (*b*) Photograph of a tracing of a 5-Hz electric voltage. The total screen width represents 1 second of time. It can be seen that five cycles occur in 1 second. (*c*) If five cycles occur in 1 *μ*s, the period is 0.2 *μ*s and the frequency is 5 MHz. In this tracing, the total screen width is 1 *μ*s. In this example, it can be seen that one cycle occurs in 0.2 *μ*s.

Frequency units include hertz (Hz) and megahertz (MHz). One hertz is one cycle per second, or one complete variation per second. *Mega* comes from the Greek *megas*, meaning great or large. Specifically, in the metric system of units, it means 1 million. Therefore, 1 MHz is 1,000,000 Hz.

Sound having a frequency of less than 20 Hz (Fig. 2.3*b*) is called infrasound because its frequency is too low for human hearing (infra meaning below). Sound with a frequency of 20,000 Hz or higher (Fig. 2.3*c*) is called ultrasound (ultra meaning beyond) because its frequency is too high for human hearing (the range of which is approximately 20 to 20,000 Hz). These cases are analogous to infrared and ultraviolet light, which are lower and higher in frequency, respectively, than the human eye can see. (In vision, light frequency is perceived as color; the lowest and highest frequency of light that we can see are perceived as red and violet, respectively). The importance of frequency will be clearer

TABLE 2.1

Common Ultrasound Periods and
Wavelengths* in Tissue

Frequency (MHz)	Period (μs)	Wavelength (mm)
2.0	0.50	0.77
3.5	0.29	0.44
5.0	0.20	0.31
7.5	0.13	0.21
10.0	0.10	0.15

*Assuming a propagation speed of 1.54 mm/μs
(1540 m/s).

later, when image resolution and imaging depth (penetration) are considered.

Period is the time that it takes for one cycle to occur (Fig. 2.3). Period units are commonly microseconds (μs). One microsecond is one millionth of a second (0.000001 second). The importance of period will become more apparent when pulsed ultrasound is considered in the next section. A list of common periods is given in Table 2.1. Period decreases as frequency increases.* As more cycles are packed into one second, there is less time (period) for each one.

> frequency ↑   period ↓ †

Wavelength is the length of space over which one cycle occurs (Fig. 2.4). If we could stop the sound wave, visualize it, and measure the distance from the beginning to the end of one cycle, the measured distance would be the wavelength. It is really the cycle length, but traditionally it has been called wavelength. It is commonly expressed in millimeters (mm). One millimeter is one thousandth of a meter (0.001 m). The importance of wavelength will be evident when image detail resolution is considered in Chapter 3. A list of common wavelengths is given in Table 2.1.

---

*The specific mathematical relationship between period and frequency is given in Appendix A, along with several other equations for the benefit of readers interested in mathematical details. Only the most basic and important equations are included within the text.

†This statement is a qualitative presentation of the relationship between variables. The up arrow represents an increase and the down arrow a decrease. Thus, this statement, as it relates to period, means that, as frequency increases, period decreases.

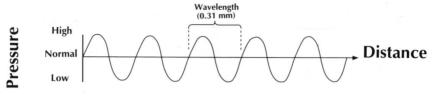

Figure 2.4. Wavelength is the length of space over which one cycle occurs. In this figure, each cycle covers 0.31 mm. Thus, the wavelength is 0.31 mm. This figure differs from Figures 2.2 and 2.3 in that the horizontal axis represents distance rather than time. For a propagation speed of 1.54 mm/μs and a frequency of 5 MHz, the wavelength is 0.31 mm (see Table 2.1).

Propagation speed* is the speed with which a wave moves through a medium. It is the speed at which a particular value of an acoustic variable moves, or with which a cycle moves. An easily identifiable value of an acoustic variable is its maximum value. The speed with which this maximum value moves through a medium is the propagation speed (Fig. 2.5). It depends on the medium but not on the frequency. Wavelength is equal to propagation speed divided by frequency.†

$$\text{wavelength (mm)} = \frac{\text{propagation speed (mm/}\mu\text{s)}}{\text{frequency (MHz)}} \qquad \lambda = \frac{c}{f}$$

$$\text{frequency} \uparrow \qquad \text{wavelength} \downarrow$$

An example of the relationship between frequency, wavelength, and propagation speed may be seen by comparing Figures 2.2b, 2.4, and 2.5 (see the legend for Fig. 2.5). Propagation speed units include meters per second (m/s) and millimeters per microsecond (mm/μs). One millimeter per microsecond equals 1000 m/s. Wavelength decreases as frequency increases (see Table 2.1).

Propagation speed is determined by the density and stiffness (hardness) of the medium. Density is the concentration of matter (mass per unit volume). Stiffness is the resistance of a material to compression. It is the opposite of compressibility. Propagation speed increases if the stiff-

---

*The word speed is used here, rather than velocity, because direction of motion is not specified. Velocity is speed with direction of motion specified.

†For the reader's convenience, symbols and equations are compiled in Appendix A. The abbreviations in parentheses represent units appropriate for each quantity.

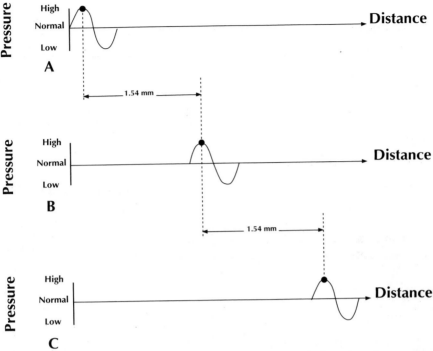

Figure 2.5. Propagation speed is the speed with which a particular value of an acoustic variable moves. The movement of a maximum (identified by the dot) is shown in this figure. Part *b* occurs 1 μs after *a*. Part *c* is 1 μs after *b* and 2 μs after *a*. The maximum (dot) moves 1.54 mm in 1μs and 3.08 mm in 2μs. The propagation speed is 1.54 mm/μs. The propagation speed in this figure (1.54 mm/μs), when divided by the frequency in Figure 2.2(*b*) (5 MHz), equals the wavelength in Figure 2.4 (0.31 mm). Propagation speeds in tissue average 1540 m/s, or, 1.54 mm/μs.

ness is increased. It decreases if the density is increased (a surprising fact for many students), assuming constant stiffness. It is generally true that media with higher densities also have higher stiffnesses. Because stiffness differences between materials generally dominate the effect of density differences, higher-density materials usually have higher sound speeds than lower-density materials.

In general, propagation speeds are low through gases, higher through liquids, and highest through solids. This increasing sequence is not caused by the increasing density (which produces a decreasing propagation speed), but by the (dominant) increasing stiffness. This is because the stiffness differences between gases, liquids, and solids are greater than the density differences. The average propagation speed in soft tissues (i.e., excluding bone) is 1540 m/s, or 1.54 mm/μs (approxi-

TABLE 2.2
Propagation Speeds in Soft Tissues

Tissue	Propagation Speed (mm/μs)
Fat	1.44
Brain	1.51
Liver	1.56
Kidney	1.56
Muscle	1.57
Soft tissue average	1.54

mately 3300 miles per hour). Values[11] for specific tissues are given in Table 2.2. In lung, because it contains gas, the propagation speed is lower than in other soft tissues. In bone, because it is a solid, the propagation speed is higher than in soft tissues. Ultrasound does not penetrate lung or bone well, so that these differing propagation speeds are normally not of concern. Values for fat (about 1.44 mm/μs) are significantly lower (by about 6 per cent) than the soft tissue average. Propagation speed is important because imaging instruments make use of it in generating the display. This is discussed later in this chapter, as well as in Chapter 4.

Impedance is equal to density multiplied by propagation speed. It will be important for the discussion of echoes later in this chapter. Its units are rayls (kg/m^3 × m/s). Impedance is determined by the density

$$\text{impedance (rayl)} = \text{density (kg/m}^3) \times \text{propagation speed (m/s)}$$
$$z = \rho c$$

$$\text{density} \uparrow \quad \text{impedance} \uparrow$$
$$\text{propagation speed} \uparrow \quad \text{impedance} \uparrow$$

and stiffness of a medium. It increases if the density is increased or if the stiffness is increased. Recall that propagation speed also depends on density and stiffness, but in a different way. Impedance does not depend on frequency.

Typical values for frequency, period, wavelength, propagation speed, and impedance are given in Table 2.8 in Section 2.5.

EXERCISES

2.1.1 A wave is a traveling variation in quantities called ___wave___ ___variables___

2.1.2 Sound is a traveling variation in quantities called ___acoustic___ ___variables___

2.1.3 Ultrasound is sound with a frequency of ___20k___ Hz or higher.

2.1.4 Acoustic variables include ___pressure___, ___density___, ___temp___, and ___particle motion___.

2.1.5 Which of the following frequencies are in the ultrasound range? (More than one correct answer.)
  a. 15 Hz
  b. 15,000 Hz
  c. 15 MHz
  d. 30,000 Hz
  e. 0.04 MHz

2.1.6 Which of the following are acoustic variables? (More than one correct answer.)
  a. pressure
  b. frequency
  c. propagation speed
  d. period
  e. particle motion

2.1.7 Frequency is a measure of how many ___cycles___ an acoustic variable goes through in a second.

2.1.8 The unit of frequency is the ___Hertz___, which is abbreviated ___Hz___.

2.1.9 Period is the ___time___ that it takes for one cycle to occur.

2.1.10 Period decreases as ___f___ increases.

2.1.11 Wavelength is the length of ___space___ over which one cycle occurs.

2.1.12 Propagation speed is the speed with which a ___wave___ moves through a medium.

2.1.13 Wavelength is equal to ___prop___ ___speed___ divided by ___freq___.

2.1.14 Propagation speed is determined by the ___density___ and ___stiffness___ of a medium.

2.1.15 Propagation speed increases if
  a. density is increased with constant stiffness
  b. density is decreased with constant stiffness

     c. stiffness is increased with constant density
     d. a and c
     e. b and c

2.1.16 The average propagation speed in soft tissues is ____ m/s
or ____ mm/μs.

2.1.17 Propagation speed is determined by
     a. frequency
     b. amplitude
     c. wavelength
     d. period
     e. medium

2.1.18 Place the following in order of increasing sound propagation
speed:
     a. gas
     b. solid
     c. liquid

2.1.19 The wavelength of 7-MHz ultrasound in soft tissues is ____
mm.

2.1.20 Wavelength in soft tissues ____ as frequency increases.

2.1.21 It takes ____ μs for ultrasound to travel 1.54 cm in soft
tissue.

2.1.22 Propagation speed in bone is ____ than in soft tissues.

2.1.23 Sound travels fastest in
     a. air
     b. helium
     c. water
     d. steel
     e. a vacuum

2.1.24 Solids have higher propagation speeds than liquids because they
have higher
     a. density
     b. stiffness

2.1.25 The propagation speeds through mercury and fat are approximately the same, even though the density of mercury is approximately 15 times that of fat. This means that the stiffness of mercury must be much ____ than that of fat.

2.1.26 Sound is a ____ ____ wave.

2.1.27 If propagation speed is doubled (a different medium) and frequency is held constant, the wavelength is ____.

2.1.28 If wavelength in a given medium at a given frequency is 2 mm
and the frequency is doubled, the wavelength becomes
____ mm.

2.1.29 If frequency in soft tissue is doubled, propagation speed is _____.

2.1.30 Waves carry _____ from one place to another. They can also carry _____ from one place to another.

2.1.31 From given values for propagation speed and frequency, which of the following can be calculated?
   a. amplitude
   b. period
   c. wavelength
   d. a and b
   e. b and c

2.1.32 If two media have the same stiffness but different densities, the one with the higher density will have the higher propagation speed. True or false?

2.1.33 If two media have the same density but different stiffnesses, the one with the higher stiffness will have the higher propagation speed. True or false?

2.1.34 If the density is 1000 kg/m³ and the propagation speed is 1.54 mm/µs, the impedance is _____ rayls.

2.1.35 If two media have the same stiffness but different densities, the one with the higher density will have the higher impedance. True or false?

2.1.36 If two media have the same density but different stiffnesses, the one with the higher stiffness will have the higher impedance. True or false?

2.1.37 Impedance is ___ρ___ multiplied by ___c___ _____.

2.1.38 What are the periods and frequencies shown in Figure 2.6?

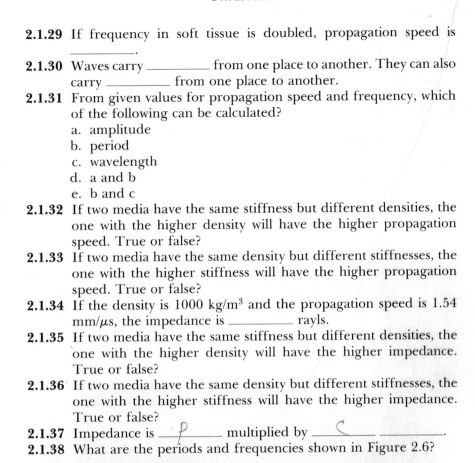

Figure 2.6. The total width of the screen in each part (*a* and *b*) represents 1 µs.

2.1.39 If the wavelength in Figure 2.6*a* is 0.154 mm, the propagation speed is _____ mm/μs.

2.1.40 If the propagation speed is 1.54 mm/μs, the wavelength in Figure 2.6*b* is _____ mm.

2.2
Pulsed Ultrasound

The terms discussed earlier (frequency, period, wavelength, and propagation speed) describe a continuous wave (cw). For sonography, continuous-wave sound is not used. Instead, short pulses of sound are used.

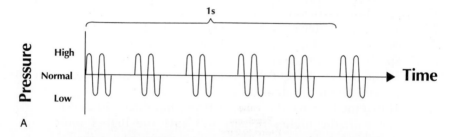

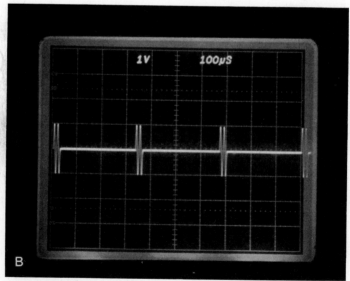

Figure 2.7. Pulse repetition frequency is the number of pulses occurring in 1 second. (*a*) Here, five pulses (containing two cycles each) occur in 1 second; thus, the pulse repetition frequency is 5 Hz. (*b*) In this photograph of a tracing of electric voltage, three pulses occur in 1 ms; thus, the pulse repetition frequency is 3 kHz. The total screen width is 1 ms.

This is called pulsed ultrasound. It is produced by applying electric pulses to the transducer (see Chapter 3). Ultrasound pulses are described by some additional parameters that have not yet been introduced.

Pulse repetition frequency (PRF) is the number of pulses occurring in 1 second (Fig. 2.7). Its units include Hz and kilohertz (kHz). One kilohertz is 1000 Hz.

Pulse repetition period is the time from the beginning of one pulse to the beginning of the next (Fig. 2.8). Its units include seconds and

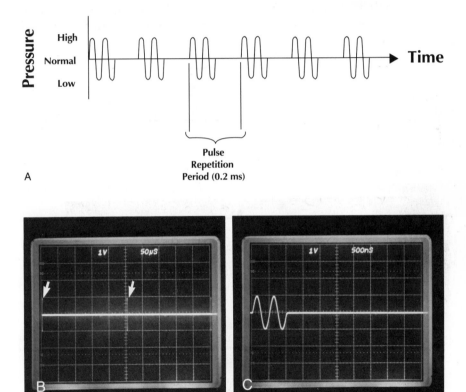

Figure 2.8. The pulse repetition period is the time from the beginning of one pulse to the beginning of the next. (*a*) Here, the pulse repetition period is 0.2 ms. Therefore, the pulse repetition frequency is 5 kHz. Pulse duration is the time that it takes for one pulse to occur. It is equal to the period multiplied by the number of cycles in the pulse. The duty factor is the fraction of time that the sound is on. (*b*) This photograph of a tracing of electric voltage shows that the pulse repetition period is 0.25 ms (pulse repetition frequency is 4 kHz); the period is 0.5 μs, as shown expanded in *c*; and the pulse duration is 1 μs. From one pulse to the next (pulse repetition period of 0.25 ms or 250 μs), the sound is on (pulse duration) 1 μs. Duty factor is, in this example, 0.004 or 0.4 per cent. Screen width is 0.5 ms in *b* and 5 μs in *c*.

milliseconds. One millisecond is one thousandth of a second (0.001 second). Pulse repetition period decreases as PRF increases. As more pulses occur in a second, there is less time (pulse repetition period) from one to the next.

PRF ↑   pulse repetition period ↓

Pulse duration is the time that it takes for a pulse to occur (see Fig. 2.8). It is equal to the period times the number of cycles in the pulse. Its units are microseconds. Sonography pulses are typically one to three cycles long.

---

period ↑   pulse duration ↑

number of cycles in the pulse ↑   pulse duration ↑

frequency ↑   pulse duration ↓

Pulse duration decreases if the number of cycles is decreased or if frequency is increased, the latter occurring as a result of period decreases.

Duty factor is the fraction of time that sound (in the form of pulses) is on. It increases with increasing pulse duration or PRF. The duty factor is unitless. Its importance will become evident when intensities are discussed in Section 2.3. It is equal to pulse duration divided by pulse repetition period. By multiplying the duty factor by 100, the result is expressed as a percentage.

$$\text{duty factor} = \frac{\text{pulse duration } (\mu s)}{\text{pulse repetition period (ms)} \times 1000}$$

$$\text{DF} = \frac{\text{PD}}{\text{PRP} \times 1000}$$

---

pulse duration ↑   duty factor ↑

pulse repetition period ↑   duty factor ↓

PRF ↑   duty factor ↑

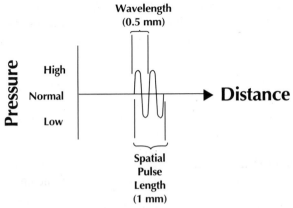

Figure 2.9. Spatial pulse length is the length of space over which a pulse occurs. It is equal to wavelength multiplied by the number of cycles in the pulse. In this figure, wavelength is 0.5 mm, there are two cycles in each pulse, and spatial pulse length is 0.5 × 2, or 1 mm. This figure differs from Figures 2.7a and 2.8a in that the horizontal axis represents distance rather than time.

Spatial pulse length is the length of space over which a pulse occurs (Fig. 2.9). It increases with wavelength and the number of cycles in the pulse. Its units are millimeters. It is an important quantity when considering axial resolution, which is discussed in Section 3.4.

wavelength ↑	spatial pulse length ↑
number of cycles in the pulse ↑	spatial pulse length ↑
frequency ↑	spatial pulse length ↓

The propagation speed for pulses is the same as that for continuous waves in a given medium. Frequency within pulses is not the same as that for continuous waves. A continuous wave may be described by a single frequency. Pulses contain frequencies in addition to the specified (operating) frequency, as discussed in Section 3.1. Pulses have many frequencies present (see Fig. 3.5 in Chapter 3). The shorter the pulse, the greater the bandwidth (range of frequencies). The dominant frequency present in the pulse is close to or equal to the frequency for the unpulsed (continuous) wave. For pulses, frequency gives the number of cycles per second, assuming continuous waves (even though this assumption is not correct for pulsed ultrasound). Therefore, 1-MHz pulsed ultrasound with a duty factor of 1 per cent will have only 10,000 cycles per second (because the quiet time between pulses eliminates 99 per cent of the cycles), even though the frequency implies that there are 1 million cycles per second.

Typical values for PRF, pulse repetition period, pulse duration, duty factor, and spatial pulse length are given in Table 2.8 in Section 2.5.

EXERCISES

2.2.1 The abbreviation cw stands for _____ _____.

2.2.2 Pulsed ultrasound is ultrasound in the form of repeated short _____.

2.2.3 Pulse repetition frequency is the number of _____ occurring in 1 second.

2.2.4 Pulsed ultrasound is produced by applying electric _____ to the transducer.

2.2.5 The pulse repetition _____ is the time from the beginning of one pulse to the beginning of the next.

2.2.6 The pulse repetition period _____ as the pulse repetition frequency increases.

2.2.7 Pulse duration is the _____ it takes for a pulse to occur.

2.2.8 Spatial pulse length is the _____ of _____ over which a pulse occurs.

2.2.9 _____ _____ is the fraction of time that pulsed ultrasound is actually on.

2.2.10 Pulse duration equals the number of cycles in the pulse times _____.

2.2.11 Spatial pulse length equals the number of cycles in the pulse times _____.

2.2.12 The duty factor of continuous-wave sound is _____.

2.2.13 If the wavelength is 2 mm, the spatial pulse length for a three-cycle pulse is _____ mm.

2.2.14 The spatial pulse length in soft tissue for a four-cycle pulse of a frequency of 3 MHz is _____ mm.

2.2.15 The pulse duration in soft tissue for a four-cycle pulse of a frequency 3 MHz is _____ μs.

2.2.16 For a 1-kHz pulse repetition frequency, the pulse repetition period is _____ ms.

2.2.17 For Exercises 2.2.15 and 2.2.16 together, the duty factor is _____.

2.2.18 How many cycles are there in 1 second of continuous-wave 5-MHz ultrasound?
   a. 5
   b. 500

c. 5000
d. 5,000,000
e. none of the above

2.2.19 How many cycles are there in 1 second of pulsed 5-MHz ultrasound with a duty factor of 0.01?
    a. 5
    b. 500
    c. 5000
    d. 5,000,000
    e. none of the above

2.2.20 In Exercise 2.2.19, how many cycles were eliminated by pulsing?
    a. 100 per cent
    b. 99.9 per cent
    c. 99 per cent
    d. 50 per cent
    e. 1 per cent

2.2.21 For pulsed ultrasound, the duty factor is always _____
_____ one.

2.3
Attenuation

The rate at which cycles occur in time (frequency), the time required for
each cycle (period), the space over which a cycle occurs (wavelength),
and the speed at which the cycles move (propagation speed) have all
been described. The magnitude of the variations will now be considered.
This will give some idea of the strength of the sound. Amplitude and
intensity are the parameters that are relevant here, as they are measures
of how loud the sound would be if it could be heard. (Because it is
ultrasound, however, it cannot be heard.)

    Amplitude is the maximum variation that occurs in an acoustic vari-
able. It is the maximum value minus the normal (undisturbed) value
(Fig. 2.10). Amplitude is expressed in units that are appropriate for the
acoustic variable considered.

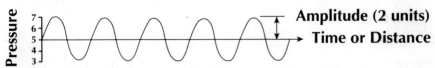

Figure 2.10. Amplitude is the maximum amount of variation that occurs in an acoustic
variable (pressure, in this case). It is equal to the maximum value of the variable minus the
normal (undisturbed) value. In this figure, the amplitude is 7 (maximum value) minus 5
(normal value), or 2 units.

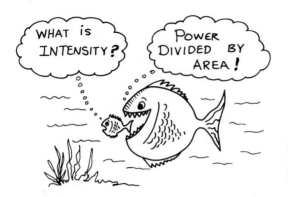

Figure 2.11. Intensity is the power in a sound wave divided by the area over which the power is spread.

Intensity is the power in a wave divided by the area over which the power is spread (Fig. 2.11).

$$\text{intensity (W/cm}^2) = \frac{\text{power (W)}}{\text{area (cm}^2)} \qquad I = \frac{P}{A}$$

power ↑	intensity ↑
area ↑	intensity ↓

Power is the rate at which work is done, or the rate at which energy is transferred. It is equal to the work done divided by the time required to do the work. It is also equal to energy transferred divided by the time required to transfer the energy. Power units include watts (W) and milliwatts (mW). If the total power across a sound beam is divided by the beam area, the spatial average intensity is calculated, as discussed later in this section. Sound beams and beam area are discussed in Section 3.2. Beam area units are centimeters squared (cm²). Intensity units include milliwatts per centimeter squared (mW/cm²) and watts per centimeter squared (W/cm²). Intensity is an important parameter in describing the sound that is produced and received by diagnostic instruments (see Chapter 4) and in discussing bioeffects and safety (see Chapter 7). It may be illustrated by analogy with the effect of sunlight on dry kindling (Fig. 2.12). Sunlight will not normally ignite the kindling, but if the same light power from the sun is concentrated in a small area (increased intensity) by focusing it with a magnifying glass, the kindling can be ignited. An effect is therefore produced by increasing the intensity, even though the power remains the same.

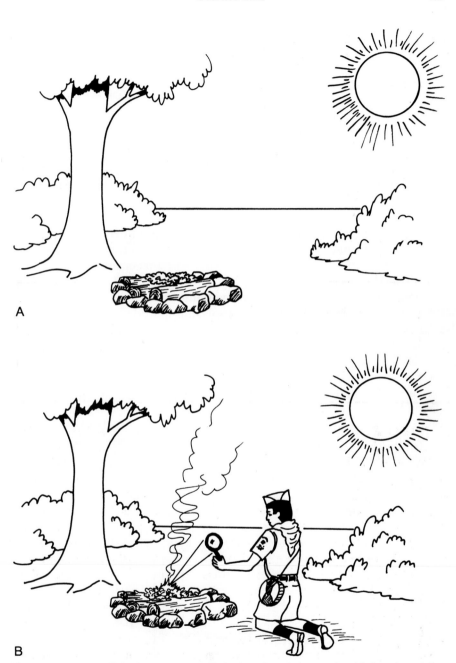

Figure 2.12. (*a*) Sunlight does not normally ignite a fire. (*b*) However, with focusing of the sunlight (increased intensity), ignition can occur.

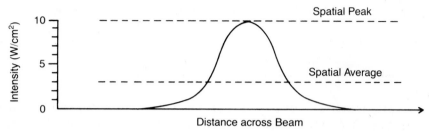

Figure 2.13. Intensity is a function of distance across the beam. In this figure, the spatial peak intensity (at the beam center) is 10 W/cm² and the spatial average is 3 W/cm². In addition to varying across the beam, intensity varies along the direction of the beam as a result of focusing and attenuation.

As discussed in Section 3.2, beam area is determined, in part, by the size and operating frequency of the sound source chosen. For a given beam power, intensity will be determined by the beam area, which is determined by the sound source.

Intensity is proportional to the amplitude squared. Thus, if amplitude is doubled, intensity is quadrupled. If amplitude is halved, intensity is quartered.

Because intensity is not uniform across a sound beam (Fig. 2.13) and, in the case of pulsed ultrasound, is not uniform in time (Fig. 2.14), several intensities are used. For spatial considerations, the spatial peak (SP) and the spatial average (SA) values are used. For temporal (time) considerations, the temporal average (TA) value or pulse average (PA) value may be used. These are related by the duty factor (fraction of time pulsed ultrasound is on). The greater the duty factor, the greater the TA intensity will be.

duty factor ↑   TA intensity ↑

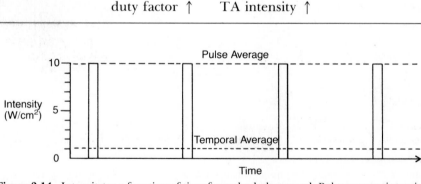

Figure 2.14. Intensity as a function of time for pulsed ultrasound. Pulse average intensity (10 W/cm²) is the intensity when the sound is actually on. Temporal average intensity (1 W/cm²) is the intensity that is averaged over time. In this figure, the duty factor is 0.1.

If the PA intensity increases, the TA intensity will increase also.

> PA intensity ↑   TA intensity ↑

If the sound is continuous instead of pulsed, the duty factor is equal to one, and the PA and TA intensities are equal to each other. The four intensities resulting from these spatial and temporal considerations are spatial average–temporal average (SATA) intensity, spatial peak–temporal average (SPTA) intensity, spatial average–pulse average (SAPA) intensity, and spatial peak–pulse average (SPPA) intensity.

The pulses shown in Figures 2.7 and 2.14 have constant amplitude and intensity within each pulse. Although pulses used in Doppler ultrasound are similar to these, pulses used in sonography are typically like that shown in Figure 2.15. In this case, the peak intensity occurring within each pulse is called the temporal peak (TP) intensity. The intensity averaged over the pulse duration is called the PA intensity. For constant amplitude pulses, such as those in Figures 2.7 and 2.14, TP and PA intensities are the same. Combining spatial considerations with the TP intensity yields spatial average–temporal peak (SATP) and spatial peak–temporal peak (SPTP) values.

EXAMPLE 2.3.1

The SAPA intensity is 500 mW/cm^2 and the duty factor is 0.002. Calculate the SATA intensity.

$$\text{SATA intensity} = \text{SAPA intensity} \times \text{duty factor} = 500 \times 0.002$$
$$= 1 \text{ mW/cm}^2$$

SATA intensity is the lowest of the six intensities introduced above. SPTP intensity is the highest. The others have intermediate values.

EXAMPLE 2.3.2

The SPTP and SPPA intensities of pulsed ultrasound are 60 and 20 W/cm^2, respectively. Calculate the SPTA intensity if the duty factor is 0.01.

$$\text{SPTA intensity} = \text{SPPA intensity} \times \text{duty factor} = 20 \times 0.01$$
$$= 200 \text{ mW/cm}^2$$

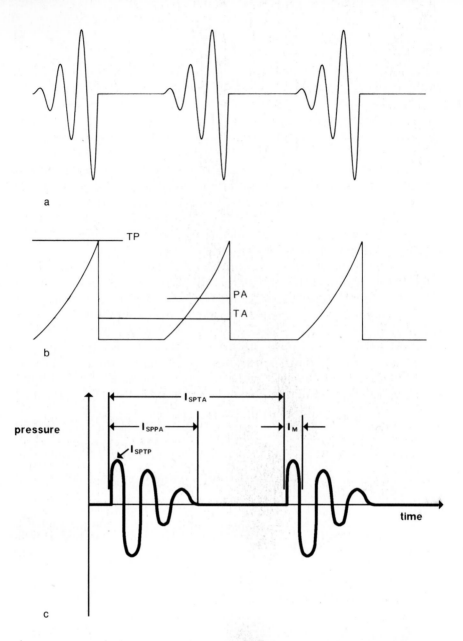

Figure 2.15. (*a*) The ultrasound pulses used in imaging have cycles of differing amplitudes. They are produced by electric excitation of a damped transducer (see Chapter 3 and Figures 3.3 and 3.4 for details). (*b*) This figure shows the intensity of the pulses in *a. TP,* temporal peak intensity; *PA,* pulse average intensity; and *TA,* temporal average intensity. The horizontal axis in both *a* and *b* represents distance. (*c*) Pressure versus time for pulses containing 2½ cycles. The relevant times for four spatial peak intensities are shown: spatial peak–temporal average (SPTA) intensity, spatial peak–pulse average (SPPA) intensity, spatial peak–temporal peak (SPTP) intensity, and I$_m$, which is the intensity averaged over the largest half-cycle.

Another intensity—maximum intensity (I_m)—is sometimes useful. It is the intensity averaged over the largest half-cycle of the pulse (Fig. 2.15c).

The terms discussed previously (frequency, period, wavelength, propagation speed, amplitude, and intensity) describe sound waves. Another term—attenuation—needs to be defined before sound reflection is considered in the next section. It is important to understand attenuation because it limits imaging depth and also must be compensated by the diagnostic instrument (see Section 4.2).

With an unfocused beam (beams and focus are discussed in Chapter 3) in any medium, such as tissue, amplitude and intensity will decrease as the sound travels through the medium. This reduction in amplitude and intensity as sound travels is called attenuation (Fig. 2.16). It encompasses absorption (conversion of sound to heat), reflection, and scattering (see Section 2.4). Absorption is normally the dominant contribution to attenuation in soft tissues. Attenuation units are decibels (dB). The attenuation coefficient is the attenuation for each centimeter of sound travel. Its units are decibels per centimeter (dB/cm). The longer the path over which the sound travels, the greater the attenuation.

Decibels are good units for comparisons. They are used for measuring attenuation (Fig. 2.16, d through g), sound levels and noise (Fig. 2.16h), gain (see Section 4.2), and dynamic range (see Section 4.3). Decibels involve logarithms. The logarithm (log) is equal to the number of tens that must be multiplied together to result in that number. More

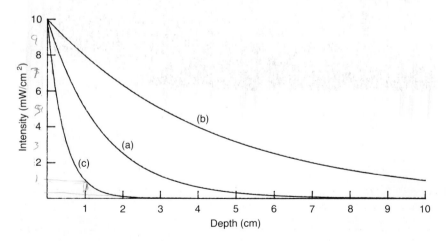

Figure 2.16. Attenuation of sound as it travels through a medium. (a) The intensity decreases by 50 per cent for each 1 cm of travel. This corresponds to an attenuation coefficient of 3 dB/cm. (b) The attenuation coefficient is 1 dB/cm. (c) The attenuation coefficient is 10 dB/cm.

Illustration continued on following page

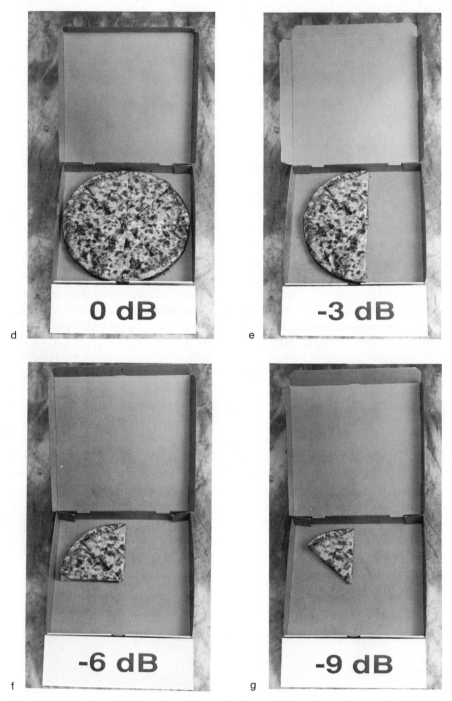

d   **0 dB**

e   **-3 dB**

f   **-6 dB**

g   **-9 dB**

Figure 2.16 *Continued.* (*d* through *g*) Each reduction of 3 dB corresponds to cutting in half.

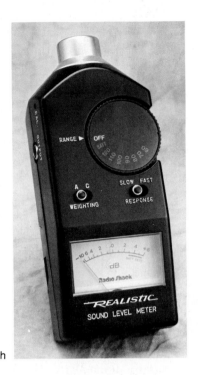

Figure 2.16 *Continued.* (*h*) A sound level meter based on dB units.   h

generally, it is the power to which 10 must be raised to give a particular
number. For example, to obtain 1000, three tens must be multiplied
together so that the logarithm of 1000 is 3. The logarithm of the reciprocal of a number is equal to the negative of the logarithm of the number.
For example, the logarithm of 0.01 is minus the logarithm of 100, or −2.

Decibels are quantities that result from taking 10 times the logarithm of the ratio of two powers or intensities.

EXAMPLE 2.3.3

Compare the following two powers in decibels: power one = 1 W; power
two = 10 W.

$$10 \log \frac{\text{power one}}{\text{power two}} = 10 \log \frac{1}{10} = 10(-\log 10) = 10(-1) = -10 \text{ dB}$$

Power one is 10 dB less than power two, or power one is 10 dB below
power two. Also,

$$10 \log \frac{\text{power two}}{\text{power one}} = 10 \log \frac{10}{1} = 10(\log 10) = 10(1) = 10 \text{ dB}$$

Power two is 10 dB more than power one, or power two is 10 dB above power one.

EXAMPLE 2.3.4

Compare intensity two with intensity one; intensity one = 10 mW/cm²; intensity two = 0.01 mW/cm.

$$10 \log \frac{\text{intensity two}}{\text{intensity one}} = 10 \log \frac{0.01}{10} = 10 \log \frac{1}{1000}$$

$$= 10(-\log 1000) = 10(-3) = -30 \text{ dB}$$

Intensity two is 30 dB less than or below intensity one.

EXAMPLE 2.3.5

As sound passes through tissue, its intensity at one point is 1 mW/cm²; at a point 10 cm farther along, it is 0.1 mW/cm². What are the attenuation and attenuation coefficient?

$$\text{attenuation (dB)} = 10 \log \frac{\text{intensity at second point}}{\text{intensity at first point}} = 10 \log \frac{0.1}{1}$$

$$= 10 \log \frac{1}{10} = 10(-\log 10)$$

$$= 10(-1) = 10 \text{ dB}$$

The minus sign results from the second intensity (in the numerator) being less than the first (in the denominator). We can then consider this to be an attenuation of 10 dB. Some authors retain the minus sign, whereas others do not. In this book, the minus sign will not be retained. The attenuation coefficient (dB/cm) is the attenuation (dB) divided by the separation between the two points (in this case, 10 dB/10 cm = 1 dB/cm). Table 2.3 lists various values of intensity ratio with corresponding decibel values of attenuation. Attenuation (dB) is attenuation coefficient (dB/cm) multiplied by the sound path (cm).

attenuation coefficient ↑ attenuation ↑

path length ↑ attenuation ↑

TABLE 2.3

Decibel (dB) Values of Attenuation
for Various Values of Intensity
Ratio*

dB Attenuation	Intensity Ratio
1	0.79
2	0.63
3	0.50
4	0.40
5	0.32
6	0.25
7	0.20
8	0.16
9	0.13
10	0.10
15	0.032
20	0.01
25	0.003
30	0.001
35	0.0003
40	0.0001
45	0.00003
50	0.00001
60	0.000001
70	0.0000001
80	0.00000001
90	0.000000001
100	0.0000000001

*The intensity ratio is the fraction of intensity
remaining after the attenuation.

The attenuation coefficient increases with increasing frequency. Persons who live in apartments or dormitories experience this fact when they hear mostly the bass notes through the wall from a neighbor's sound system. For soft tissues, average attenuation coefficients[11] are given in Table 2.4. A simple proportional approximation is that soft tissue, on the average, has 0.5 dB of attenuation per centimeter for each megahertz of frequency (Table 2.5). Therefore, the average attenuation coefficient in decibels per centimeter for soft tissues is approximately equal to one half the frequency in megahertz. This rule, although a good description of attenuation values experienced in normal ultrasound imaging practice, yields attenuation values that are lower than those found in some laboratory measurements (Table 2.4). As attenuation measurement techniques have improved, attenuation values have decreased. The more recent (lower) values are the most accurate. The

TABLE 2.4
Average Attenuation Coefficients in
Tissues at 1 MHz

Tissue	Attenuation Coefficient (dB/cm)
Fat	0.6
Brain	0.6
Liver	0.5
Kidney	0.9
Muscle	1.0
Heart	1.1

inclusion of the factor of one half appears to better approximate the most recent data than do previous (larger) values. To calculate the attenuation in decibels, simply multiply one half the frequency in megahertz (which is approximately equal to the attenuation coefficient in dB/cm) by the path length in centimeters.

$$\text{attenuation (dB)} = \tfrac{1}{2} \times \text{frequency (MHz)} \times \text{path length (cm)}$$
$$a = \tfrac{1}{2}fL$$

frequency ↑   attenuation coefficient ↑

frequency ↑   attenuation ↑

The intensity ratio corresponding to that number of decibels may be obtained from Table 2.3. This ratio is equal to the fraction of the inten-

TABLE 2.5
Average Attenuation Coefficients in Tissue

Frequency (MHz)	Average Attenuation Coefficient for Soft Tissue (dB/cm)	Intensity Reduction in 1-cm Path (%)	Intensity Reduction in 10-cm Path (%)
2.0	1.0	21	90
3.5	1.8	34	98
5.0	2.5	44	99.7
7.5	3.8	58	99.98
10.0	5.0	68	99.999

sity (at the beginning of the path) that remains at the end of the path. If the intensity at the beginning is known, the intensity at the end may be found by multiplying by the intensity ratio. A summary of this four-step process follows:

1. Multiplying the frequency (MHz) by one half yields the approximate attenuation coefficient (dB/cm).
2. Multiplying the attenuation coefficient (dB/cm) by the path length (cm) yields attenuation (dB).
3. The intensity ratio is then determined for the decibel value calculated in step 2 (Table 2.3).
4. Multiplying the intensity ratio by the intensity at the start of the path equals the intensity at the end of the path.

EXAMPLE 2.3.6

If 4-MHz ultrasound at 10 mW/cm^2 SATA intensity is applied to a soft tissue surface, what is the SATA intensity 1.5 cm into the tissue? Multiplying one half by the frequency yields an attenuation coefficient of 2 dB/cm. Multiplying the attenuation coefficient (2 dB/cm) by the path length (1.5 cm) yields 3 dB. The attenuation, then, is 3 dB. From Table 2.3, it can be found that 3 dB corresponds to an intensity ratio of 0.5. Thus, 50 per cent of the intensity remains after the sound travels through this path. Multiplying the intensity ratio (0.5) by the SATA intensity at the beginning of the path (10 mW/cm^2) gives the SATA intensity at the end of the path (5 mW/cm^2).

Attenuation is higher in lung than in other soft tissues, and it is higher in bone than in soft tissues. Lung and bone attenuations are not proportionally dependent on frequency. Therefore, the four-step process just described cannot be used for them (specifically, step one fails).

A practical consequence of attenuation is that it limits the depth at which images can be obtained. The imaging depth decreases as frequency increases (Figs. 2.17 to 2.19). Table 2.6 lists attenuation coefficients and imaging depths for various frequencies in soft tissue.

frequency ↑   imaging depth ↓

Note that Table 2.6 shows that imaging depths are approximately 400 wavelengths. For example, at 10 MHz, wavelength is 0.15 mm and imaging depth is about 60 mm, or 60/0.15, or 400 wavelengths.

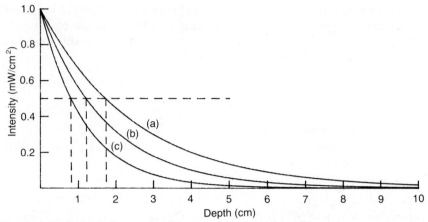

Figure 2.17. Intensity versus depth in soft tissue for 3.5 MHz (*a*), 5.0 MHz (*b*), and 7.5 MHz (*c*). The depth at which half-intensity (3-dB attenuation) occurs (1.7, 1.2, and 0.8 cm, respectively) is indicated for each.

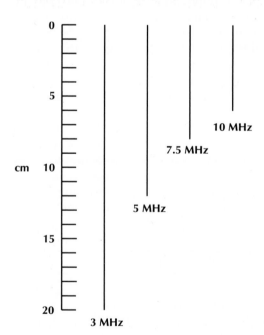

Figure 2.18. Typical imaging depths for several frequencies in soft tissues. Imaging depth decreases as frequency increases because attenuation increases.

Figure 2.19. Examples of imaging depth in a tissue-equivalent phantom at 3 MHz (*a*), 5 MHz (*b*), and 7 MHz (*c*). Imaging depth decreases as frequency increases.

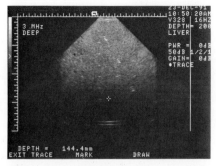

a

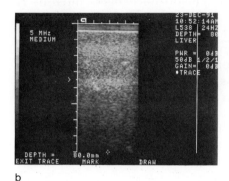

b

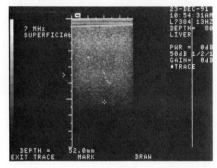

c

TABLE 2.6

Common Values for Various Diagnostic Ultrasound Terms

Frequency (MHz)	Wavelength (mm)	Attenuation Coefficient (dB/cm)	Imaging Depth (cm)
2.0	0.77	1.0	30
3.5	0.44	1.8	17
5.0	0.31	2.5	12
7.5	0.21	3.8	8
10.0	0.15	5.0	6

EXERCISES

2.3.1 Amplitude is the maximum _____ that occurs in an acoustic variable.

2.3.2 Intensity is the _____ in a wave divided by _____.

2.3.3 The unit for intensity is _____.

2.3.4 Intensity is proportional to the square of _____.

2.3.5 If power is doubled and area remains unchanged, intensity is _____.

2.3.6 If area is doubled and power remains unchanged, intensity is _____.

2.3.7 If both power and area are doubled, intensity is _____.

2.3.8 If amplitude is doubled, intensity is _____.

2.3.9 If a sound beam has a power of 10 mW and a beam area of 2 cm², the spatial average intensity is _____ mW/cm².

2.3.10 If the beam in Exercise 2.3.9 is focused to a beam area of 0.1 cm², the intensity becomes _____ mW/cm².

2.3.11 Multiplying pulse-average intensity by duty factor yields _____ _____ intensity.

2.3.12 Which of the following intensities are equal for continuous-wave sound?
  a. spatial peak and spatial average
  b. temporal peak and temporal average
  c. spatial peak and temporal average
  d. spatial average and temporal average
  e. none of the above

2.3.13 If the SPTA intensity is 1 mW/cm² and the duty factor is 0.01, calculate the SPPA intensity in mW/cm².

2.3.14 If pulsed ultrasound is on 50 per cent of the time (duty factor = 0.5) and pulse average intensity is 4 mW/cm², temporal average intensity is _____ mW/cm².

2.3.15 If the maximum value of an acoustic variable is 10 units and the normal (undisturbed) value is 7 units, the amplitude is _____ units. The minimum value of the acoustic variable is _____ units.

2.3.16 Attenuation is the reduction in _____ and _____ as a wave travels through a medium.

2.3.17 Attenuation consists of _____, _____, and _____.

2.3.18 The attenuation coefficient is attenuation per _____ of sound travel.

2.3.19 The attenuation and attenuation coefficient are given in the units ___dB___ and ___dB/cm___, respectively.

2.3.20 For soft tissues, there is approximately ___0.5 dB cm___ dB of attenuation per centimeter for each megahertz of frequency.

2.3.21 For soft tissues, the attenuation coefficient at 3 MHz is approximately ___1.5___.

2.3.22 The attenuation coefficient in soft tissue ___↑___ as frequency increases.

2.3.23 For soft tissue, if frequency is doubled, attenuation is ___doble___; if path length is doubled, attenuation is ___doble___; if both frequency and path length are doubled, attenuation is ___quadruple___.

2.3.24 If frequency is doubled and path length is halved, attenuation is ___unchse___.

2.3.25 Absorption is the conversion of _____ to _____.

2.3.26 Can the absorption be greater than the attenuation in a given medium at a given frequency? _____

2.3.27 Is attenuation in bone higher or lower than in soft tissue? ___high___

2.3.28 For average soft tissue, the attenuation is such that for each 1.5 cm traveled, a 4-MHz sound intensity is reduced by _____ per cent. For 1 cm and 6 MHz, the reduction is _____ per cent. For 4 cm and 3.5 MHz, the reduction is _____ per cent. (Use Table 2.3).

2.3.29 The attenuation coefficient for soft tissue at 10 MHz is _____ dB/cm.

2.3.30 The attenuation coefficient for soft tissue at 5 MHz is _____ dB/cm.

2.3.31 The attenuation coefficient in soft tissue is approximately one half the _____.

2.3.32 The imaging depth ___decrease___ as frequency increases.

2.3.33 If the intensity of 4-MHz ultrasound entering soft tissue is 2 W/cm, the intensity at a depth of 4 cm is _____ W/cm^2.

2.3.34 If the intensity of 40-MHz ultrasound entering soft tissue is 2 W/cm, the intensity at a depth of 4 cm is _____ W/cm^2.

2.3.35 The depth at which half-intensity occurs in soft tissues at 7.5 MHz is
 a. 0.6 cm
 b. 0.7 cm
 c. 0.8 cm
 d. 0.9 cm
 e. 1.0 cm

2.3.36 Give the logarithms of the following numbers:
   a. 10 _____
   b. 0.1 _____
   c. 100 _____
   d. 0.001 _____

2.3.37 If the intensity at point A is 40 mW/cm² and at point B it is 10 mW/cm², the attenuation from A to B is _____ dB.

2.3.38 If the intensities of traveling sound are 10 mW/cm² and 0.1 mW/cm² at two points 5 cm apart, the attenuation between the two points is _____ dB. The attenuation coefficient is _____ dB/cm.

2.3.39 If the intensity at the start of a path is 3 mW/cm² and the attenuation over the path is 2 dB, the intensity at the end of the path is _____ mW/cm². (Use Table 2.3.)

2.4
Echoes

Thus far in this chapter, the propagation of ultrasound through homogeneous media has been considered. The usefulness of ultrasound as an imaging tool is primarily the result of reflection and scattering at organ and tissue boundaries and scattering within heterogeneous tissues. These phenomena will be considered in this section.

Perpendicular incidence (called normal incidence in geometry) occurs when the direction of travel of the ultrasound is perpendicular to the boundary between two media (Fig. 2.20). If the incidence is not perpendicular, it is called oblique incidence (Fig. 2.21).

When there is perpendicular incidence, the incident sound may be reflected or transmitted, or both (see Fig. 2.20). Reflected sound travels through medium one in a direction opposite to the incident sound (i.e., the reflected sound returns to the sound source). Transmitted sound moves through medium two in the same direction as the incident sound. The intensities of the reflected sound and transmitted sound depend on the incident intensity and the impedances (see Section 2.1) of the media.

Dividing the reflected intensity by the incident intensity yields the intensity reflection coefficient. Dividing the transmitted intensity by the incident intensity yields the intensity transmission coefficient. These coefficients can then be used to determine the fractions of incident sound intensity that are reflected and transmitted, respectively. They must add up to one in order to account for all the incident sound intensity (i.e., what is not reflected must be transmitted).

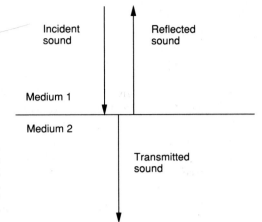

Figure 2.20. Reflection and transmission at a boundary with perpendicular incidence. The lateral offset of transmitted and reflected sound with respect to incident sound is solely for figure clarity. In practice, a lateral shift does not occur.

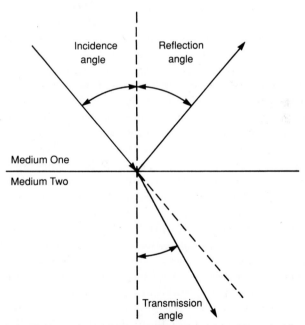

Figure 2.21. Reflection and transmission at a boundary with oblique incidence. Incidence and reflection angles are equal. The transmission angle depends on the incidence angle and the media propagation speeds.

$$\text{intensity reflection coefficient} = \frac{\text{reflected intensity (W/cm}^2)}{\text{incident intensity (W/cm}^2)}$$

$$= \left[\frac{\text{medium two impedance} - \text{medium one impedance}}{\text{medium two impedance} + \text{medium one impedance}}\right]^2$$

$$\text{IRC} = \frac{I_r}{I_i} = \left[\frac{z_2 - z_1}{z_2 + z_1}\right]^2$$

---

impedance difference ↑   intensity reflection coefficient ↑

$$\text{intensity transmission coefficient} = \frac{\text{transmitted intensity (W/cm}^2)}{\text{incident intensity (W/cm}^2)}$$

$$= 1 - \text{intensity reflection coefficient}$$

$$\text{ITC} = \frac{I_t}{I_i} = 1 - \text{IRC}$$

---

intensity reflection coefficient ↑ intensity transmission coefficient ↓

For perpendicular incidence, if the media impedances are the same, there is no reflected sound, and the transmitted intensity is equal to the incident intensity. If there is no reflection, the media impedances are equal. The reflected and transmitted intensities depend not only on the (subtraction) difference between the media impedances, but also on their sum. (Compare Exercises 2.4.4 and 2.4.5, in which the impedance differences are the same but the answers are different; then compare Exercises 2.4.4 and 2.4.6, in which the impedance differences are different but the answers are the same).

Recall that impedance is density times propagation speed (see Section 2.1). For perpendicular incidence, an echo is generated at a boundary if the impedances are different. An echo may be generated when the densities are the same if the propagation speeds are different (see Exercise 2.4.10). By contrast, no reflection may be generated, even when the densities are different (see Exercise 2.4.11). If there is a large difference between the impedances, there will be almost total reflection (an intensity reflection coefficient of close to one; an intensity transmission coefficient of close to zero). An example of this is an air–soft tissue boundary (see Exercise 2.4.17). For this reason, a gel coupling medium is used to provide a good sound path from the transducer to the skin (eliminating the thin layer of air) during the diagnostic use of ultrasound.

EXAMPLE 2.4.1

For impedances of 40 and 60 rayls, calculate the intensity reflection and transmission coefficients.

$$\text{intensity reflection coefficient} = \left[\frac{60 - 40}{60 + 40}\right]^2$$

$$= \left[\frac{20}{100}\right]^2 = 0.2^2 = 0.2 \times 0.2 = 0.04$$

$$\text{intensity transmission coefficient} = 1 - 0.04 = 0.96$$

The intensity reflection coefficient can be expressed as 4 per cent and the intensity transmission coefficient as 96 per cent. The sum of the two coefficients is 100 per cent, underscoring the fact that all of the incident intensity must be either reflected or transmitted.

If the incident intensity is known, the reflected and transmitted intensities can be calculated by multiplying the incident intensity by the intensity reflection coefficient and the intensity transmission coefficient, respectively.

EXAMPLE 2.4.2

For Example 2.4.1, if the incident intensity is 10 mW/cm^2, calculate the reflected and transmitted intensities.

From Example 2.4.1, the intensity reflection and transmission coefficients are 0.04 and 0.96, respectively, so that:

$$\text{reflected intensity} = 10 \times 0.04 = 0.4 \text{ mW/cm}^2$$
$$\text{transmitted intensity} = 10 \times 0.96 = 9.6 \text{ mW/cm}^2$$

The coefficients give the fraction of the incident intensity that is reflected or transmitted. By multiplying the coefficients by 100, these fractions are expressed in percentages. They must always add up to 1 (or 100 per cent). In Example 2.4.2, all of the incident intensity is accounted for (0.4 mW/cm^2 reflected, 9.6 mW/cm^2 transmitted, for a total of 10 mW/cm^2, or 100 per cent).

Oblique incidence occurs when the direction of travel of the incident ultrasound is not perpendicular to the boundary between two media (see Fig. 2.21). This is a common situation in diagnostic ultrasound. The

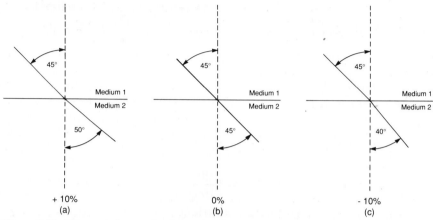

Figure 2.22. Transmission angles for an incidence angle of 45 degrees and propagation speeds through medium two that are (*a*) 10 per cent greater than, (*b*) equal to, and (*c*) 10 per cent less than propagation speed through medium one.

direction of travel with respect to the boundary is given by the incidence angle (for perpendicular incidence, the incidence angle is zero). The reflected and transmitted directions are given by the reflection angle and transmission angle, respectively (see Fig. 2.21). The incidence angle equals the reflection angle. This is observed in optics also (e.g., a laser beam reflecting off a mirror). The transmission angle depends on the propagation speeds in the media. A change in direction of sound (transmission angle unequal to incidence angle) when crossing a boundary is called refraction (from Latin, meaning to turn aside). The transmission angle is greater than the incidence angle if the propagation speed through medium two is greater than the propagation speed through medium one (Fig. 2.22*a*). The changes are approximately proportional. For example, if the speed increases by 5 per cent as the sound enters medium two, the transmission angle will be about 5 per cent greater than the incidence angle. There is no refraction if the propagation speeds are equal (Fig. 2.22*b*), or if the incidence angle is zero (perpendicular incidence). Refraction is important because, when it occurs, lateral position errors occur on an image. This is discussed further in Section 6.1.

EXAMPLE 2.4.3

If the incidence angle is 20 degrees, the propagation speed in medium one is 1.7 mm/μs, and the propagation speed in medium two is 1.6 mm/μs, calculate the reflection and transmission angles.

The incidence and reflection angles are equal, so that the reflection angle is 20 degrees. The speed decreases by 6 per cent $\left(\frac{1.6}{1.7} = 0.94\right)$, so that the transmission angle is 6 per cent less than the incidence angle ($0.94 \times 20 = 19$ degrees).

Refraction occurs with light as well as with sound. It is the principle on which lenses operate. It is also the cause of distortion when viewing objects in a fish bowl. As with sound, when light crosses a boundary obliquely and a change in light speed occurs, the direction of the light changes.

Expressions for calculating oblique reflection and transmission coefficients are more complicated than those that apply when there is perpendicular incidence, and they are not addressed here. For given media, the reflection coefficient for oblique incidence may be smaller than, equal to, or greater than that for normal incidence, depending on incidence angle. If the propagation speeds through the media are the same, the intensity reflection coefficient is the same as that for perpendicular incidence and is independent of incidence angle. For oblique incidence, it is possible for a reflection to occur even if the media have equal impedances. This will occur if the propagation speeds are different. Conversely, it is possible that no reflection will occur even when the media impedances are different. Therefore, absence of reflection with oblique incidence does not necessarily mean that the media impedances are equal (as it does with perpendicular incidence).

It is sometimes stated by authors that reflection amplitude decreases with increasing incidence angle. Whether this is true or not depends on the densities and propagation speeds involved. It is possible, with certain values of propagation speed and density, for the reflection amplitude to increase, decrease, or remain constant as angle increases. The reflection amplitude may pass through a minimum and then increase, or start at zero (equal impedances) and increase.

Thus far in this section, it has been assumed that wavelength is small as compared to the boundary dimensions, and that the boundary is smooth. The resulting reflections are called specular (from Latin, meaning mirror-like) reflections. If, on the other hand, the boundary dimensions are comparable in size or small as compared to the wavelength, or if the boundary is not smooth (surface irregularities comparable in size or large as compared to the wavelength), the incident sound will be scattered (diffused). Scattering is the redirection of sound in many directions by rough surfaces or by heterogeneous media, such as (cellular) tissues, or particle suspensions, such as blood (Fig. 2.23). These cases are

Figure 2.23. A sound pulse may be scattered by a rough boundary between tissues (*a*) or within tissues due to their heterogeneous character (*b*).

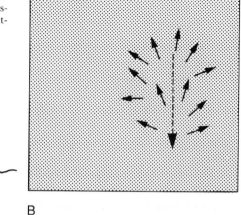

Tissue 1

Tissue 2

A   B

analogous to light in which specular reflections occur at mirrors. For a rougher surface, such as a white wall, although virtually all the light is reflected (that is why the wall is white) a reflected image is not observed (as in a mirror) because the light is scattered at the surface and mixed up as it travels back to the viewer's eyes. When light passes through a suspension of water droplets in air (fog), it is scattered as well. This limits the viewer's ability to see through fog. Although scattering inhibits vision (we cannot see ourselves reflected in a wall and we cannot see well through fog), it is of great benefit in ultrasound imaging. This is because, with ultrasound, the goal is to see the "wall" (tissue interface), not a reflection of "oneself" (the sound source). There is also a desire to see the "fog" (tissue parenchyma), not just objects beyond it.

Backscatter (sound scattered back in the direction from which it originally came) intensities from rough surfaces and heterogeneous media vary with frequency and scatterer size. These intensities may be comparable to or less than specular reflection intensities from tissue boundaries. Normally, scatter intensities are much less than boundary specular reflection intensities. The roughness of a tissue boundary or heterogeneity of a medium (such as tissue) effectively increases as frequency is increased (increased backscatter). This is because wavelength decreases as frequency increases, thus making wavelength smaller relative to roughness or scatterer dimensions. This is why the sky is blue. Light with higher frequencies is scattered more strongly by particles suspended in the atmosphere than that with lower frequencies (low-frequency light is red, high-frequency light is blue).

The intensity received by the sound source from specular reflections is highly angle-dependent. Scattering from boundaries helps to make echo reception less dependent on incidence angle. Because diagnostic ultrasound is confined to beams (see Section 3.2), there are conditions under which all or part of the reflected sound may not return to the transducer and will thus be missed. Again, scattering helps to reduce this effect.

Scattering, then, permits ultrasound imaging of tissue boundaries that are not necessarily perpendicular to the direction of the incident sound. It also allows imaging of tissue parenchyma as well as organ boundaries. Scattering is relatively independent of the direction of the incident sound and, therefore, is more characteristic of the scatterers. Most surfaces in the body are rough for our purposes. Reflections from smooth boundaries (e.g., vessel intima) depend not only on the acoustic properties at the boundaries but also on the angles involved.

Because the ultrasound pulse encounters several scatterers at any point in its travel, several echoes are generated simultaneously. These may arrive at the transducer in such a way that they reinforce (constructive interference) or partially or totally cancel (destructive interference) each other. This results in a displayed dot pattern that does not directly represent scatterers, but rather represents an interference pattern of the scatterer distribution scanned. This phenomenon is called acoustic speckle. It is analogous to the speckle phenomenon observed with lasers.

Now that sound propagation, reflection, and scattering have been considered, a very important aspect of pulse-echo diagnostic ultrasound—the range equation—can be studied. The aim in pulse-echo diagnostic ultrasound is (1) to generate short pulses of sound that travel through the body, producing reflections (echoes) that travel back to the source; and (2) to detect and display the returning echoes. The method that the instruments use to position the echo properly on the display is described in Chapter 4. The two items of information required are (1) the direction from which the echo came (which is assumed to be the direction in which the emitted pulse is launched), and (2) the distance to the boundary (reflector or scatterer) where the echo was produced. The underlying principle can be illustrated as follows. The instrument cannot measure distance directly; rather, it measures time and determines distance from it. Similarly, measuring the distance from one city to another directly might be inconvenient (a very long tape measure might be required!), but we could determine the distance by asking someone to drive from one city to the other and observe the time required. Of course we would not know when the person arrived at the other city if we were not riding along, so we would ask the driver to return immediately after arriving at the destination (Fig. 2.24). Let's say that the round trip took 4 hours. What was the distance traveled? We cannot, of course, calculate the answer unless we know the speed traveled. If the driver

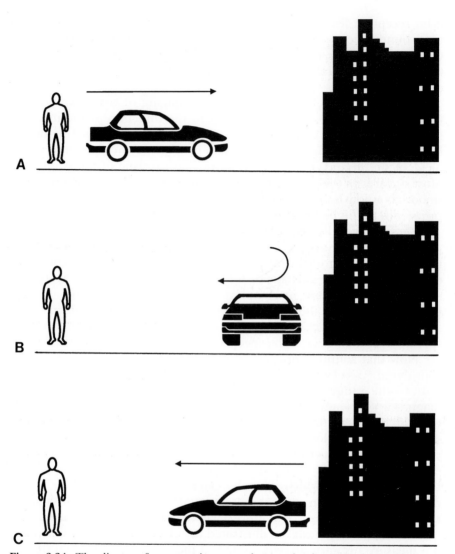

Figure 2.24. The distance from one city to another can be determined by multiplying speed by one-half the round-trip travel time.

says he was traveling at a speed of 60 mph, then we can determine that the distance traveled was 240 miles (60 mph × 4 hours). Therefore, the distance to the city is 120 miles. Note that the total distance was halved because round trip mileage was used to determine a one-way distance. The same principle is used with the ultrasonic tape measure (Fig. 2.25).

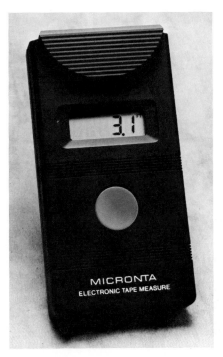

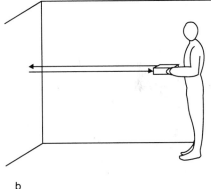

Figure 2.25. (*a*) Ultrasonic tape measure. (*b*) This device uses the round-trip travel time of ultrasound to determine the dimensions of a room.

a   b

Thus, the distance of ultrasound is calculated from the range (distance to reflector) equation:

distance to reflector (mm)
= ½[propagation speed (mm/μs)   d = ½ ct
× pulse round-trip time (μs)]

round-trip time ↑   reflector distance ↑

To determine the distance from the source to the reflector, the propagation speed in the intervening medium must be known or assumed, and the pulse round-trip time must be measured. The reason that the factor ½ appears is that the round-trip time is the time for the pulse to travel to the reflector and return. However, only the distance *to* the reflector is desired. The soft tissue average propagation speed (1.54 mm/μs) is usually assumed in using the range equation (unless another speed is known). For this case, the distance (mm) to the reflector can be calculated by multiplying 0.77 by round-trip time (μs). The figure 0.77 is derived from dividing 1.54 by 2.

   In the city distance problem presented earlier, we can also consider the fact that 60 mph is also equivalent to 1 mile/minute. Thus, at this speed, 2 minutes of round trip travel are required for each mile of

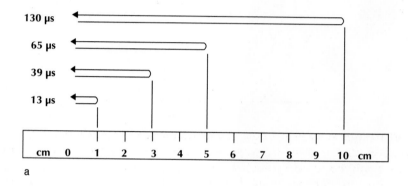

a

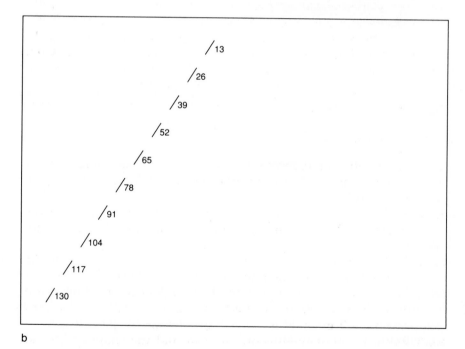

b

Figure 2.26. (*a*) Echo arrival times for 1-, 3-, 5-, and 10-cm reflector distances. (*b*) Echoes from 1-, 2-, 3-, 4-, 5-, 6-, 7-, 8-, 9-, and 10-cm depths arrive at the times (μs) indicated.

TABLE 2.7
Pulse Round-Trip Travel Time for
Various Reflector Depths

Depth (cm)	Travel Time (μs)
0.5	6.5
1	13
2	26
3	39
4	52
5	65
10	130
15	195
20	260

distance separating the cities. Similarly, sound speed in tissue is 1.54 mm/μs so that 0.65 μs are required for each millimeter of travel. Also, 6.5 μs would be required for 1 cm of travel. Therefore, 13 μs of round-trip travel time are required for each centimeter of distance from the transducer to the reflector. If the pulse round-trip time is 13 μs, substitution in the range equation above yields a reflector distance of 10 mm (1 cm). All this leads to the important 13 μs/cm rule. That is, pulse round-trip travel time is 13 μs for each centimeter of distance from source to reflector (Table 2.7). Figure 2.26 illustrates the correspondence between echo arrival time and reflector depth.

EXERCISES

2.4.1 When ultrasound encounters a boundary with perpendicular incidence, the _____ of the tissues must be different to produce a reflection.

2.4.2 With perpendicular incidence, two media _____ and the incident _____ must be known to calculate reflected intensity.

2.4.3 With perpendicular incidence, two media _____ must be known to calculate the intensity reflection coefficient.

2.4.4 For an incident intensity of 2 mW/cm² and impedances of 49 and 51 rayls, the reflected intensity is _____ mW/cm², and the transmitted intensity is _____ mW/cm².

2.4.5 For an incident intensity of 2 mW/cm² and impedances of 99 and 101 rayls, the reflected and transmitted intensities are _____ and _____ mW/cm², respectively.

2.4.6 For an incident intensity of 2 mW/cm² and impedances of 98 and 102 rayls, the reflected and the transmitted intensities are _____ and _____ mW/cm², respectively.

2.4.7 For an incident intensity of 5 mW/cm² and impedances of 45 and 55 rayls, the intensity reflection coefficient is _____, or _____ per cent.

2.4.8 For impedances of 45 and 55 rayls, the intensity transmission coefficient is _____, or _____ per cent.

2.4.9 For impedances of 45 and 55 rayls, the intensity reflection coefficient is _____ dB.

2.4.10 Given the following, calculate the reflected intensity (mW/cm²):
incident intensity = 1 mW/cm²
medium one:
   density = 1.0 kg/m³
   propagation speed = 1350 m/s
medium two:
   density = 1.0 kg/m³
   propagation speed = 1650 m/s

2.4.11 Given the following, calculate the reflected intensity (mW/cm²):
incident intensity = 5 mW/cm²
medium one:
   density = 1.00 kg/m³
   propagation speed = 1515 m/s
medium two:
   density = 1.01 kg/m³
   propagation speed = 1500 m/s

2.4.12 Given the following, calculate the reflected _____ and transmitted _____ intensities (mW/cm²):
incident intensity = 5 mW/cm²
medium one impedance = 2 rayls
medium two impedance = 0 rayls

2.4.13 If the impedances of the media are equal, there is no reflection. True or false?

2.4.14 If the densities of the media are equal, there is no reflection. True or false?

2.4.15 If propagation speeds of the media are equal, there is no reflection. True or false?

2.4.16 The intensity reflection and transmission coefficients depend on whether the sound is traveling from medium one into medium two, or vice versa. True or false?

2.4.17 The intensity reflection coefficient at a boundary between soft tissue (impedance of 1,630,000 rayls) and air (impedance of 400 rayls) is _____.

2.4.18 A coupling medium is used to eliminate _____ between the sound source and the skin, thus eliminating a strong _____ at the air–skin boundary.

2.4.19 The intensity reflection coefficient at a boundary between fat (impedance of 1,380,000 rayls) and muscle (impedance of 1,700,000 rayls) is _____.

2.4.20 The intensity reflection coefficient at a boundary between soft tissue (impedance of 1,630,000 rayls) and bone (impedance of 7,800,000 rayls) is _____.

2.4.21 With perpendicular incidence, the reflected intensity depends on
  a. density difference
  b. acoustic impedance difference
  c. acoustic impedance sum
  d. both b and c
  e. both a and b

2.4.22 Refraction is a change in _____ of sound when it crosses a boundary. It is caused by a change in _____ _____ at the boundary.

2.4.23 If the propagation speed through medium two is greater than the propagation speed through medium one, the transmission angle will be _____ _____the incidence angle, and the reflection angle will be _____ _____the incidence angle.

2.4.24 If the propagation speed through medium two is less than the propagation speed through medium one, the transmission angle will be _____ _____the incidence angle, and the reflection angle will be _____ _____the incidence angle.

2.4.25 If the propagation speed through medium two is equal to the propagation speed through medium one, the transmission angle will be _____ _____the incidence angle, and the reflection angle will be _____ _____the incidence angle.

2.4.26 If the incidence angle is 30 degrees, the propagation speed through medium one is 1 mm/μs, and the propagation speed through medium two is 0.7 mm/μs, the reflection angle is _____ degrees and the transmission angle is _____ degrees.

2.4.27 If the incidence angle is 30 degrees, the propagation speed through medium one is 1 mm/μs, and the propagation speed through medium two is 1 mm/μs, the reflection angle is _____ degrees and the transmission angle is _____ degrees.

2.4.28 If the incidence angle is 30 degrees and the propagation speed through medium two is 30 per cent higher than the propagation speed through medium one, the reflection angle is _____ degrees and the transmission angle is _____ degrees.

2.4.29 Given the following, calculate the reflection coefficient:
incidence angle = 20 degrees
incident intensity = 5 mW/cm²
propagation speed through medium one = 1.5 mm/μs
impedance of medium one = 8 rayls
propagation speed through medium two = 1.5 mm/μs
impedance of medium two = 12 rayls

2.4.30 Given the following, calculate the reflected intensity (mW/cm²):
incidence angle = 20 degrees
incident intensity = 5 mW/cm²
transmission angle = 20 degrees
impedance of medium one = 8 rayls
impedance of medium two = 12 rayls

2.4.31 Under what two conditions does refraction *not* occur?
a. _____
b. _____

2.4.32 Under what condition is the reflection coefficient not dependent on incidence angle?

2.4.33 When ultrasound encounters a boundary with oblique incidence, either _____ or _____ _____ must change to generate a reflection.

2.4.34 The low speed of sound in fat is a source of image degradation because of refraction. If the incidence angle at a boundary between fat (1440 m/s) and kidney (1560 m/s) is 30 degrees, the transmission angle is _____ degrees.

2.4.35 For Exercise 2.4.34, the lateral shift of the sound path 5 cm beyond the boundary because of refraction is _____ mm. Proceed as follows: The difference between the incidence and transmission angles is 2 degrees. The tangent of 2 degrees is 0.0349. The tangent multiplied by the distance (5 cm) yields the lateral shift.

2.4.36 Redirection of sound in many directions as it encounters rough media junctions or particle suspensions (heterogeneous media) is called _____.

2.4.37 With specular reflection, wavelength is small compared with boundary dimensions. True or false?

2.4.38 Scattering occurs when boundary dimensions are large compared with wavelength or when the boundary is smooth. True or false?

2.4.39 As frequency increases, backscatter strength
   a. increases
   b. decreases
   c. does not change
   d. refracts
   e. infarcts
2.4.40 Backscatter helps make echo reception less dependent on incidence angle. True or false?
2.4.41 As frequency increases, specular reflections
   a. increase
   b. decrease
   c. do not change
   d. refract
   e. infarct
2.4.42 The approach in pulse-echo ultrasound is (1) to generate _____ of sound that travel through the body, producing _____ that travel back to the source, and (2) to detect and _____ the returning echoes.
2.4.43 To calculate the distance to a reflector, the _____ _____ and the pulse round-trip _____ must be known.
2.4.44 If the propagation speed is 1.6 mm/μs and the pulse round-trip time is 5 μs, the distance to the reflector is _____ mm.
2.4.45 If the propagation speed is 1.4 mm/μs and the time for a pulse to travel to the reflector is 5 μs, the distance to the reflector is _____ mm.
2.4.46 When the pulse round-trip time is 10 μs, the distance to a reflector in soft tissue is _____ mm.
2.4.47 When the pulse round-trip time is 13 μs, the distance to a reflector in soft tissue is _____ cm.
2.4.48 If an echo arrives 39 μs after a pulse was emitted, at what depth should the echo be placed on its scan line?
2.4.49 When the pulse round-trip time is 130 μs, the distance to a reflector in soft tissue is _____ cm.
2.4.50 How long after a pulse is sent out by a transducer does an echo from an object at a depth of 5 cm return?

2.5
Review

Ultrasound is sound (a wave of traveling acoustic variables, including pressure, density, temperature, and particle motion) having a frequency of greater than 20 kHz. It is described by frequency, period, wavelength,

propagation speed, amplitude, intensity, and attenuation. Pulsed ultrasound is described by additional terms: PRF, pulse repetition period,
pulse duration, duty factor, and spatial pulse length. Propagation speed
and impedance are characteristics of the medium that are determined by
density and stiffness. Attenuation increases with frequency and path
length. Imaging depth decreases with increasing frequency. Six intensities (SATA, SPTA, SAPA, SPPA, SATP, and SPTP) are used to describe
pulsed ultrasound. The soft tissue propagation speed is 1.54 mm/μs, and
the attenuation coefficient is 0.5 dB/cm for each megahertz of frequency. Table 2.8 gives typical values for several parameters of diagnostic ultrasound. Table 2.9 indicates how various parameters change with
frequency.

With perpendicular incidence, when sound encounters boundaries
between media with different impedances, part of the sound is reflected
and part is transmitted. If the two media have the same impedance,
there is no reflection. With oblique incidence, the sound is refracted at a
boundary between media where propagation speeds are different. Incidence and reflection angles are always equal. For oblique incidence,
there may be a reflection when the impedances are equal (if the propagation speeds are different), and there may not be a reflection even if the
impedances are different. Scattering occurs at rough media boundaries

TABLE 2.8
Diagnostic Ultrasound Parameters in Tissue

Parameter	Symbol or Abbreviation	Typical Value	Range of Common Values
Frequency	f	3.5 MHz	2–10 MHz
Period	T	0.3 μs	0.1–0.5 μs
Wavelength	λ	0.4 mm	0.1–0.8 mm
Propagation speed	c	1.54 mm/μs	1.4–1.7 mm/μs
Impedance	z	1,630,000 rayls	1,300,000– 1,700,000 rayls
Pulse repetition frequency	PRF	5 kHz	2–10 kHz
Pulse repetition period	PRP	0.2 ms	0.1–0.5 ms
Cycles per pulse	n	2	1–3
Pulse duration	PD	1 μs	0.5–3 μs
Spatial pulse length	SPL	0.4 mm	0.1–1 mm
Duty factor	DF	0.005	0.001–0.01
Spatial peak temporal aver- age intensity	I_{SPTA}	1 mW/cm^2	0.01–100 mW/cm^2
Spatial peak pulse average intensity	I_{SPPA}	1 W/cm^2	0.01–100 W/cm^2
Attenuation coefficient	a_c	3 dB/cm	1–5 dB/cm

TABLE 2.9
Dependence of Various Factors on
Increasing (↑) Frequency

Period ↓
Wavelength ↓
Pulse duration ↓
Duty factor ↓
Spatial pulse length ↓
Attenuation ↑
Imaging depth ↓

and within heterogeneous media. The range equation is used to determine distance to reflectors.

The definitions for terms discussed in this chapter are as follows:

Absorption. Conversion of sound to heat.

Acoustic. Having to do with sound.

Acoustic propagation properties. Characteristics of a medium that affect the propagation of sound through it.

Acoustic variables. Pressure, density, temperature, and particle motion—things that vary with space and time in a sound wave.

Amplitude. Maximum variation of an acoustic variable or voltage.

Anechoic. Echo-free.

Attenuation. Decrease in amplitude and intensity as a wave travels through a medium.

Attenuation coefficient. Attenuation per centimeter of wave travel.

Backscatter. Sound scattered back in the direction from which it originally came.

Compressibility. Ability of a material to be reduced to a smaller volume under external pressure.

Continuous wave. A wave in which cycles repeat indefinitely; not pulsed.

Continuous-wave mode. Mode of operation in which continuous-wave sound is used.

Coupling medium. Gel used to provide a good sound path between the transducer and the skin.

cw. Abbreviation for continuous wave.

Cycle. Complete variation of an acoustic variable.

dB. Abbreviation for decibel.

Decibel. Unit of power or intensity ratio; the number of decibels is 10 times the logarithm (to the base 10) of the power or intensity ratio.

Density. Mass divided by volume.

Displacement. Distance that an object has moved.

Duty factor. Fraction of time that pulsed ultrasound is actually on.

Echo. Reflection.

Energy. Capability of doing work.

Force. That which changes the state of rest or motion of an object.

Frequency. Number of cycles per unit of time.

Hertz. Unit of frequency, one cycle per second; unit of pulse repetition frequency, one pulse per second.

Hz. Abbreviation for hertz.

Impedance. Density multiplied by sound propagation speed.

Incidence angle. Angle between incident sound direction and a line perpendicular to the boundary of a medium.

Intensity. Power divided by area.

Intensity reflection coefficient. Reflected intensity divided by incident intensity.

Intensity transmission coefficient. Transmitted intensity divided by incident intensity.

Interference. Combination of positive and negative pressures.

kHz. Abbreviation for kilohertz.

Kilohertz. One thousand hertz.

Log. Abbreviation for logarithm.

Logarithm. The logarithm (to the base of 10) of a number is equal to the number of tens that must be multiplied together to result in that number.

Longitudinal wave. Wave in which the particle motion is parallel to the direction of wave travel (compressional wave).

Medium. Material through which a wave travels.

Megahertz. One million hertz.

MHz. Abbreviation for megahertz.

Oblique incidence. Sound direction that is not perpendicular to media boundaries.

Particle. Small portion of a medium.

Particle Motion. Oscillatory movement of particles as a sound wave travels through a medium.

Penetration. Imaging depth.

Period. Time per cycle.

Perpendicular. Geometrically related by 90 degrees.

Perpendicular incidence. Sound direction that is perpendicular to media boundaries.

Power. Rate at which work is done; rate at which energy is transferred.

Pressure. Force divided by area in a fluid.

PRF. Abbreviation for pulse repetition frequency.

Propagation. Progression or travel.

Propagation speed. Speed with which a wave moves through a medium.

Pulse. A brief excursion of a quantity from its normal value; a few cycles.

Pulse duration. Time from beginning to end of a pulse.

Pulse repetition frequency. Number of pulses per second. Sometimes called pulse repetition rate.

Pulse repetition period. Time from the beginning of one pulse to the beginning of the next.

Pulsed ultrasound. Ultrasound produced in pulse form by applying electrical pulses to the transducer.

Range equation. Relationship between round-trip pulse travel time and distance to a reflector.

Rarefaction. Region of low density and pressure in a compressional wave.

Rayl. Unit of impedance; equal to kg/m^2-second.

Reflection. Portion of sound returned from a boundary of a medium.

Reflection angle. Angle between reflected sound direction and a line perpendicular to the boundary of a medium.

Reflector. Medium boundary that produces a reflection; reflecting surface.

Refraction. Change of sound direction upon passing from one medium to another.

Scatterer. An object that scatters sound because of its small size or its surface roughness.

Scattering. Diffusion or redirection of sound in several directions upon encountering a particle suspension or a rough surface.

Sound. Traveling wave of acoustic variables.

Spatial pulse length. Length of space over which a pulse occurs.

Specular reflection. Reflection from a large, flat, smooth boundary.

Speed. Displacement divided by the time over which displacement occurs.

Stiffness. Property of a medium; applied pressure divided by fractional volume change produced.

Strength. Nonspecific term referring to amplitude or intensity.

Temperature. Condition of a body that determines transfer of heat to or from other bodies.

Transmission angle. Angle between transmitted sound direction and a line perpendicular to the boundary of a medium.

Ultrasound. Sound having a frequency greater than 20 kHz.

Velocity. Speed with direction of motion specified.

Wave. Traveling variation of wave variables.

Wavelength. Length of space over which a cycle occurs.

Wave variables. Things that are functions of space and time in a wave.

Work. Force multiplied by displacement.

EXERCISES

   2.5.1 Which of the following is a characteristic of a medium through which sound is propagating?
     a. impedance
     b. intensity
     c. amplitude
     d. frequency
     e. period

   2.5.2 Which of the following applies to continuous-wave sound?
     a. pulse duration
     b. pulse repetition frequency
     c. frequency
     d. intensity
     e. c and d

2.5.3 Match the following:

a. frequency: _____
b. period: _____

c. wavelength: _____
d. propagation speed: _____
e. amplitude: _____

1. time per cycle
2. maximum variation per cycle
3. length per cycle
4. cycles per second
5. speed of a wave through a medium

2.5.4 Match the following:

a. wavelength: _____

b. duty factor: _____

c. intensity: _____

1. $\dfrac{\text{propagation speed}}{\text{frequency}}$

2. $\dfrac{\text{pulse duration}}{\text{pulse repetition period}}$

3. $\dfrac{\text{power}}{\text{beam area}}$

2.5.5 Match the following:

a. period: _____

b. pulse repetition period: _____
c. impedance: _____

d. propagation speed: _____

e. pulse duration: _____

f. spatial pulse length: _____

1. density × propagation speed
2. frequency × wavelength
3. $\dfrac{1}{\text{frequency}}$

4. $\dfrac{1}{\text{pulse repetition frequency}}$

5. number of cycles in pulse × wavelength
6. number of cycles in pulse × period

2.5.6 Match the following quantities with their units (answers may be used more than once):

a. frequency: _____
b. wavelength: _____
c. period: _____
d. propagation speed: _____
e. pulse duration: _____
f. pulse repetition frequency: _____
g. pulse repetition period: _____
h. intensity: _____

1. μs
2. mm/μs
3. MHz
4. mm
5. mW/cm^2
6. W
7. dB/cm
8. dB
9. cm^2
10. kHz

   i. attenuation: _____   11. ms
   j. attenuation coefficient: _____
   k. power: _____
   l. beam area: _____
2.5.7 Match the following (each answer should be used twice):
   a. attenuation coefficient of
      0.5 dB/cm at 1 MHz: _____   1. soft tissues
   b. high attenuation: _____, _____   2. lung
   c. high propagation speed: _____   3. bone
   d. propagation speed of 1.54
      mm/μs: _____
   e. low propagation speed: _____
2.5.8 Given the following values:
   frequency = 2 MHz
   pulse repetition frequency = 1 kHz
   4 cycles per pulse
   SATA intensity = 1 mW/cm^2
   density = 1058 kg/m
   Apply these values to a soft tissue surface in order to find the
   following:
   a. propagation speed: _____ mm/μs
   b. wavelength: _____ mm
   c. spatial pulse length: _____ mm
   d. period: _____ μs
   e. pulse duration: _____ μs
   f. pulse repetition period: _____ ms
   g. duty factor: _____
   h. SAPA intensity at the surface: _____ mW/cm
   i. attenuation coefficient: _____ dB/cm
   j. depth for 3 dB of attenuation: _____ cm
   k. attenuation from surface to 3 cm depth: _____ dB
   l. intensity ratio corresponding to dB in k: _____
   m. SATA intensity at 3-cm depth: _____ mW/cm^2
   n. SATA intensity at 6-cm depth: _____ mW/cm^2
   o. SAPA intensity at 3-cm depth: _____ mW/cm^2
   p. SAPA intensity at 6-cm depth: _____ mW/cm^2
   q. impedance: _____ rayls
2.5.9 Which of the following cannot be determined from the others?
   a. frequency
   b. period
   c. amplitude
   d. wavelength
   e. propagation speed

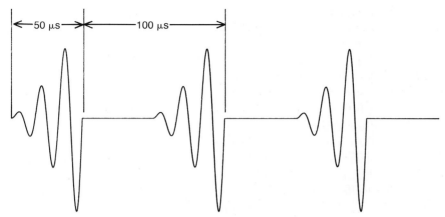

Figure 2.27. Pressure versus time for three-cycle pulses.

2.5.10 Which of the following cannot be determined from the others?
  a. frequency
  b. amplitude
  c. intensity
  d. power
  e. beam area

2.5.11 If stiffness is increased, impedance is _____.

2.5.12 In Figure 2.27, give the pulse repetition period, pulse duration, duty factor, pulse repetition frequency, period, and frequency.

2.5.13 If no refraction occurs as an oblique sound beam passes through the boundary between two materials, the _____ _____ of the materials are known to be _____.

2.5.14 What must be known to calculate distance to a reflector?
  a. attenuation, speed, density
  b. attenuation, impedance
  c. attenuation, absorption
  d. travel time, speed
  e. density, speed

2.5.15 With perpendicular incidence, if the impedances of two media are the same, there will be no
  a. inflation
  b. reflection
  c. refraction
  d. calibration
  e. both b and c

2.5.16 What is the transmitted intensity if the incident intensity is 1 mW/cm² and the impedances are 1.00 and 2.64 units?

    a. 0.2

    b. 0.4

    c. 0.6

    d. 0.8

    e. 1.0

2.5.17 If the incident intensity is 1 mW/cm² and the impedances are 3 and 2 units, the reflected intensity is _____.

2.5.18 No reflection will occur with perpendicular incidence if the media _____ are equal.

2.5.19 No reflection will occur with oblique incidence if the media _____ are equal and the media _____ _____ are equal.

2.5.20 If the incidence angle is 20 degrees and the propagation speeds of media one and two are 1.7 and 1.5 mm/μs, respectively, the transmission angle is _____ degrees.

2.5.21 If the incidence angle is 20 degrees and propagation speeds of media one and two are 1.5 and 1.7 mm/μs, respectively, the transmission angle is _____ degrees.

2.5.22 Scattering occurs at smooth boundaries and within homogeneous media. True or false?

2.5.23 A 3-MHz instrument with an SPTA output intensity of 10 mW/cm² images to a maximum depth of 12 cm. To image to a depth of 18 cm, the output intensity of the instrument must be increased to _____ mW/cm².

CHAPTER 3

Transducers

In this chapter, we consider the following questions: What is a transducer? How does a transducer generate ultrasound pulses? How does a transducer receive echoes? How are sound beams described and on what do they depend? How are sound beams automatically focused and scanned through tissue cross sections? What is the difference between a linear phased array and a phased linear array? How is detail resolution described and on what does it depend? The following terms are discussed in this chapter:

annular
annular array
aperture
apodization
array
axial
axial resolution
bandwidth
beam
beam area
burst-excited mode
channel
composite
continuous mode
convex array
crystal
Curie point
damping
detail resolution
disk
dynamic aperture

electric pulse
electric voltage
element
far zone
f number
focal length
focal region
focal zone
focus
fractional bandwidth
Fraunhofer zone
Fresnel zone
grating lobes
internal focus
lateral
lateral resolution
lens
linear
linear array
linear phased array
linear sequenced array

matching layer
mechanical transducer
near zone
operating frequency
phased array
phased linear array
piezoelectricity
probe
pulsed mode
PVDF
PZT
quality factor (Q factor)
resolution
resonance frequency

scanhead
sector
sensitivity
shock-excited mode
side lobes
sound beam
transducer
transducer array
transducer assembly
transducer element
ultrasound transducer
vector array
voltage pulse

The characteristics of ultrasound that are important for diagnosis have been described in Chapter 2. In this chapter, the devices that generate and receive ultrasound are described. They form the connecting link between the ultrasound–tissue interactions of Chapter 2 and the instruments described in Chapters 4 and 5. Except for a brief mention of sound beams in Chapter 2, the confining of sound to beams has not yet been covered. The devices described in this chapter do not produce sound that travels uniformly in all directions away from the source. Rather, the sound is confined in beams, which are described in Section 3.2.

3.1
Construction and Operation

Transducers convert one form of energy to another. The most general definition of a transducer is a device through which energy can flow from one medium or system to another. The energy conducted by these devices may be of the same or of different forms. The latter case conforms to the transducer definition given here. Examples are given in Table 3.1. Ultrasound transducers are sometimes called probes or scanheads. They convert electric energy into ultrasound energy and vice versa. Electric voltages applied to them are converted to ultrasound. Ultrasound incident on them produces electric voltages. Loudspeakers (Fig. 3.1a), microphones (Fig. 3.1b), and intercoms accomplish similar functions with audible sound.

Ultrasound transducers operate according to the principle of piezoelectricity (from the Greek πιεζώ, to press; and ηλεκτρον, meaning am-

TABLE 3.1
Transducer Examples

Transducer	Energy Converted	Resulting Form of Energy
Light bulb	Electricity	Light and heat
Automobile engine	Chemical energy	Motion and heat
Ear	Sound	Electric impulses
Oven	Electricity	Heat
Motor	Electricity	Motion
Generator	Motion	Electricity
Battery	Chemical energy	Electricity
Human body	Chemical energy	Heat, motion, and sound
Microphone	Audible sound	Electricity
Loudspeaker	Electricity	Audible sound

ber, which was the organic resin that was used in early electrical studies), which was discovered in 1880. This principle states that some materials (ceramics, quartz, polyvinylidene fluoride [PVDF], and others) produce a voltage when deformed by an applied pressure. Piezoelectricity also results in production of a pressure when these materials are deformed by an applied voltage. Various formulations of lead zirconate titanate

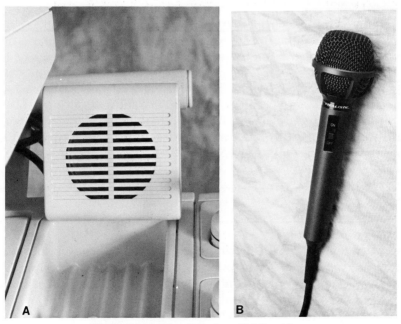

Figure 3.1. (*a*) Loudspeaker. (*b*) Microphone.

(PZT) are commonly used as materials for production of modern transducer elements. Ceramics such as these are not *naturally* piezoelectric (as quartz is). They are made piezoelectric during their production by placing them in a strong electric field while they are at a high temperature. They are often combined with a nonpiezoelectric polymer to create materials that are called piezocomposites. These composites have improved bandwidth, sensitivity, and resolution (characteristics discussed later in this chapter and in Chapter 4).

Single-element transducers take the form of disks (Fig. 3.2a). Linear-array transducers (discussed in Section 3.3) contain numerous elements that have a rectangular shape (Fig. 3.2b). When an electric voltage is applied to the faces, the thickness of the element increases or decreases, depending on the polarity of the voltage. The term transducer element (also called piezoelectric element, active element, or crystal) refers to the piece of piezoelectric material that converts electricity to ultrasound and vice versa. The element, with its associated case and damping and matching materials (discussed later in this section), is called the transducer assembly, probe, or scanhead (Fig. 3.2d). Both the transducer element and the transducer assembly are commonly referred to as the transducer. Typical diagnostic ultrasound elements are 0.2 to 1 mm thick.

Transducers operated in the burst-excited mode are driven by a cycle or two of alternating voltage (see Section 4.1). This produces an alternating pressure that propagates as a sound pulse (Fig. 3.3a). The frequency of the sound produced is equal to the frequency of the driving voltage. The operating frequency (sometimes called resonance frequency) of the transducer is its preferred frequency of operation. Operating frequency is determined by the propagation speed of the transducer material (typically 4 to 6 mm/μs) and the thickness (Table 3.2) of the transducer element. It is such that the thickness corresponds to half a wavelength in the element material. Because wavelength decreases as frequency increases (Section 2.1),

---

thickness ↓   operating frequency ↑

The returning echo encountering the transducer is converted into an alternating voltage burst (Fig. 3.3b).

Transducers operated in the shock-excited mode are driven by voltage pulses (see Section 4.1) and produce ultrasound pulses (Fig. 3.4). These transducers convert received echoes into voltage bursts.

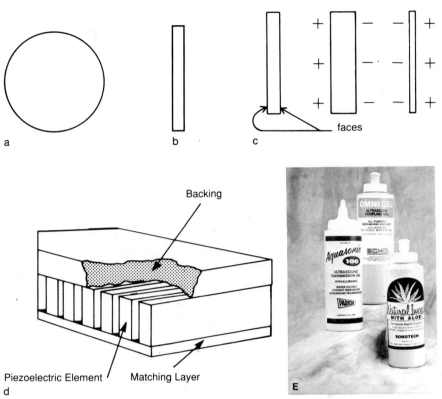

a   b   c

faces

Backing

Piezoelectric Element   Matching Layer
d

E

Figure 3.2. (*a*) Front view of a disk transducer element. (*b*) Front view of a rectangular element. (*c*) Side view of either element with no voltage applied to faces (normal thickness), with voltage applied (increased thickness), and with opposite voltage applied (decreased thickness). (*d*) A transducer assembly (scanhead or probe). The damping material reduces pulse duration, thus improving axial resolution. The matching layer increases sound transmission into the tissues. (*e*) Coupling gel improves sound transmission into the patient by eliminating air reflection.

The pulse repetition frequency (PRF) is equal to the voltage burst (or pulse) repetition frequency, which is determined by the instrument driving the transducer. The pulse duration is equal to the period multiplied by the number of cycles in the pulse (see Section 2.2).

Damping material (usually a mixture of metal powder and a plastic or epoxy) is attached to the rear face of the transducer element to reduce the number of cycles in each pulse (see Figs. 3.2*d* and 3.5). This reduces pulse duration and spatial pulse length and thus results in improved axial resolution (see Section 3.4). This method of damping is analogous to packing foam rubber around a bell that is rung by a tap with a

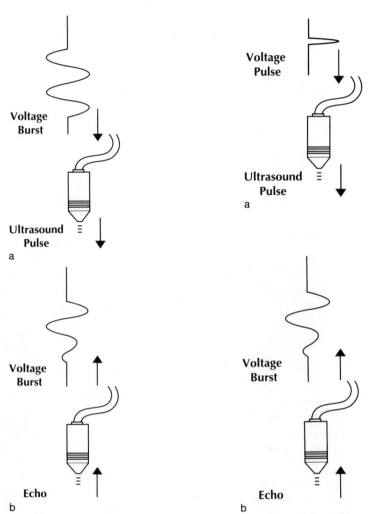

Figure 3.3. A transducer operating in the burst-excited mode. This device converts electric voltage bursts into ultrasound pulses (*a*) and converts received echoes into electric voltage bursts (*b*).

Figure 3.4. A transducer assembly operating in the shock-excited mode. This device converts electric voltage pulses into ultrasound pulses (*a*) and converts received echoes into electric voltage bursts (*b*).

hammer (mechanical shock excitation). The rubber reduces the time that the bell rings following the tap. It also reduces the loudness or intensity of the ringing.

For ultrasound transducers, the damping material additionally reduces the ultrasound amplitude and thus decreases the efficiency and sensitivity of the system (undesired effect). This is the price paid for

TABLE 3.2
Transducer Element Thickness* for
Various Operating Frequencies

Frequency (MHz)	Thickness (mm)
2.0	1.0
3.5	0.6
5.0	0.4
7.5	0.3
10.0	0.2

* Assuming an element propagation speed of 4 mm/μs.

reduced spatial pulse length (a desired effect resulting in improved axial resolution). Some damping may also be accomplished electrically within the instrument and within the element. If this type of damping is sufficiently large, the backing material is not required. Typically, pulses of one to three cycles are generated with diagnostic ultrasound transducers.

Because the transducer element is a solid (having high density and sound speed), it has an impedance that is about 20 times that of tissues. Without being compensated, this would cause about 90 per cent of the emitted intensity to be reflected at the skin boundary. Thus, most of the sound energy would not enter the body. A returning echo would have about 90 per cent of its intensity reflected also, so that only a small portion would enter the transducer. To solve this problem, a matching layer is commonly placed on the transducer face (Fig. 3.2d). This material has an impedance of intermediate value between that of the transducer element and that of the tissue. It reduces the reflection of ultrasound at the transducer element surface, thereby improving sound transmission across it. This is analogous to the coating layer on eyeglasses or camera lenses, which reduces light reflection at the air–glass boundary. The optimum thickness for this matching layer is one quarter of a wavelength. Because many frequencies and wavelengths are present in short ultrasound pulses (see the discussion of bandwidth later in this section), multiple matching layers provide a greater improvement in sound transmission across the element–tissue boundary than does a single layer.

Because of its very low impedance, even a very thin layer of air between the transducer and the skin surface will reflect virtually all the sound, preventing any penetration into the tissue. For this reason, a coupling medium, usually an aqueous gel (see Fig. 3.2e), is applied to the

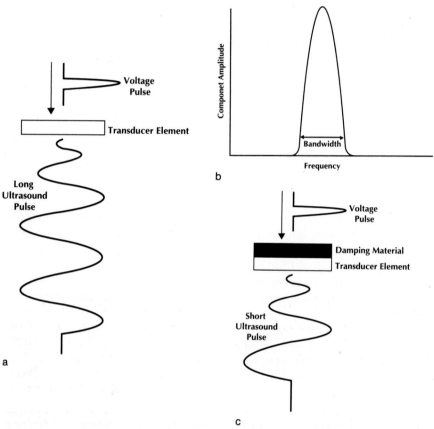

Figure 3.5. Without damping (*a*), a voltage pulse applied to a transducer element results in a long ultrasound pulse of many cycles. With damping material on the rear face of the transducer element (*c*), application of a voltage pulse results in a short ultrasound pulse of a few cycles. This figure shows each pulse traveling (down) away from the transducer in space so that the bottom end is the beginning or leading edge of the pulse as it travels down. (*b* and *d*) Plot of the frequencies present in the ultrasound pulses (from *a* and *c*). Component amplitude is the amplitude of each frequency component present. Bandwidth is the frequency range within which the amplitudes exceed some reference value. Plot *d* represents a broad-band, low-Q factor, damped pulse (*c*). Plot (*b*) represents a narrow-band, high-Q factor, undamped pulse (*a*).

skin before transducer contact. This eliminates the air layer and facilitates sound passage into and out of the tissue.

A transducer preferentially produces a frequency equal to its operating frequency (introduced earlier in this section). However, the ultrasound pulses produced contain frequencies in addition to this. The shorter the pulse (the fewer the number of cycles), the more frequencies that are present. The range of frequencies involved in a pulse is called its

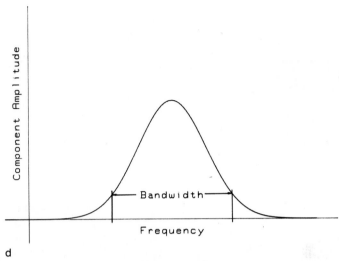

d

Figure 3.5 *Continued*

bandwidth (see Fig. 3.5). Bandwidth must be specified by some definition of where in the frequency range to stop. For example, a 6-dB
bandwidth refers to a range of frequencies, including those that have
half or greater the amplitude (one quarter or greater the power) of the
strongest one (operating frequency). Fractional bandwidth is the bandwidth divided by the operating frequency. Quality factor (Q factor) is the
operating frequency divided by the bandwidth, or $\dfrac{1}{\text{fractional bandwidth}}$.

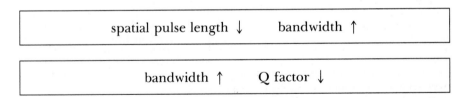

Q factor is unitless. The inclusion of damping material in the transducer assembly increases the bandwidth and decreases the Q factor. For
short pulses (those having one to three cycles), the Q factor is approximately equal to the number of cycles in the pulse. The overall system
bandwidth is determined not only by the transducer, but also by the
instrument electronics.

For wide-bandwidth transducers (e.g., those having a fractional
bandwidth of 70 per cent or a Q factor of 1.4), burst excitation (see **Fig.**

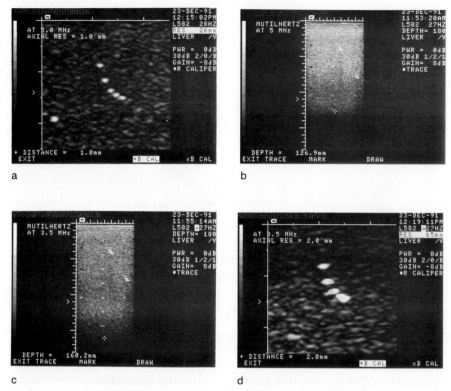

a   b

c   d

Figure 3.6. Multihertz operation allows the transducer to selectively provide (at a higher frequency) better detail resolution (*a*) with reduced penetration (*b*), or (at a lower frequency) deeper penetration (*c*) with some loss of resolution (*d*).

3.3) can be used selectively to operate the same transducer at more than one frequency (Fig. 3.6). The transducer is driven at one of two selectable frequencies by voltage bursts of the selected frequency. The two frequencies must fall within the transducer bandwidth. Choosing the higher frequency yields better detail resolution (see Section 3.4). If the resulting penetration is not sufficient for the study at hand, however, the lower frequency can be selected (resulting in some degradation in detail resolution). Push-button frequency switching is quicker and more convenient than a change in transducers would be.

Some transducers are designed to enter the body (Fig. 3.7) via the vagina,[12] rectum, esophagus, or blood vessel (catheter-mounted type). These approaches allow the transducer to be placed closer to the anatomy of interest, thus avoiding intervening tissues (e.g., lung or gassy bowel) and reducing the sound transmission path. This reduction in

Figure 3.7. (*a*) Several endovaginal transducers. (*b*) Transvaginal view of uterus. (*c*) Transesophageal probe for echocardiography. (*d*) Catheter-mounted transducer for viewing the interior of a blood vessel. (*e*) Close-up view of a catheter-mounted transducer.

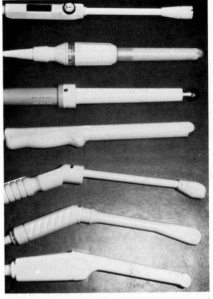

a

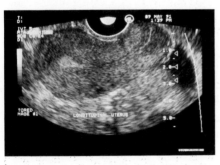

b

c

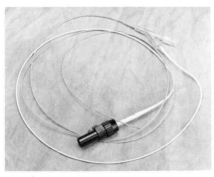

d

e

79

path length (less attenuation) allows higher frequencies to be used with improved resolution.

EXERCISES

3.1.1 A transducer converts one form of _____ to another.

3.1.2 Ultrasound transducers convert_____energy into_____ energy and vice versa.

3.1.3 Ultrasound transducers operate on the _____ principle.

3.1.4 Single-element transducers are in the form of _____.

3.1.5 The _____ of a transducer element changes when a voltage is applied to the faces.

3.1.6 The term transducer is often used to refer to either a transducer _____ or a transducer _____.

3.1.7 A transducer _____ is part of a transducer _____.

3.1.8 Electric voltage bursts, when applied to a transducer, produce ultrasound _____ of a _____ that is equal to that of the bursts.

3.1.9 Electric voltage pulses applied to a transducer produce ultrasound _____ of a frequency determined by element _____.

3.1.10 Operating frequency _____ as transducer element thickness is increased.

3.1.11 Addition of damping material to a transducer reduces the number of _____ in the pulse, thus improving _____ _____. It increases the _____ and decreases the _____ _____.

3.1.12 Addition of damping material reduces the _____ and _____ of the diagnostic system.

3.1.13 Ultrasound transducers typically generate pulses of _____ to _____ cycles.

3.1.14 For a particular transducer element material, if a thickness of 0.4 mm yields an operating frequency of 5 MHz, the thickness required for an operating frequency of 10 MHz is _____ mm.

3.1.15 A transducer with which frequency would have the thinnest element(s) in it?
a. 2 MHz
b. 3 MHz
c. 5 MHz
d. 7 MHz
e. 10 MHz

3.1.16 The matching layer on the transducer surface reduces _____ caused by impedance differences.

3.1.17 A coupling medium on the skin surface eliminates reflection caused by _____.

3.1.18 Quality (Q) factor is expressed in
   a. MHz
   b. mm/μs
   c. W/cm^2
   d. all of the above
   e. none of the above

3.1.19 Increasing the bandwidth increases the Q factor. True or false?

3.1.20 The range of _____ involved in an ultrasound pulse is called its bandwidth.

3.1.21 A two-cycle pulse has a Q factor of approximately _____.
   a. 0.2
   b. 0.5
   c. 2
   d. 5
   e. 20

3.1.22 If bandwidth is 1 MHz and operating frequency is 3 MHz, calculate the following:
   a. Q factor_____
   b. fractional bandwidth_____
   c. lowest frequency_____
   d. highest frequency_____
   e. approximate number of cycles per pulse_____

3.1.23 Elements in linear arrays are in the form of _____.

3.1.24 Transducer assemblies are also called _____ or _____.

3.1.25 Operating frequency is also called _____ _____.

3.1.26 Mixtures of a piezoelectric ceramic and nonpiezoelectric polymer are called _____.

3.1.27 To operate a transducer at more than one frequency requires _____ _____.

3.1.28 Is it practical to attempt to operate a 5-MHz transducer with a Q factor of 2 at 3 and 7 MHz?

3.2
Beams and Focusing

The ultrasound pulse generated by the (flat) disk transducer in Figure 3.2*a* is contained within in a tear-drop shape, as shown in Figure 3.8. Spatial pulse length was previously discussed in Sections 2.2 and 3.1.

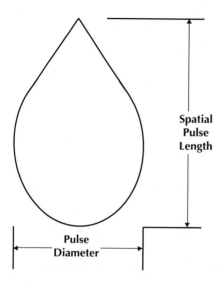

**Spatial
Pulse
Length**

**Pulse
Diameter**

Figure 3.8. An ultrasound pulse generated by a single-element disk transducer driven by an electric voltage pulse, as shown in Figures 3.3 and 3.4, has a tear-drop shape. The pulse diameter is equal to the beam diameter, which varies according to the distance from the transducer (see Fig. 3.9). (Spatial pulse length is described in Figure 2.9.)

This section is concerned with the pulse width or diameter. The sound beam is a description of this diameter as the pulse travels away from the transducer. For a disk element and cylindrical beam, the beam widths in the scan plane and perpendicular to it (the section-thickness dimension discussed in Sections 3.4 and 6.1) are both equal to the beam diameter. This is also true for the annular array discussed in the next section. In the case of linear arrays (discussed in the next section), these two beam widths are not generally the same. The width in the scan plane determines the lateral resolution (see Section 3.4), whereas the width perpendicular to the scan plane determines the extent of section-thickness artifacts (see Section 6.1).

A single-element (flat) disk transducer operating in the continuous-wave mode produces a sound beam with a beam diameter that varies according to the distance from the transducer face, as shown in Figure 3.9. The intensity is not uniform throughout the beam (see Section 2.3). The beam diameter shown in Figure 3.9 approximately bounds that portion of the sound beam that has an intensity of greater than 4 per cent of the spatial peak value (at the center of the beam). This particular value, corresponding to 14 dB, was chosen because it gives a simple picture of the beam.

The 6-dB and 20-dB beam diameters that are sometimes used are narrower and wider, respectively, than that pictured in Figure 3.9. They include that portion of the sound that is greater than 25 per cent and

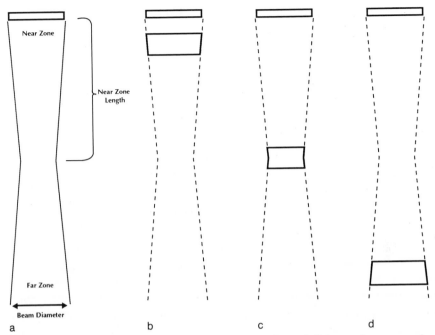

Figure 3.9. (*a*) Beam diameter for a single-element unfocused disk transducer operating in the continuous-wave mode. This diameter approximates the region of that portion of the sound produced that is greater than 4 per cent of the spatial peak intensity. The near zone is the region between the disk and the minimum beam diameter. The far zone is the region beyond the minimum beam diameter. Intensity varies within the beam, with intensity variations being greatest in the near zone. The beam diameter in *a* approximates the changing pulse diameter as an ultrasound pulse travels away from the transducer. (*b*) An ultrasound pulse shortly after leaving the transducer. (*c*) Later, the ultrasound pulse is located at the end of the near-zone length, where its diameter is at a minimum. (*d*) Still later, the pulse is in the far zone, where its diameter is increasing as it travels. (This figure assumes a nonscattering, nonrefracting medium, such as water.)

greater than 1 per cent, respectively, of the spatial peak intensity. Sometimes, significant intensity travels out in some directions not included in the beam, as pictured. These additional beams are called side lobes. They are really cone or ring beams for a disk transducer (see Section 6.1).

The region extending from the element out to a distance of one near-zone length is called the near zone, near field, or Fresnel zone. Near-zone length (also called near-field length) is determined by the size and operating frequency of the element. It increases proportionally with increasing frequency. It also increases with diameter squared.

diameter ↑   near-zone length ↑

frequency ↑   near-zone length ↑

Table 3.3 lists near-zone lengths for various disk element frequencies and diameters.

The region that lies beyond a distance of one near-zone length is called the far zone, far field, or Fraunhofer zone.

The beam diameter depends on the following:

1. wavelength (and, therefore, frequency)
2. transducer diameter
3. distance from the transducer

In the approximation of Figure 3.9, at a distance of one near-zone length from the transducer, the beam diameter is equal to one half the transducer diameter (Fig. 3.10). At a distance of two times the near-zone length, the beam diameter is equal to the transducer diameter. Beyond this distance, the beam diameter increases in proportion to the distance.

The diameter of an ultrasound pulse (see Fig. 3.8) is equal to the beam diameter (see Fig. 3.9) for the distance from the transducer face at which the pulse is located at any given time. As the pulse travels through the near zone, its diameter decreases; as it travels through the far zone, its diameter increases.

A beam description differing from that presented in Figure 3.9 is often seen (Fig. 3.11). As beam characteristics in the near zone are complicated,[13] they may be depicted in a simplified, albeit approximate, way, of which Figure 3.11 is one example. However, a more accurate descrip-

TABLE 3.3
Near-zone Length (NZL) for
Unfocused Transducers

Frequency (MHz)	Diameter (mm)	NZL (cm)
2.0	19	12
3.5	13	10
3.5	19	20
5.0	6	3
5.0	10	8
5.0	13	14
7.5	6	4
10.0	6	6

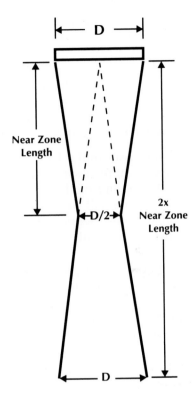

Figure 3.10. Sound beam from a flat disk transducer. The beam diameter narrows to half the disk diameter (D) at the near-zone length and then widens to the disk diameter at twice the near-zone length.

tion is given in Figure 3.10, which indicates that the beam narrows to a minimum diameter at approximately the site of transition from the near to the far zone. It is important to realize that, even for flat, unfocused transducer elements (see Figs. 3.9 and 3.10), there is some beam narrowing or "focusing."

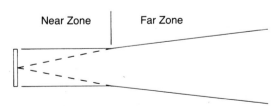

Figure 3.11. Traditional presentation of the beam for a flat disk transducer element. A more accurate view, using a beam diameter with an intensity of 4 per cent of the peak value, is presented in Figure 3.10.

Sound beams produced by disk transducers have beam areas that vary according to the diameter squared.

---

beam diameter ↑   beam area ↑

EXAMPLE 3.2.1

For soft tissue and a 10-mm, 5-MHz disk transducer, what are the beam diameters at the near-zone length and at two times the near-zone length? At the end of the near zone, the beam diameter is approximately equal to one half the diameter of the transducer element, or 5 mm. At double the near-zone length, the beam diameter is approximately equal to the diameter of the transducer element, or 10 mm.

The effect of frequency on near-zone length is shown in Figure 3.12. The effect of transducer diameter is shown in Figure 3.13. An

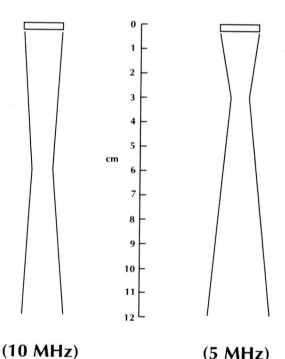

(10 MHz)   (5 MHz)

Figure 3.12. Beams for disk transducers having a diameter of 6 mm at two frequencies. Higher frequencies produce smaller beam diameters (at a distance greater than 4 cm in this case) and longer near-zone lengths.

increase in frequency or in transducer size increases the near-zone length. At a sufficient distance from the transducer, increasing the frequency or the transducer size can decrease the beam diameter (see Figs. 3.12 and 3.13).

The beam in Figure 3.9a is for continuous-wave mode, but is used to describe pulses in the rest of the figure. The beam for pulses is similar to, but not exactly the same as, that for continuous sound. One important reason for this is that the beam is a result of Huygens' principle, which states that each small portion of the surface of a transducer may be considered as a separate (omnidirectional) source. The beam is a result of combining the resulting sound emanating from all the small sources. For short pulses, this combination process is altered. Another reason why pulse beams are different is because pulses contain many frequencies. Because a beam depends on frequency, many beams are produced for a wide-bandwidth pulse. The combination of all of these yields the resultant pulse beam. Because lateral resolution depends on beam diameter, which depends on pulse duration, axial and lateral resolutions are

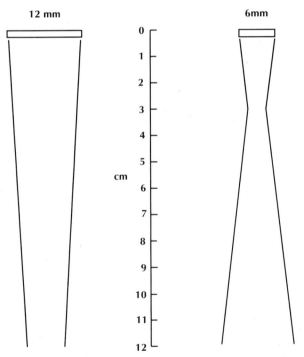

Figure 3.13. Beams for 5-MHz disk transducers of two diameters. The larger transducer (*left*) produces the larger near-zone length. A smaller transducer (*right*) can produce a larger-diameter beam. These beam diameters are equal at a distance of 8 cm.

not independent. However, for simplicity, these complications are usually ignored.

For improved lateral resolution (see Section 3.4), beam diameter may be reduced by focusing the sound in a manner similar to that used to focus light. Sound may be focused (Fig. 3.14) by using a curved (rather than a flat) transducer element, a curved reflector in the transducer assembly, a lens, or a phased array (see Section 3.3). Internal focus refers to the use of a curved transducer element. Beam diameter is decreased in the focal region and in the area between it and the transducer, but it is widened in the region beyond (Fig. 3.15). Focal length is the distance from the transducer to the center of the focal region or to the location of the spatial peak intensity. Qualitative terms used to describe focus, such as short, medium, or long, indicate the length of focal regions, or focal length. For comparably sized elements, the two normally go together; that is, long focal lengths are associated with long

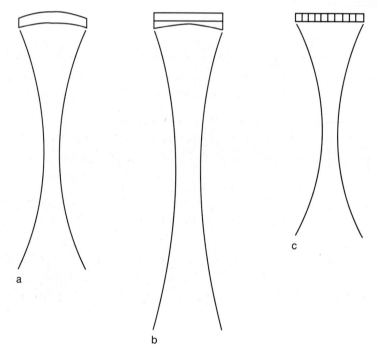

Figure 3.14. Sound focusing by a curved transducer (*a*), a lens (*b*), and a phased array (*c*). Lenses focus because the propagation speed through them is higher than that through tissues. Refraction (see Section 2.4) at the surface of the lens forms the beam in such a way that a focal region occurs. The operation of phased arrays is described in Section 3.3. The degree to which the beam diameter is reduced by focusing is described qualitatively as either weak or strong focusing.

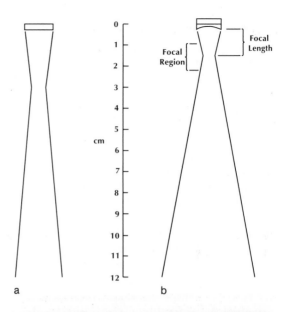

Figure 3.15. Beam diameter for a 6-mm 5-MHz transducer of Figures 3.12 and 3.13 without (*a*) and with (*b*) a focusing lens. Focusing reduces the minimum beam diameter compared to that produced without focusing. However, beyond the focal region, the diameter of the focused beam is greater than that of the unfocused beam. (*c*) A focused beam from a 5-MHz transducer with a 19-mm diameter. This is an ultrasound image of a beam profile test object (see Chapter 7), containing a thin vertical scattering layer down the center. Scanning this object generates a picture of the beam profile (the pulse width at all depths). In this case, the focus occurs at a depth of about 4 cm (this image has a total depth of 15 cm). Depth markers (in 1-cm increments) are indicated on the left edge of the figure.

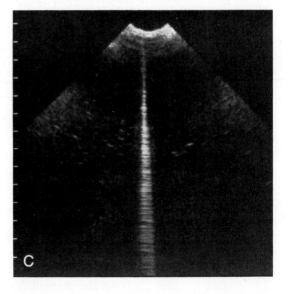

focal regions. The focal length cannot be greater than the near-zone length of comparable (same transducer diameter and operating frequency) unfocused transducers. That is, focusing can only be accomplished in the near-zone of a transducer. Focal zone (called depth of field in photography) is specified as the distance between two points at

TABLE 3.4
f-Number Ranges

Focus	f Number
Weak	Greater than 6
Moderate	2 to 6
Strong	Less than 2

the center of the beam at which the intensity is some fraction (commonly 25 per cent, 6 dB) of the peak intensity at the focus. Another way of defining focal zone is the distance between equal beam widths or diameters that are some multiple (e.g., ×2) of the minimum value (at the focus). Most diagnostic transducers are focused to some degree.

As the element or lens is increasingly curved (or phase-delay curvature in a phased array is increased), the focus moves closer to the transducer and becomes "tighter" (i.e., the beam width at the focus decreases). The limit to which a beam can be narrowed depends on the wavelength, transducer size, and focal length. An approximation of the minimum beam width (at the focus) can be calculated by multiplying the wavelength by the f number, which is the focal length divided by the aperture (transducer size). As the aperture is increased, the focus narrows and the focal zone shortens (for a given focal length). Table 3.4 shows f number ranges in use.

EXERCISES

3.2.1 The beam diameter in Figure 3.9 includes that portion of the sound produced that is greater than _____ per cent of the spatial peak intensity.

3.2.2 The beam is divided into two regions called the _____ zone and the _____ zone.

3.2.3 The dividing point between the two regions is at a distance from the transducer equal to one _____ length.

3.2.4 Beam diameter depends on _____, transducer _____, and _____ from the transducer.

3.2.5 Near-zone length increases with increasing _____ _____ and _____.

3.2.6 Near-zone length decreases with increasing _____.

3.2.7 At a distance of one near-zone length from the transducer, beam diameter is equal to _____ the transducer diameter.

3.2.8 At a distance of _____ times the near-zone length, beam diameter is equal to transducer diameter.

3.2.9 In the near zone, beam diameter _____ as distance from the transducer increases.

3.2.10 In the far zone, beam diameter _____ as distance from the transducer increases.

3.2.11 If a 5-MHz transducer with a near-zone length of 10 cm is increased in size, the near-zone length _____.

3.2.12 Which transducer has the longest near zone?
   a. 6 mm, 5 MHz
   b. 6 mm, 7 MHz
   c. 8 mm, 7 MHz

3.2.13 A 6-mm 10-MHz transducer has a near-zone length of 60 mm. If frequency is reduced to 5 MHz, near-zone length is _____ mm.

3.2.14 For Exercise 3.2.13 (10 MHz), the beam diameters at 60, 120, and 180 mm from the transducer are _____, _____, and _____ mm, respectively.

3.2.15 A higher-frequency transducer produces a _____ near-zone length.

3.2.16 A smaller transducer produces a _____ near-zone length.

3.2.17 A transducer with a near-zone length of 10 cm can be focused at 12 cm. True or false?

3.2.18 Which of the following transducer(s) can focus at 6 cm?
   a. 5 MHz, near-zone length of 5 cm
   b. 4 MHz, near-zone length of 6 cm
   c. 4 MHz, near-zone length of 10 cm
   d. b and c
   e. none of the above

3.2.19 Doubling the transducer diameter _____ the near-zone length.

3.2.20 Doubling the frequency _____ the near-zone length.

3.2.21 If transducer diameter is doubled and frequency is halved, the near-zone length is _____.

3.2.22 Sound may be focused by employing a
   a. curved element
   b. curved reflector
   c. lens
   d. phased array
   e. more than one of the above

3.2.23 Focusing reduces the beam diameter at all distances from the transducer. True or false?

3.2.24 The distance from a transducer to the location of the spatial peak intensity produced by a focused transducer is called the _____ _____.

3.2.25 For a wavelength of 0.5 mm and an f number of 4, the focal beam width is _____ mm.
    a. 0.5
    b. 1
    c. 2
    d. 4
    e. 8

3.2.26 For a 5-MHz transducer with an aperture of 25 mm and a focal length of 5 cm, the focal beam width is _____ mm.
    a. 0.3
    b. 0.6
    c. 1.0
    d. 2.0
    e. 3.0

3.2.27 Match the following f numbers with the appropriate description of the resulting focus:

a. 1: _____	1. weak
b. 3: _____	2. moderate
c. 5: _____	3. strong
d. 7: _____	
e. 9: _____	

3.3
Automatic Scanning

Not only must the transducer emit ultrasound pulses and receive echoes (as discussed in Section 3.1), it is also responsible for sending the pulses through the many paths required to generate a cross-sectional image. This is sometimes called scanning or steering the beam through the tissue cross section to be imaged. This is done rapidly and automatically so that many images can be acquired and presented within 1 second. Presenting images in a rapid sequential format is commonly called real-time sonography.

There are two ways in which automatic scanning or steering of a sound beam can be performed: mechanical and electronic. Both of these methods provide a means for sweeping the sound beam through the tissues rapidly and repeatedly. Mechanical scanning may be accomplished by oscillating a transducer in angle, by rotating a transducer or a group of transducers, by oscillating a reflector, or by linearly translating

Figure 3.16. (*a*) An oscillating mechanical transducer. (*b*) A rotating mechanical transducer. (*c*) An image generated by a mechanical transducer.

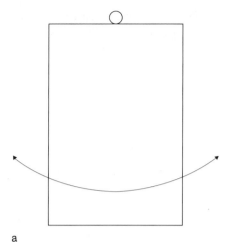

a

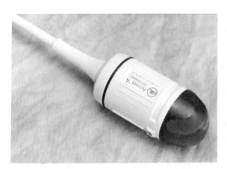

b

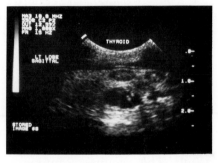

c

a transducer. In most mechanical transducers, the rotating or oscillating component is immersed in an acoustic coupling liquid within the transducer assembly. The sound beam is thus swept at a rapid rate without movement of the entire transducer assembly. The most common methods of mechanical scanning currently used are the oscillating transducer and the rotating group driven by a motor (Fig. 3.16).

Electronic scanning is performed with arrays. An array is a grouping or arrangement of parts forming a complete unit. This textbook is composed of an array of pages. Transducer arrays are transducer assemblies with several transducer elements. The elements may be rectangular in shape and arranged in a line (linear array), or they may be ring-shaped and arranged concentrically (annular array) (Fig. 3.17). Linear is the adjectival form of line. Annular is the adjectival form of annulus, meaning ring.

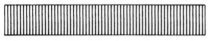

a

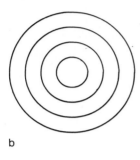

b

Figure 3.17. Front views of a linear array with 64 rectangular elements (*a*) and an annular array with four elements (*b*).

A linear sequenced array (sometimes called a linear switched array and commonly called simply a linear array) is operated by applying voltage pulses to groups of elements in succession (Fig. 3.18). In this case, each group of elements acts like a larger transducer element. The origin of the sound beam moves across the face of the transducer assembly, thus producing the same effect as would manual linear scanning with a single-element transducer. Such electronic scanning, however, can be done in a rapid and consistent manner without involving moving parts or a coupling liquid. If this electronic scanning is repeated rapidly enough, a real-time presentation (see Section 4.4) of information can result. This requires scanning across the transducer assembly several times per second. The aperture is the size of the group of elements energized to produce one pulse. The width of the image is approximately equal to the length of the array (Fig. 3.19). The linear image consists of parallel scan lines produced by pulses originating at different points across the surface of the array but all traveling in the same direction (parallel). This produces a rectangular image (see Figs. 1.7, 1.8, and 3.18*g*).

The firing sequence described in Figure 3.18 (eight elements, fired in groups of four) yields only five scan lines to make up the image. This would certainly be a poor-quality image. A 128-element array fired in groups of four would yield a 125-line display. Firing these elements individually (rather than in groups of four) would yield a 128-line display, but the small aperture (a single element approximately 1 mm in size) would cause excessive beam divergence and poor resolution (see Section 3.4). If the firing sequence alternated groups of three and four elements (e.g., elements 1 through 3, then 1 through 4, then 2 through

Figure 3.18. A linear sequenced array (side view). Voltage pulses are applied simultaneously to all elements in a small group: first to elements 1 through 4 (for example) as a group (*a*), next to elements 2 through 5 (*b*), and so on across the transducer assembly (*c* through *e*). The process is then repeated (*f*). (*g*) An image generated from a linear sequenced array. (*h*) A linear array.

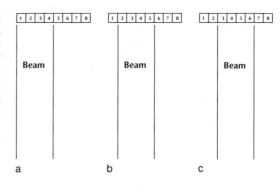

a   b   c

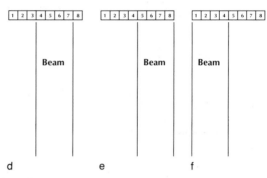

d   e   f

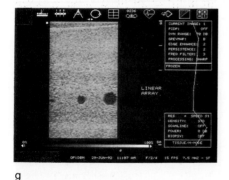

g

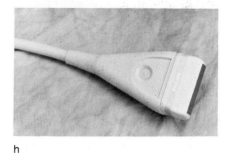

h

4, 2 through 5, 3 through 5, 3 through 6, 4 through 6, 4 through 7, etc.), 250 scan lines would be produced, improving the line density and quality of the image.

A convex sequenced array (curved or curvilinear array) is constructed as a curved line of elements rather than a straight one (convex means bowed out). Its operation is identical to that of the linear se-

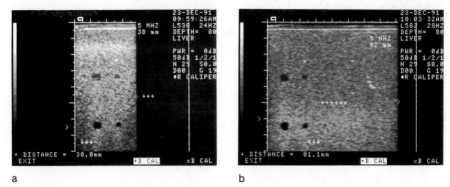

Figure 3.19. The linear image width is determined by the length of the linear array used. (*a*) A 5-MHz, 38-mm linear array (L538) produces an image that is 38 mm wide. (*b*) A 5-MHz, 82-mm linear array (L582) produces an image that is 81 mm wide.

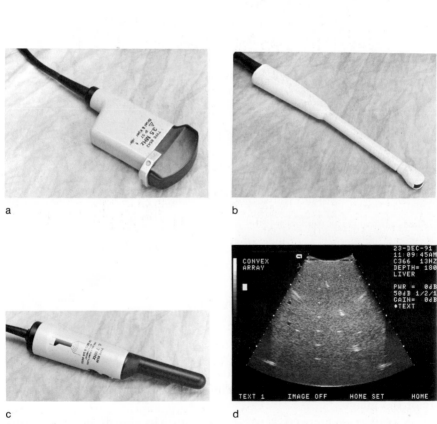

Figure 3.20. (*a* through *c*) Convex arrays send pulses out in different directions from different points across the curved array surface. (*d*) A sector-type image with a curved top is produced by a convex array.

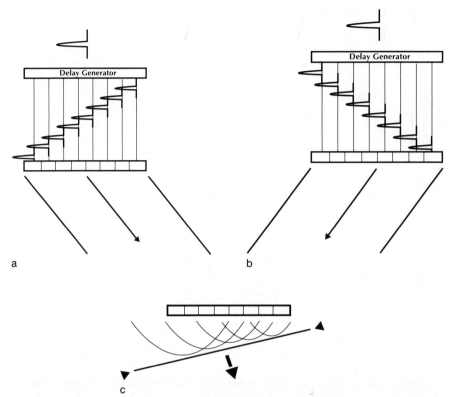

Figure 3.21. A linear phased array (side view). (*a*) By applying voltage pulses in rapid progression from left to right, one ultrasound pulse is produced that is directed to the right. (*b*) Similarly, by applying voltage pulses in rapid progression from right to left, one ultrasound pulse is produced that is directed to the left. The delays in part *a* produce a pulse whose combined pressure wavefront (*arrowheads*) is angled from lower left to upper right, as shown in part *c*. A wave always travels perpendicular to its wavefront, as indicated by the arrow.

quenced array (sequencing groups of elements), but because of the curved construction, the pulses travel out in different directions, producing a sector-type image (Fig. 3.20).

A linear phased array (commonly called a phased array) is operated by applying voltage pulses to all elements (not a small group) in the assembly as a complete group, but with small (less than 1 μs) time differences (phasing), so that the resulting sound pulse may be sent out in a specific path direction (Fig. 3.21). If the same time differences were used each time the process was repeated, the same direction would result repeatedly. However, the time differences (phasing) are changed with each successive repetition so that the beam direction can continually

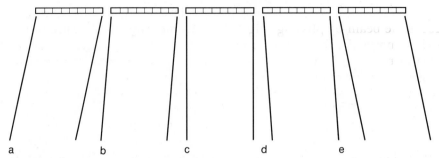

Figure 3.22. A five-pulse sequence in which each pulse travels out in a different direction. (*a*) The firing pattern is from right to left across the array. (*b*) A right-to-left pattern with shorter time delays. (*c*) No delays (all elements fire simultaneously). (*d*) A left-to-right pattern. (*e*) A left-to-right pattern with longer delays.

change (Fig. 3.22); that is, each pulse travels out in a slightly different direction. This can then result in sweeping of the beam (with beam direction changing with each pulse) to produce a sector image (see Figs. 1.9, 1.10, and 3.23). The phased array is sometimes called an electronic sector transducer.

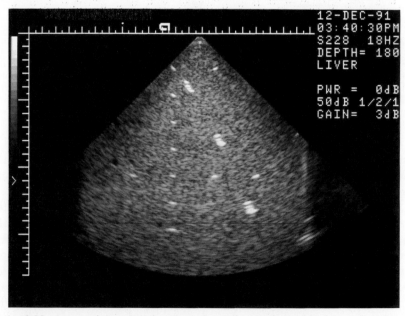

Figure 3.23. A sector image (coming to a point at the top) is produced by a phased array.

In addition to steering the beam by phasing, the phased array can focus the beam by phasing (Fig. 3.24). An increase in curvature in the delays moves the focus closer to the transducer, whereas a decrease in curvature moves it deeper. Thus, phasing provides electronic control of the location of the focus (Fig. 3.25). Multiple focuses can be employed to effectively achieve a long focus (Fig. 3.26). A pulse can be focused at only one depth. Therefore, multiple focuses require multiple pulses, each focused at a different depth (Fig. 3.27). Echoes from the focal region of each pulse are imaged and the rest are discarded. The resulting image is a montage of the focal regions of the different pulses. However, using multiple pulses per scan line takes more time, and the frame rate (see Section 4.4) is reduced. Thus, temporal resolution (see Section 4.4) is sacrificed for an improvement in detail resolution (see Section 3.4).

Phasing can also be applied to linear sequenced arrays to provide electronic focal control (Fig. 3.28). The name phased linear array indicates that phased focus control has been added to a linear sequenced

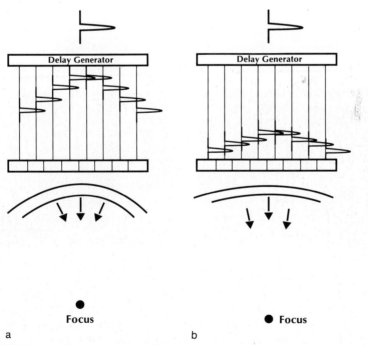

Figure 3.24. By putting curvature in the phase delay pattern, a pulse is focused. (*a*) Greater curvature places the focus closer to the transducer. (*b*) Less curvature moves the focus deeper.

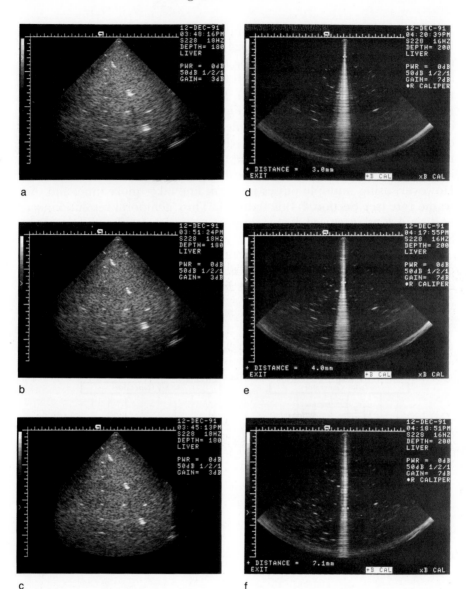

Figure 3.25. Phase control of focal length. Focus located at 3 (*a*), 7 (*b*), and 11 cm (*c*). The arrowhead on the left shows the location of the focus. Beam profiles show focuses located at 3 (*d*), 7 (*e*), and 13 cm (*f*).

array. For example, in Figure 3.18, rather than each group of four elements being fired simultaneously, the outer two elements are fired slightly ahead of the inner two. This produces a curved pulse that is focused at a depth determined by the delay between outer and inner

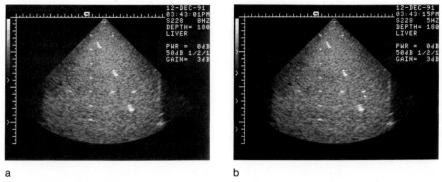

a   b

Figure 3.26. (*a*) Triple focuses at 3, 9, and 15 cm. (*b*) Five focuses at 2, 5, 8, 12, and 16 cm. Note the reduced frame rates (8 and 5 Hz, compared to 18 and 16 Hz in Figure 3.25).

element firing. The pulses are focused, but not steered, by phasing. They still travel straight down to produce parallel scan lines and a rectangular display.

As mentioned in Section 3.2, the beam width at the focus is limited by the aperture size, focal length, and wavelength. To maintain the same beam width at the focus for increasing focal lengths, the aperture must be increased also. This is called dynamic aperture. It means that, in fact, not all elements of a phased array are used to generate all pulses.

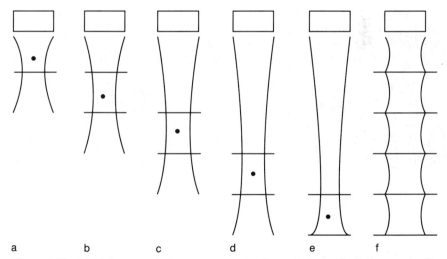

a   b   c   d   e   f

Figure 3.27. Multiple-transmit focus uses a pulse for each focus. In this example, five pulses focused at different depths (*a* through *e*) are needed to produce a montage image (*f*) with an effectively long focus (narrow beam). Only the echoes from the focal region of each pulse are used to produce the image. The rest are discarded.

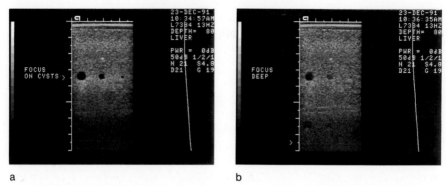

a   b

Figure 3.28. (*a*) Phased linear array with the focus located at 3.5 cm. (*b*) The focus is located at 7.5 cm (less phase delay curvature).

Smaller groups are used for short focal lengths, whereas incrementally larger groups are used for focuses of increasing depth (Fig. 2.29).

A single line of elements can focus or steer electronically only in the scan plane (in the plane of Fig. 3.21). Focus (fixed at one depth) can be achieved in the third dimension with a lens or with curved elements. With an odd number of rows (more than 1), phasing can be applied to focus the third dimension electronically. This dimension is called the slice thickness or section-thickness dimension. It is also called z axis or elevation axis. Beam width in this dimension is important with regard to section-thickness artifacts (see Section 6.1).

In addition to side lobes, which single-element transducers have (see Section 3.2), arrays have grating lobes, which are additional beams resulting from their multielement structure (see Section 6.1). Grating lobes

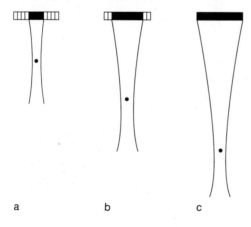

a   b   c

Figure 3.29. Dynamic aperture. To maintain comparable focal beam width, more array elements are used (increasing the aperture) as the focus is moved deeper. (*a*) Four elements. (*b*) Eight elements. (*c*) Twelve elements.

can be reduced by driving the elements nonuniformly (i.e., with different voltage amplitudes). This is called apodization. Because optimum apodization changes continually with focusing and steering, it is called dynamic apodization.

Phasing can be applied to a linear sequenced array to steer pulses in various directions. Vector array is the name applied to this type of transducer (Fig. 3.30). Scan lines originate from different points across the top of the display and travel out in different directions. The image format is similar to that for the convex array except that the contact surface (footprint) is smaller and the top of the display is flat. More elements can be used at a time, allowing for larger apertures than can be achieved with convex arrays.

Annular phased arrays consist of several concentric rings. They are operated as phased arrays to provide electronic focal control. Because the elements are ring-shaped, the focused beam is cone-shaped, reducing the beam width both in the scan plane and perpendicular to it (Fig. 3.31). The latter reduces section-thickness artifacts (Section 6.1). Because steering a beam with phasing requires that elements be fired in rapid progression from one end of the array to the other, annular arrays

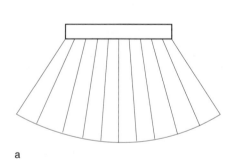

a

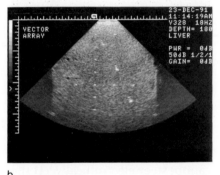

b

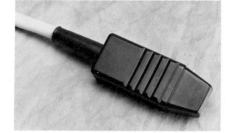

Figure 3.30. (*a*) A vector array sends pulses out in different directions from different starting points across the flat surface of the array. (*b*) A scan produced by a vector array. (*c*) A vector array.

c

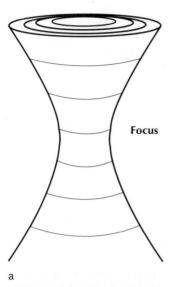

Focus

Figure 3.31. Annular phased array. (*a*) Ring elements produce a cone-shaped beam that is focused not only in the scan plane (improving lateral resolution), but also perpendicular to it (reducing section-thickness artifacts). (*b*) Image of liver. The thin section thickness allows echo-free imaging of the lumen of a small vessel at a distance of only 3.5 cm from transducer, whereas other types of transducers often have section thickness luminal fill-in. (*c*) Annular array.

a

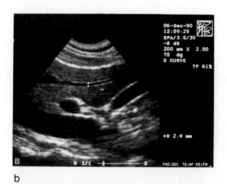

b

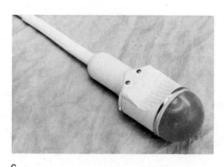

c

cannot steer electronically. (If the left end element is fired first, the right end element is fired first also, as they are the same ring.) Therefore, annular arrays can only fire in an outside-inward progression (for focusing) and must be steered mechanically.

When an array is receiving echoes, the electric outputs of the elements can be timed so that the array "listens" in a particular direction with a listening focus at a particular depth (Fig. 3.32). This receiving focus depth may be continually increased as the transmitted pulse travels through the tissues. This continually changing receiving focus is called dynamic focusing. It is similar to the continual change in focusing that occurs in a camcorder when filming a child riding away on a bicycle. The combination of transmit focus (particularly, multizone focusing) and

Figure 3.32. (*a*) A spherical echo arrives at array elements at different times, producing noncoincident voltages in the various channels. If simply combined, a long voltage (with poor resolution) would result. However, with proper delays, the voltages are made to coincide, producing a short (good resolution) voltage. As echoes return from deeper and deeper locations, their curvature is reduced. Thus, the delay correction must be reduced as echoes return. This is called dynamic focusing. (*b*) Dynamic focus off. (*c*) When the dynamic focus is on, resolution improves.

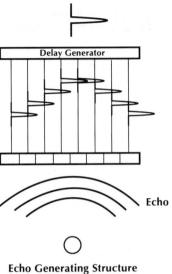

a

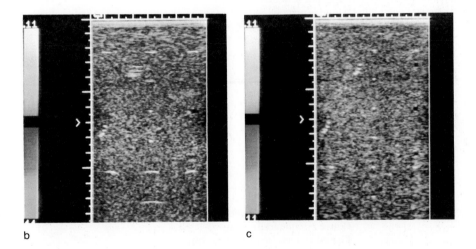

b   c

dynamic receiving focus greatly improves detail resolution over large depth ranges in images. Each independent element, delay, and amplifier path constitutes a channel. An increased number of channels allows improved phase correction in dynamic focus.

The terms used to describe the arrays in this section describe construction and function, as shown in Table 3.5. Tables 3.6 through 3.9 summarize transducer types, terminology, characteristics, and display formats.

TABLE 3.5
Terms Used to Describe Arrays

| | Parameter Described | | |
| | Construction | Function | |
Term		Scanning	Focusing
Mechanical		×	×
Array	×		
Linear	×		
Sequenced		×	
Convex	×		
Phased		×	×
Annular	×		

TABLE 3.6
Transducer Types

Mechanical sector
Annular array
Linear array
Phased linear array
Convex array
Phased convex array
Electronic sector (phased array)
Vector array

TABLE 3.7
Array Terminology*

Linear (sequenced) array
Phased linear (sequenced) array
Convex (sequenced) array
Phased convex (sequenced) array
(Linear) phased array
(Phased and sequenced) (linear) vector array
Annular (phased) array

* The words in parentheses are implied in the abbreviated common terminology.

TABLE 3.8
Transducer Characteristics

Type	Scanned or Steered by			Focused by	
	Motor Drive	Electronic Sequencing	Electronic Phasing	Curved Element or Lens	Electronic Phasing
Mechanical sector	×			×	
Linear array		×			
Phased linear array		×			×
Convex array		×			
Phased convex array		×			×
Annular array	×				×
Phased array			×		×
Vector array		×	×		×

TABLE 3.9
Display Formats

	Rectangular	Parallelogram	Sector	Flat Top	Curved Top	Pointed Top
Mechanical			×		×	
Phased array			×			×
Annular array			×		×	
Linear array	×			×		
Phased linear array	×	×		×		
Convex array			×		×	
Vector array			×	×		

EXERCISES

3.3.1 Transducer arrays are transducer assemblies with more than one transducer _____.

3.3.2 Three types of array construction are _____, _____, and _____.

3.3.3 Linear arrays scan beams by _____ element groups.

3.3.4 Match the following (answers may be used more than once):

a. A linear sequenced array can _____ the beam.

b. Without phasing, a linear sequenced array cannot _____ or _____ the beam.

c. A linear phased array can _____ and _____ the beam.

d. An annular phased array can _____ the beam, but cannot _____ or _____ the beam.

e. A phased linear sequenced array can _____ and _____ the beam.

f. A convex array can _____ the beam.

g. A phased convex array can also _____ the beam.

h. A vector array can _____, _____, and _____ the beam.

1. scan (slide beam across array surface)

2. electronically steer

3. electronically focus

3.3.5 A single-line phased linear array can focus in _____ dimension(s).

3.3.6 An annular array can focus in _____ dimension(s).

3.3.7 An annular array can steer a beam with the aid of a _____ _____.

3.3.8 Match the following (answers may be used more than once).

a. linear switched array:

_____

b. linear phased array:

_____

c. annular phased array:

_____

1. Voltage pulses are applied in succession to groups of elements across the face of a transducer.

2. Voltage pulses are applied to all elements as a group, but with small time differences.

3.3.9 In Figure 3.21, if elements are pulsed in rapid succession from right to left, the resulting beam is

a. steered right

b. steered left

c. focused

3.3.10 In Figure 3.21, if elements are pulsed in rapid succession from left to right, the resulting beam is
a. steered right
b. steered left
c. focused

3.3.11 In Figure 3.21, if elements are pulsed in rapid succession from outside in, the resulting beam is
a. steered right
b. steered left
c. focused

3.3.12 _____, _____, and _____ describe how arrays are constructed.
a. linear
b. phased
c. annular
d. sequenced
e. vector
f. convex

3.3.13 _____, _____, and _____ describe how arrays are operated.
a. linear
b. phased
c. annular
d. sequenced
e. vector

3.3.14 Shorter time delays between elements fired from outside in results in _____ curvature in the emitted pulse and a _____ focus.
a. no, weak
b. less, shallower
c. less, deeper
d. greater, shallower
e. greater, deeper

3.3.15 A rectangular image is a result of linear scanning of the beam. This means that pulses travel in _____ _____ direction from _____ starting points across the transducer face.

3.3.16 A sector image is a result of sector (angular) scanning (steering) of the beam. This means that pulses travel in _____ directions from the transducer face.

3.3.17 In _____ and _____ arrays, pulses travel out in different directions from different starting points on the transducer face.

3.4
Detail Resolution

There are three aspects to resolution in imaging: detail, contrast, and temporal resolution. Contrast and temporal resolution are discussed in Chapter 4. If two reflectors are not sufficiently separated, they will not produce separate echoes and thus will not be separated on the instrument display. Characteristics of the instrument electronics and display may further degrade this detail resolution. It is apparent, however, that if separate echoes are not initially generated, the reflectors will not be separated on the display. In ultrasound imaging, there are two aspects to detail resolution: axial and lateral. They depend on different characteristics of the ultrasound pulses as they travel through the tissues. A related aspect, section thickness, is discussed in Sections 3.3 and 6.1.

The important parameter in determining the required separation for resolution along the direction of the sound travel (along scan lines: axial resolution) is the spatial pulse length (see Section 2.2). The axial

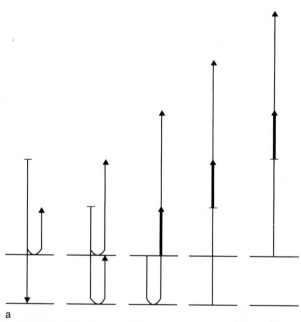

a

Figure 3.33. Axial resolution. (*a*) The separation of the reflectors is less than half the spatial pulse length, so that echo overlap occurs. Separate echoes are not produced. The reflectors are not resolved on the display.

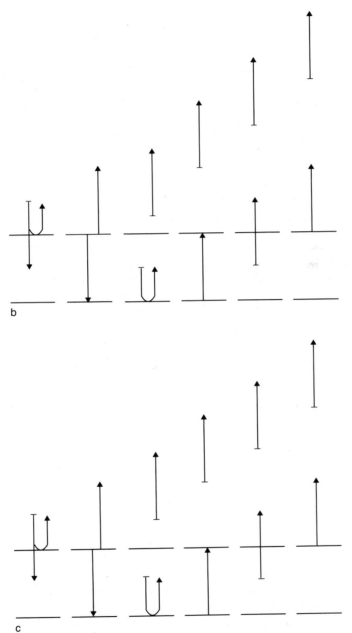

Figure 3.33 *Continued.* (*b*) The reflector separation is increased so that it is greater than half the spatial pulse length. Therefore, echo overlap does not occur. Separate echoes are produced and the reflectors are resolved on the display. (*c*) The reflector separation is the same as in part *a*, but resolution is achieved by shortening the pulse so that separate echoes are produced. Action proceeds in time from left to right in each part of the figure.

resolution is the minimum reflector separation required along the direction of sound travel (along the scan line) to produce separate echoes (Figs. 3.33 and 3.34). It is also called longitudinal, range, or depth resolution. It is equal to half the spatial pulse length.

$$\text{axial resolution (mm)} = \frac{\text{spatial pulse length (mm)}}{2} \qquad R_A = \frac{SPL}{2}$$

spatial pulse length ↑   axial resolution ↑ (worsened)

cycles per pulse ↑   axial resolution ↑ (worsened)

frequency ↑   axial resolution ↓ (improved)

Note that the down arrow for axial resolution in the last box indicates that the numerical value for this resolution *decreases* as frequency increases. Axial resolution is like a golf score—the smaller the better. The smaller the axial resolution, the more detail that can be displayed and the closer two reflectors can be along the sound path and still be seen distinctly, thereby allowing tinier objects to be displayed. To improve axial resolution, spatial pulse length must be reduced. Because spatial pulse length is wavelength multiplied by the number of cycles in the pulse (see Section 2.2), one or both of these must be reduced. For a given propagation speed (such as 1.54 mm/µs in soft tissue), wavelength is reduced as frequency is increased (see Section 2.1). The number of cycles in each pulse may be reduced by transducer damping, as previously discussed in Section 3.1. If the number of cycles per pulse is reduced to a minimum (one to three), the only way to improve axial resolution further is to increase frequency. When this is done, however, there is a price to be paid. Specifically, there is a reduction in penetration (imaging depth) (see Section 2.3) because attenuation increases as frequency increases.

frequency ↑   imaging depth ↓

Figure 3.34. Axial resolution improves as frequency increases: 3.5 MHz, with a resolution of 2.0 mm (*a*); 5.0 MHz, with a resolution of 1.0 mm (*b*); 7.0 MHz, with a resolution of 0.5 mm (*c*). Detail resolution is like a golf score (*d*); that is, smaller is better.

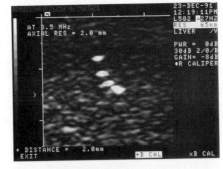

a

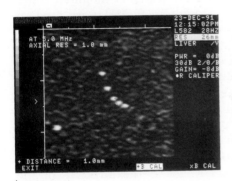

b

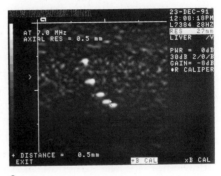

c

d

To reasonably meet resolution and imaging depth requirements, the useful frequency range is 2 to 10 MHz. The lower portion of the range is useful when increased depth (e.g., in an obese subject) or high attenuation (e.g., in transcranial studies) is encountered. The higher portion of the frequency range is useful when little penetration is required (e.g., in imaging the breast, eye, thyroid, or superficial vessels, or in pediatric imaging). In most large patients, 3.5 MHz is a satisfactory frequency, whereas in thin patients and in children, 5 and 7.5 MHz can often be used. If frequencies less than 2 MHz are used, axial resolution is insufficient. In most applications, if frequencies higher than 10 MHz (less than 10 MHz in many applications) are used, the depth is not sufficient. In the case of ophthalmologic or intravascular (catheter-mounted transducer) imaging, higher frequencies (as high as 40 MHz) are used, as penetration of only a few millimeters is needed.

Table 3.10 lists values for imaging depth (from Table 2.6) and (two-cycle pulse) axial resolution for various frequencies. Imaging depth expressed in centimeters, is equal to 60 divided by the frequency (MHz). Axial resolution (mm) for a two-cycle pulse in soft tissue is equal to one wavelength and, therefore, is equal to 1.54 divided by the frequency (MHz). Therefore, for a two-cycle pulse in soft tissue, imaging depth (cm) is approximately 40 times axial resolution (mm).

Lateral resolution is the minimum separation (in the direction perpendicular to the direction of sound travel or the direction of the beam—that is, across scan lines) between two reflectors such that when the beam is scanned across them, two separate echoes are produced (Fig. 3.35). Lateral resolution is equal to beam width in the scan plane.

beam width ↓   lateral resolution ↓ (improved)

TABLE 3.10
Imaging Depth and Axial Resolution (Two-Cycle Pulse) in Tissue

Frequency (MHz)	Imaging Depth (cm)	Axial Resolution (mm)
2.0	30	0.77
3.5	17	0.44
5.0	12	0.31
7.5	8	0.20
10.0	6	0.15

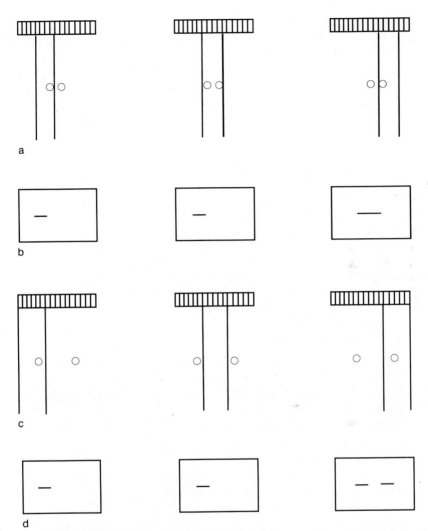

Figure 3.35. Lateral resolution. Reflector separation (perpendicular to beam direction) is less than beam diameter in parts *a* and *b*, whereas in parts *c* and *d*, reflector separation is greater than beam diameter. Action proceeds in time from left to right in each part of the figure. The beam first encounters the left reflector, then is reflected by both reflectors, and finally is reflected by the right reflector. (*b*) This scanning sequence results in continual reflection from one or both of the reflectors. Separate echoes are not produced, and the reflectors are not resolved. (*c*) The beam encounters the left reflector, then fits between both reflectors (yielding no echo), and finally is reflected by the right reflector. (*d*) Separate echoes are produced, and the reflectors are resolved.

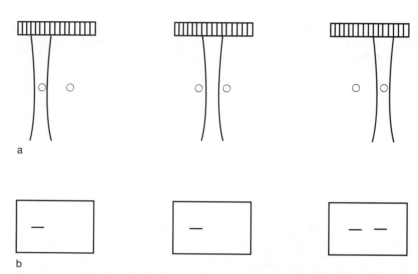

Figure 3.36. (*a*) With the same reflector separation and a similar scanning sequence as in Figure 3.35*a*, two separate echoes are generated because the beam is focused and is narrower than the reflector separation. (*b*) The two reflectors are resolved on the display.

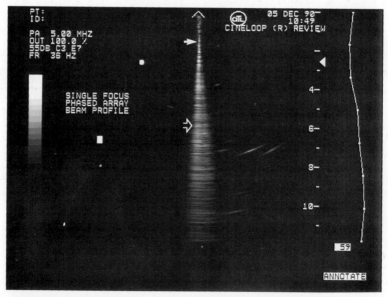

Figure 3.37. Beam width is shown as lateral smearing of a thin vertical scattering layer in a test object. The beam indicates the lateral resolution at each depth. It is about 2 mm at the focus (*closed arrow*) and about 10 mm at a depth of 6 cm (*open arrow*) in this example.

Figure 3.38. Imaging of small cysts improves at various depths as the focus is located there. Focus at 3 cm (*a*), 7 cm (*b*), 11 cm (*c*), and 17 cm (*d*). With multiple focuses (*e*), resolution is improved throughout depth.

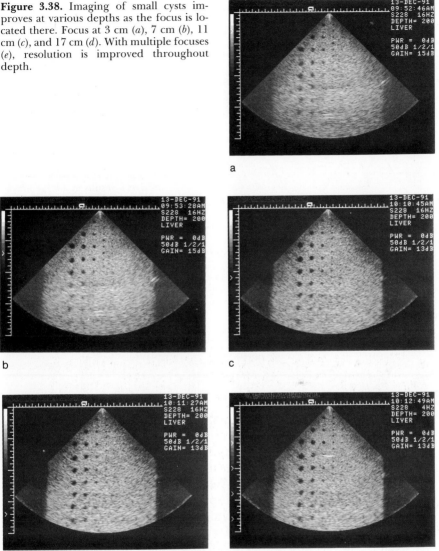

As with axial resolution, lateral resolution is like a golf score—that is, smaller is better. A smaller value indicates an improvement (finer detail and the ability to image smaller objects). Recall that beam diameter varies with distance from the transducer; so, too, does lateral resolution. If the lateral separation between two reflectors is greater than the beam

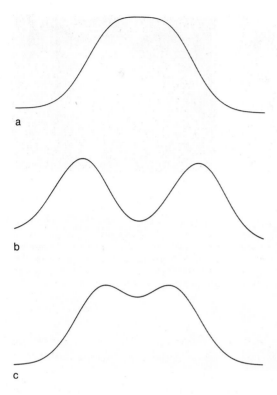

a

b

c

Figure 3.39. (*a*) These two echoes overlap enough so that there
is no amplitude dip between
them. As these cannot be distinguished by the instrument, they
will be presented as one and will
remain unresolved. (*b*) Significantly less overlap (significantly
greater reflector separation) than
in part *a* results in a large amplitude dip so that the echo pulses
can be resolved easily, even with
poor contrast resolution. (*c*) With
an overlap that is intermediate
between that in parts *a* and *b*, a
moderate amplitude dip occurs.
This may or may not be detected
(depending on the contrast resolution of the instrument [see Section 4.3]). Therefore, these echoes (and the reflectors from
which they originated) may or
may not be resolved on the display.

diameter, two separate echoes are produced when the beam is scanned
across them. Thus they are resolved, or detected as separate reflectors.

Lateral resolution is also called transverse, angular, and azimuthal
resolution. Lateral resolution is improved by reducing the beam diameter. The primary means for reducing beam diameter and improving
lateral resolution is focusing (see Section 3.2) (Fig. 3.36). Figure 3.37
shows a focused beam. The lateral smearing of a thin layer of scatterers
indicates the beam width and lateral resolution at various depths. The
best resolution is obtained at the focus (see Figs. 3.28 and 3.38).

Because ultrasound pulses used in imaging do not have constant
amplitude (see Fig. 2.15), the overlapping and separation concept of
resolution in this section needs further discussion. How much can the
pulses overlap and still be distinguished? This depends on the contrast
resolution of the imaging system (see Section 4.3). The better it is, the
better the detail (axial and lateral) resolution. This is because even with
overlap, pulses can have a dip in their combined amplitude (Fig. 3.39). If
the contrast resolution of the system can sense this dip, the echoes can be
resolved. Thus, contrast resolution and detail resolution interact and are

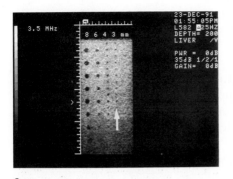 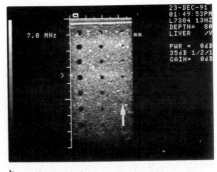

a b

Figure 3.40. (*a*) An image of a resolution penetration phantom (see Section 7.1) that contains circular anechoic regions ("cysts") in tissue-equivalent material. From left to right, the "cysts" are 8, 6, 4, 3, and 2 mm in diameter, and occur every 1 or 2 cm in depth of the image. Close examination reveals that the 3-mm "cysts" are the smallest that can be resolved. This image was produced using a 3.5-MHz transducer. (*b*) The same phantom is imaged with a 7.0-MHz transducer. In this instance, the 2-mm "cysts" can be seen. Note the loss of penetration compared to that in part *a* (8 cm versus 20 cm). Detail resolution can be improved by increasing the frequency of the ultrasound beam, but at the expense of decreasing the imaging depth.

not independent. This also means that, strictly, detail resolutions are *related to*, not necessarily *equal to*, half the spatial pulse length and beam diameter.

Diagnostic ultrasound transducers sometimes have better axial resolution than lateral resolution, although the two may be comparable in the focal region of strongly focused beams. Imaging system resolution is normally not quite as good as transducer (acoustic) resolution (discussed in this section). The resolution of the imaging system (ability to display detail) will be no better than the acoustic resolution. In fact, it may be slightly worse, because electronics and the display can degrade resolution. Figure 3.40 shows examples of typical detail resolution.

EXERCISES

3.4.1 Axial resolution is the minimum reflector separation required along the direction of the _____ _____ to produce separate _____.

3.4.2 Axial resolution depends directly on _____ _____ _____.

3.4.3 The smaller the axial resolution is, the better it is. True or false?

3.4.4 If there are three cycles of 1-mm wavelength in a pulse, the axial resolution is _____ mm.

3.4.5 For pulses traveling through soft tissue in which the frequency is 3 MHz and there are 4 cycles per pulse, the axial resolution is _____ mm.

3.4.6 If there are two cycles per pulse, the axial resolution in soft tissue at the extremes of the useful frequency range for diagnostic ultrasound are _____ and _____ mm.

3.4.7 Doubling the frequency causes axial resolution to be _____.

3.4.8 Doubling the number of cycles per pulse causes axial resolution to be _____.

3.4.9 When studying an obese subject, a higher frequency will likely be required. True or false?

3.4.10 If better resolution is desired, a lower frequency will help. True or false?

3.4.11 If frequencies less than _____ MHz are used, axial resolution is not sufficient.

3.4.12 If frequencies higher than _____ MHz are used, penetration is not sufficient in most applications.

3.4.13 Increasing the frequency improves resolution because _____ is reduced, thus reducing _____ _____ _____.

3.4.14 Increasing the frequency decreases the penetration because _____ is increased.

3.4.15 Lateral resolution is the minimum _____ between two reflectors at the same depth such that when a beam is scanned across them, two separate _____ are produced.

3.4.16 Lateral resolution is equal to _____ _____ in the scan plane.

3.4.17 Lateral resolution is also called (more than one correct answer):
   a. axial resolution
   b. longitudinal resolution
   c. angular resolution
   d. azimuthal resolution
   e. range resolution
   f. transverse resolution
   g. depth resolution

3.4.18 For a transducer element of given size, increasing the frequency improves lateral resolution. True or false?

3.4.19 Lateral resolution varies with distance from the transducer. True or false?

3.4.20 For a given frequency, a smaller transducer always yields improved lateral resolution. True or false?

3.4.21 Lateral resolution is determined by (more than one correct answer):

a. damping
b. frequency
c. transducer size
d. number of cycles in the pulse
e. distance from the transducer
f. focusing

3.5
Review

Transducers convert energy from one form to another. Ultrasound transducers convert electric energy to ultrasound energy and vice versa. They operate on the piezoelectricity principle. Transducers may be operated in burst-excited mode or shock-excited mode. The preferred operating frequency depends on the element thickness. Axial resolution is equal to one half the spatial pulse length. Pulsed transducers have damping material to shorten the spatial pulse length. Transducers produce sound in the form of beams with near and far zones. Lateral resolution is equal to beam width. Beam width may be reduced by focusing. Linear, convex, and annular are all types of array construction. Sequenced, phased, and vector are types of array operation. Phasing provides electronic control of focus.

Definitions for the terms discussed in this chapter are listed below:

Annular. Ring-shaped.

Annular array. Array made up of ring-shaped elements arranged concentrically.

Aperture. Size of transducer.

Apodization. Nonuniform (involving different voltage amplitudes) driving of elements in an array to reduce grating lobes.

Array. Transducer array.

Axial. In the direction of the transducer axis (sound-travel direction).

Axial resolution. Minimum reflector separation along the sound path required to produce separate echoes.

Bandwidth. Range of frequencies contained in an ultrasound pulse.

Beam. Region containing continuous-wave sound; region through which a sound pulse propagates.

Beam area. Cross-sectional area of a sound beam.

Burst-excited mode. A transducer driven by a cycle or two of alternating driving voltage.

Channel. An independent element, delay, and amplifier path.

Composite. Combination of piezoelectric ceramic with nonpiezoelectric polymer.

Continuous mode. Continuous-wave mode.

Convex array. Curved linear array.

Crystal. Element.

Curie point. Temperature at which element material loses its piezoelectric properties.

Damping. Material placed behind the rear face of a transducer element to reduce pulse duration; also, the process of reducing pulse duration.

Detail resolution. Ability to image fine detail and to distinguish closely spaced reflectors.

Disk. A thin, flat, circular object.

Dynamic aperture. Aperture that increases with increasing focal length (to maintain constant focal width).

Electric pulse. A brief excursion of electric voltage from its normal value.

Electric voltage. Electric potential or potential difference expressed in volts.

Element. The piezoelectric component of a transducer assembly.

Far zone. The region of a sound beam in which the beam diameter increases as the distance from the transducer increases.

f number. Focal length divided by transducer size (aperture).

Focal length. Distance from the focused transducer to the center of the focal region or to the location of the spatial peak intensity.

Focal region. Region of minimum beam diameter and area.

Focal zone. Length of the focal region.

Focus. Concentration of the sound beam into a smaller beam area than would exist otherwise.

Fractional bandwidth. Bandwidth divided by operating frequency.

Fraunhofer zone. Far zone.

Fresnel zone. Near zone.

Grating lobes. Additional minor beams of sound traveling out in directions different from the primary beam; these result from the multielement structure of transducer arrays.

Internal focus. A focus produced by a curved transducer element.

Lateral. Perpendicular to the direction of sound travel.

Lateral resolution. Minimum reflector separation perpendicular to the sound path required to produce separate reflections.

Lens. A curved material that focuses a sound beam.

Linear. Adjectival form of line.

Linear array. Array made up of rectangular elements arranged in a line.

Linear phased array. Linear array operated by applying voltage pulses to all elements, but with small time differences.

Linear sequenced array. Linear array operated by applying voltage pulses to groups of elements sequentially.

Matching layer. Material placed in front of the front face of a transducer element to reduce reflections at the transducer surface.

Mechanical transducer. A transducer that scans the beam by moving the element(s) with a motor drive.

Near zone. The region of a sound beam in which the beam diameter decreases as the distance from the transducer increases.

Operating frequency. Preferred (maximum efficiency) frequency of operation of a transducer.

Phased array. An array that steers and focuses the beam electronically (with short time delays).

Phased linear array. Linear array with phased focusing added.

Piezoelectricity. Conversion of pressure to electric voltage.

Probe. Transducer assembly.

Pulsed mode. Mode of operation in which pulsed ultrasound is used.

PVDF. Polyvinylidene fluoride, a piezoelectric thin film material.

PZT. Lead zirconate titanate.

Quality (Q) factor. Operating frequency divided by bandwidth.

Resolution. The ability to separate echoes in space, time, or strength (called detail, temporal, and contrast resolutions, respectively).

Resonance frequency. Operating frequency.

Scanhead. Transducer assembly.

Sector. A geometric figure bounded by two radii and the arc of a circle included between them.

Sensitivity. Ability of an imaging system to detect weak echoes.

Shock-excited mode. A transducer excited by a brief excursion of driving voltage.

Side lobes. Minor beams of sound traveling out from a single-element transducer in directions different from the primary beam.

Sound beam. The region of a medium that contains virtually all of the sound produced by a transducer.

Transducer. Device that converts energy from one form to another.

Transducer array. Transducer assembly containing more than one transducer element.

Transducer assembly. Transducer element and damping and matching materials assembled in a case.

Transducer element. Piece of piezoelectric material in a transducer assembly.

Ultrasound transducer. Device that converts electric energy to ultrasound energy and vice versa.

Vector array. Linear sequenced array that emits pulses from different starting points and (by phasing) in different directions.

Voltage pulse. Brief excursion of voltage from its normal value.

Exercises

3.5.1 Match the following transducer assembly parts with their functions:

a. cable: _____
b. damping material: _____
c. piezoelectric element: _____
d. matching layer: _____

1. reduces reflection at transducer surface
2. converts voltage pulses to sound pulses
3. reduces pulse duration
4. conducts voltage pulses

3.5.2 Which of the following improve sound transmission from the transducer element into the tissue (more than one correct answer)?

a. matching layer
b. Doppler effect

    c. damping material

    d. coupling medium

    e. refraction

3.5.3 A 5-MHz unfocused transducer with a thickness of 0.4 mm, an element size of 13 mm, and a near zone length of 14 cm produces two-cycle pulses. Given this information, calculate the following:

    a. operating frequency if thickness is reduced to 0.2 mm: _____ MHz

    b. axial resolution in the case of (a): _____ mm

    c. depth at which lateral resolution is best: _____ cm

    d. lateral resolution at 14 cm: _____ mm

    e. lateral resolution at 28 cm: _____ mm

    f. transducer can be focused at depths less than _____ cm.

3.5.4 Lateral resolution is improved by

    a. damping

    b. pulsing

    c. focusing

    d. reflecting

    e. absorbing

3.5.5 For an unfocused transducer, the best lateral resolution (minimum beam diameter) is _____ times the transducer diameter. This value of lateral resolution is found at a distance from the transducer face that is equal to the _____ length.

3.5.6 For a focused transducer, the best lateral resolution (minimum beam diameter) is found in the _____ region.

3.5.7 An unfocused 3.5-MHz 13-mm transducer will yield a minimum beam diameter (best lateral resolution) of _____ mm.

3.5.8 An unfocused 3.5-MHz 13-mm transducer produces three-cycle pulses. The axial resolution in soft tissue is _____ mm.

3.5.9 In Exercises 3.5.7 and 3.5.8, axial resolution is better than lateral resolution. True or false?

3.5.10 Axial resolution is often not as good as lateral resolution in diagnostic ultrasound. True or false?

3.5.11 The two resolutions may be comparable in the _____ region of a strongly focused beam.

3.5.12 Beam diameter may be reduced in the near zone by focusing. True or false?

3.5.13 Beam diameter may be reduced in the far zone by focusing. True or false?

3.5.14 Match each transducer characteristic with the sound beam characteristic it determines (answers may be used more than once):

a. element thickness: _____,   1. axial resolution
_____, and _____.   2. lateral resolution
b. element size: _____   3. operating frequency
c. element shape (flat or
curved): _____
d. damping: _____

3.5.15 The axial resolution of a transducer can be improved by
a. increasing the damping
b. increasing the diameter
c. decreasing the damping
d. decreasing the frequency
e. decreasing the diameter

3.5.16 The principle on which ultrasound transducers operate is the
a. Doppler effect
b. acousto-optic effect
c. acoustoelectric effect
d. cause and effect
e. piezoelectric effect

3.5.17 Which of the following is *not* decreased by damping?
a. refraction
b. pulse duration
c. spatial pulse length
d. efficiency
e. sensitivity

3.5.18 Which three things determine beam diameter for a disk transducer?
a. pulse duration
b. frequency
c. disk diameter
d. distance from disk face
e. efficiency

3.5.19 A two-cycle pulse of 5-MHz ultrasound produces separate echoes from reflectors in soft tissue separated by 1 mm. True or
false?

3.5.20 The lower and upper limits of the frequency range useful
in diagnostic ultrasound are determined by _____ and
_____ requirements, respectively.

3.5.21 The range of frequencies useful for most applications of diagnostic ultrasound is _____ to _____ MHz.

3.5.22 Because diagnostic ultrasound pulses are usually one to three
cycles long, axial resolution is usually equal to _____ to
_____ wavelengths.

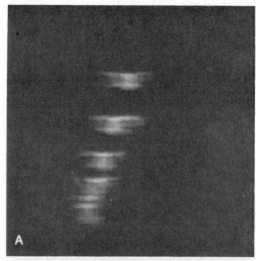

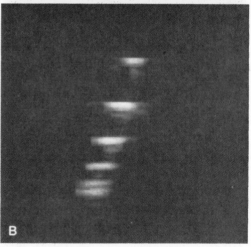

Figure 3.41. (*a*) An image of a set of six rods in a test object (see Section 7.1). They are separated by 5, 4, 3, 2, and 1 mm from top to bottom. This scan was made using a transducer that produces 3.5-MHz ultrasound. The first three rods have been separated, whereas the images of the last three rods have merged. This image also shows small reverberation echoes behind each rod. This artifact is discussed in Chapter 6. (*b*) The same rods imaged with a 5-MHz transducer. Higher-frequency transducers produce shorter pulse lengths and, therefore, provide improved axial resolution.

3.5.23 What is the axial resolution in Figures 3.41*a* and 3.41*b*?

3.5.24 The best lateral resolution in Figure 3.15*c* is at what depth?

3.5.25 At the bottom of Figure 3.15*c* (15-cm depth), the pulse width is about 1 cm. What is the pulse width at the focus?

3.5.26 Match the transducer type with the display formats in Figure 3.42.

    a. mechanical _____

    b. linear array _____

    c. convex array _____

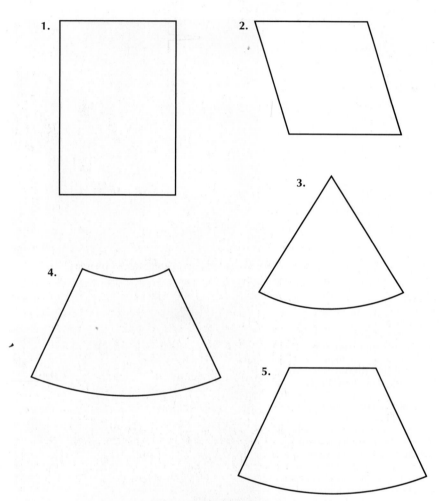

Figure 3.42. Display formats.

d. phased array _____
e. vector array _____
f. annular array _____
g. phased linear array_____

CHAPTER 4

Imaging Instruments

In the preceding chapters, the means by which ultrasound is generated and how it interacts with tissues were described. The instruments that receive and present the information resulting from this interaction are considered in this chapter. The pulse-echo method (see Figs. 1.1 and 1.2) uses received echoes. This method consists of ultrasound generation, propagation, and reflection in tissues, together with reception of returning echoes. Diagnostic ultrasound systems in use today are pulse-echo instruments. These instruments determine both the strength and the location of arriving echoes. The location of echo generation sites is determined by the direction and arrival time of echoes occurring within the tissues. This chapter describes what the instruments do with these echoes.

Imaging systems produce visual displays from the electric voltages received from the transducer. The voltages represent the echoes received by the transducer. Figure 4.1 is a diagram of the components of a pulse-echo imaging system. Several parameters that describe ultrasound were presented in Chapters 2 and 3. What determines these parameters is detailed in Table 4.1.

In this chapter, we consider the following questions: How do ultrasound imaging instruments work? What are the primary components in such instruments? What is the purpose of attenuation compensation? How are images stored electronically? What is contrast resolution and on what does it depend? How do displays work? What are the common display modes in imaging? What is temporal resolution and on what does it depend? The following terms are discussed in this chapter:

amplification
amplifier
analog

analog-to-digital converter
(ADC)
B mode

B scan
beam former
bit
burst
cathode ray tube (CRT)
compensation
compression
contrast resolution
demodulation
depth gain compensation (DGC)
digital
digital scan converter
digital-to-analog converter
  (DAC)
dynamic focusing
dynamic imaging
dynamic range
frame
frame rate
freeze frame
gain

gray scale
gray-scale display
impulse
M mode
noise
pixel
postprocessing
preprocessing
radio frequency (RF)
real-time
real-time display
rectification
rejection
scan converter
scan line
scanning
temporal resolution
time gain compensation (TGC)
variable focusing
video

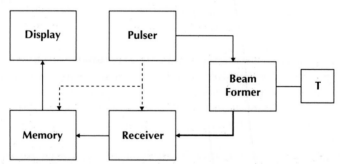

Figure 4.1. The components of a pulse-echo imaging system. The pulser produces electric pulses (see Fig. 4.2) that drive the transducer (T) through the beam former. It also produces pulses that tell (*dashed line*) the receiver and memory when the transducer has been driven. The transducer (acting as a source) produces an ultrasound pulse (see Fig. 4.2) for each electric pulse applied. For each echo received from the tissues, an electric voltage is produced by the transducer (acting as a receiving transducer). These voltages go through the beam former to the receiver, where they are processed to a form suitable for input to the memory. Electric information from memory drives the display, which produces a visual image of the cross-sectional anatomy interrogated by the system. (*Note:* Some authors consider a clock or timing circuit separately in a diagram such as this. The clock determines the pulse repetition frequency and synchronizes the various components of the instrument so that they work together properly. In this figure and in Section 4.1, the clock is considered to be part of the pulser.)

TABLE 4.1
Determination of Ultrasound Parameters*

Ultrasound Parameter	Determining Component
Frequency	Transducer, pulser
Period	Transducer, pulser
Wavelength	Transducer, pulser, tissue
Propagation speed	Tissue
Pulse repetition frequency	Pulser
Pulse repetition period	Pulser
Pulse duration	Transducer
Duty factor	Pulser, transducer
Spatial pulse length	Transducer
Axial resolution	Transducer, receiver, memory, display
Amplitude	Pulser, transducer
Intensity	Pulser, transducer
Attenuation	Transducer, tissue
Imaging depth	Transducer, tissue
Beam diameter	Transducer, pulser
Lateral resolution	Transducer, pulser, memory, display

* The ultrasound parameters described in Chapters 2 and 3 are determined by imaging system components described in Chapters 3 and 4 (see Fig. 4.1). The beam former is considered to be part of the pulser in this table.

4.1
Pulser and Beam Former

The pulser is where the action originates. It produces electric voltage pulses (Fig. 4.2) that drive the transducer. These are in the form of short impulses for shock excitation or a cycle or two of voltage for burst excitation, as discussed in Section 3.1. In response, the transducer produces ultrasound pulses. Voltages from the pulser also inform the receiver and memory (dashed lines in Fig. 4.1) when ultrasound pulses are produced. The pulse repetition frequency (PRF) of the pulser is the number of electric pulses or bursts produced per second. It ranges from about 1 to 10 kHz. The ultrasound PRF is equal to the voltage PRF because one ultrasound pulse is produced for each voltage pulse (see Fig. 4.2). Similarly, the ultrasound pulse repetition period is equal to the voltage pulse repetition period. The voltage impulse duration for shock excitation is less than the period of the cycles in the ultrasound pulses. To receive information for display at a rapid rate, it is necessary to use a high PRF. PRF, however, must be limited to provide an unambiguous display of returning echoes, as described in Section 6.1. The timing sequence that is initiated by the pulse is shown in Figure 4.3. To avoid

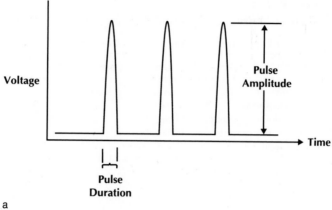

a

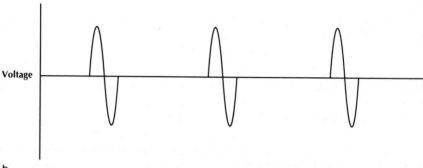

b

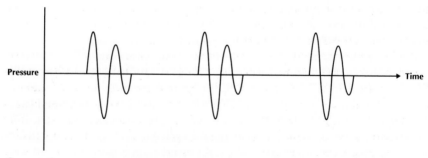

c

Figure 4.2. With every voltage impulse (*a*) or burst (*b*) applied, an ultrasound pulse (*c*) is produced by the transducer.

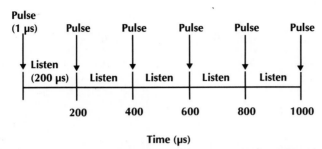

Time (μs)

Figure 4.3. Timing sequence for pulse-echo ultrasound imaging. The sequence is initiated by the production of a 1-μs pulse of ultrasound when the pulser sends a voltage pulse to the transducer. This is followed by a period of up to 250 μs, during which echoes are received from the tissue by the transducer. The length of this time is determined by the maximum depth from which the echoes return. For example, at a frequency of 5 MHz, echoes can return from as deep as 15 cm. The round-trip travel time (13 μs/cm × 15 cm) to this depth is 195 ms. This listening period is followed (5 ms later) by the next pulse. In this illustration, the listening period is 200 μs; that is, the pulse repetition period is 200 μs (pulse repetition frequency [PRF] is 5 kHz). If the PRF were greater, the pulse repetition period would be decreased, resulting in emission of the next pulse prior to the reception of all the (deeper) echoes from the previous pulse. This would produce range-ambiguity artifact (see Section 6.1) and thus should be avoided. The PRF is adjusted to avoid this problem: higher PRFs are used for superficial imaging and lower PRFs are used for deep imaging (a longer time required for arrival of deeper echoes). The latter causes a reduction in frame rate (see Section 4.4).

ambiguity, all echoes from one pulse must be received before the next pulse is emitted. For deeper imaging, this forces a reduction in the PRF and the frame rate, as discussed in Section 4.4.

Although the pulser's job appears simple, we must remember that, for arrays, complicated sequencing and phasing operations are involved. Therefore, when array transducers are used, the switching, delays, and variations in pulse amplitudes that are necessary for the electronic control of beam scanning, steering, transmit focusing, and dynamic aperture and apodization (described in Section 3.3) must be accomplished. The beam former carries out these tasks. It may be considered either as part of the pulser or as a separate component.

The greater the voltage amplitude produced by the pulser, the greater the amplitude and intensity of the ultrasound pulses produced by the transducer. Ultrasound pulse amplitude and intensity depend also on transducer efficiency. Pulser voltage amplitudes are generally a few tens or hundreds of volts. Output level is often shown on the display in terms of a percentage or decibels relative to maximum (100 per cent or 0 decibels) output (Fig. 4.4). Recent standard output display indexes relevant to risk mechanisms are discussed in Section 7.4. Acoustic outputs of diagnostic instruments are discussed further in Sections 7.2 and 7.4.

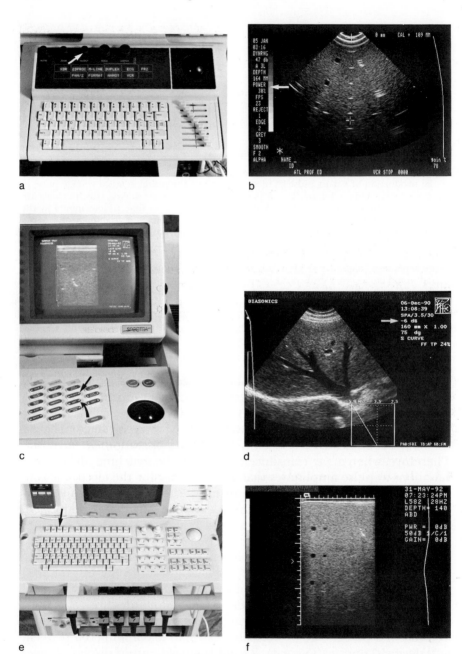

Figure 4.4. (*a, c,* and *e*) Output controls (*arrows*) on three instruments. (*b*) Output indicator (*arrow*) shows a percentage relative to the maximum (30 per cent in this example). (*d*) Output indicator (*arrow*) shows decibels relative to maximum. In this example, the value is −6 dB, which corresponds to 25 per cent of maximum. (*f*) An output of 0 dB is compared with one of −9 dB (*g*), in which the weaker echoes produce a darker image. The straight arrow in *c* shows the reject control (see Section 4.2).

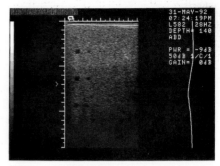

Figure 4.4 *Continued*   g

Reduction of acoustic output reduces received echo amplitude (Fig. 4.4*g*). This can be compensated for by increasing receiver gain (see Section 4.2). There will also be a reduction in imaging depth, but it is surprisingly small.[14] For example, a reduction of 50 per cent in output (−3 dB) from a 5-MHz transducer corresponds to only a 5 per cent penetration reduction (from about 12.0 to 11.4 cm).

EXERCISES

4.1.1 The ultrasound pulse repetition frequency is equal to the voltage _____ repetition frequency of the pulser.

4.1.2 Increased voltage amplitude produced by the pulser increases the _____ and _____ of ultrasound pulses produced by the transducer.

4.1.3 If a 6-MHz transducer images to a depth of 10 cm, the maximum PRF the pulser can produce (while avoiding range ambiguity) is:
   a. 7.7 kHz
   b. 6.0 kHz
   c. 10.0 kHz
   d. 1.54 MHz
   e. 13.0 Hz

4.2
Receiver

Electric voltages produced in the transducer by returning echoes are sent through the beam former to the receiver for processing. The beam former performs the receiving dynamic focus, steering, apodization, and aperture functions discussed in Section 3.3. The receiver performs the following functions:

1. amplification
2. compensation
3. compression
4. demodulation
5. rejection

Although all receivers perform these functions, they do not necessarily perform them in this order. Indeed, some are not separate functions in a given design; that is, some amplification may be incorporated into the compensation and compression functions. However, it is useful to think of these functions as distinct to promote our understanding of them.

Amplification is the conversion of the small voltages received from the transducer to larger ones suitable for processing and storage (Fig. 4.5). Gain is the ratio of output to input electric power. The power ratio, which may be expressed in decibels (see Section 2.3), is equal to the voltage ratio squared. For example, if the input voltage amplitude to an amplifier is 2 mV and the output voltage amplitude is 200 mV, the voltage ratio is 200/2 or 100. The power ratio is $(100)^2$ or 10,000 (electric power depends on voltage squared). From Table 4.2, the power ratio or gain is found to be 40 dB. Receiver amplifiers usually have 60 to 100 dB of gain. Voltages applied to these amplifiers range from a few microvolts (μV) (e.g., from blood) to a few hundred millivolts (e.g., from bone or gas). If a 10 μV-voltage input is applied to a 60-dB gain amplifier, the output power is 1,000,000 times the input power. Therefore, the output voltage is 1000 times the input, or 10 mV. If the gain of this amplifier is increased to 100 dB, the output voltage increases to 1 V.

The gain control (Fig. 4.6) determines how much amplification is accomplished in the receiver. It is similar in function to the volume or level control on your sound system at home. With too little gain, weak echoes are not imaged. With too much gain, saturation occurs; that is, most echoes appear bright and differences in echo strength (contrast resolution) are lost.

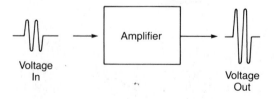

Voltage
In

Amplifier

Voltage
Out

Figure 4.5. Amplification (gain) increases both voltage amplitude and electric power.

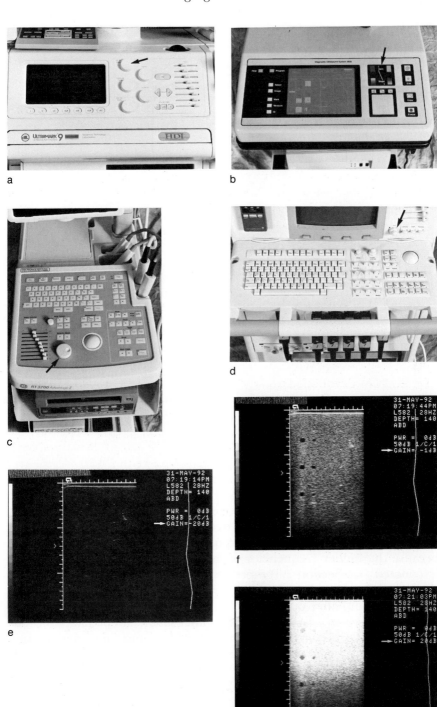

Figure 4.6. (*a* through *d*) Gain controls (*arrows*) on several control panels. (*e*) Gain is too low. (*f*) Proper gain. (*g*) Gain is too high, causing saturation.

TABLE 4.2
Gain (Expressed in Decibels) for
Various Power Ratios*

Gain (dB)	Power Ratio
0	1.0
1	1.3
2	1.6
3	2.0
4	2.5
5	3.2
6	4.0
7	5.0
8	6.3
9	7.9
10	10.0
15	32.0
20	100.0
25	320.0
30	1000.0
35	3200.0
40	10,000.0
45	32,000.0
50	100,000.0
60	1,000,000.0
70	10,000,000.0
80	100,000,000.0
90	1,000,000,000.0
100	10,000,000,000.0

* The ratio is equal to output power divided by input power.

Tuned amplifiers are often used to reduce noise in the electronics (discussed later). Some tuned receivers change the frequency range of the receiver to follow (track) the decreasing frequency content of the returning series of echoes from a pulse. The echo frequency decreases because the higher frequencies in the bandwidth (see Section 3.1) are attenuated (see Section 2.3) more than are the lower ones. The box in the lower right-hand corner of Figure 4.4*d* describes such a tracking-filter tuned amplifier operation.

Compensation (also called gain compensation, swept gain, time-varied gain [TVG], sensitivity-time control [STC], time gain compensation [TGC], or depth gain compensation [DGC]) equalizes differences in received echo amplitudes because of reflector depth. Reflectors with equal reflection coefficients (see Section 2.4) will not result in equal amplitude echoes arriving at the transducer (Fig. 4.7) if their travel distances are

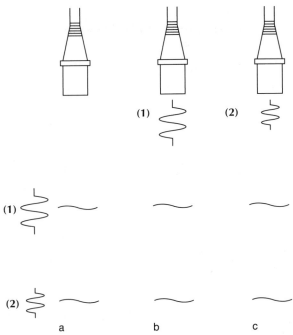

Figure 4.7. Two identical reflectors are located at different distances from the transducer. (*a*) The echo at the second reflector is weaker because the incident pulse had to travel farther to get there, thus experiencing more attenuation. (*b*) The echo from the first reflector arrives at the transducer. It is weaker than it was in *a* because of attenuation on the return trip. (*c*) The echo from the second reflector arrives at the transducer later and in a weaker form than the first one did. This is because of the longer path to the second reflector.

different (i.e., if the distance between the transducer and the reflectors is different). This is because attenuation depends on path length (see Section 2.3). It is desirable to display echoes from similar reflectors in a similar way. As these echoes may not arrive with the same amplitude because of different path lengths, their amplitudes must be adjusted to compensate for path length differences. Longer path lengths result in later arrival times (see Section 2.4). Therefore, if voltages from echoes arriving later are correctly amplified to a greater degree than are earlier ones, attenuation compensation is accomplished. This is what compensation does (Figs. 4.8 and 4.9).

The rate of increase of gain with depth is commonly called the DGC slope because it is often displayed graphically as a line with increasing deflection to the right (Fig. 4.9). This slope is expressed in decibels (gain) per centimeter of depth. When properly adjusted, the slope should correspond to the attenuation in the tissue in decibels per centimeter of depth. Remember that each centimeter of depth corresponds to 2 cm of sound travel (see Section 2.4), so that the resulting slope should be about 1 dB/cm-MHz. Because the attenuation depends upon the frequency of the ultrasound beam, the DGC is adjusted by the operator to compen-

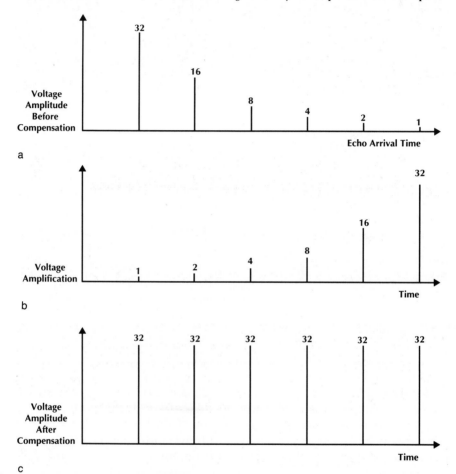

Figure 4.8. Compensation for attenuation by varying amplification. The time scale represents the arrival time of echoes. (*a*) Arriving echoes from six *identical* reflectors produce different echo amplitudes ranging from 32 to 1 mV because of attenuation. Each echo amplitude is one half that of the previous one in this example. (*b*) Amplification must compensate for this by doubling during each time interval from one echo to the next. Multiplying each arriving echo amplitude (*a*) by the gain or amplification (*b*) existing at the time the echo voltage arrives at the amplifier equals the echo amplitude out of the amplifier (*c*). Following this process, all the amplitudes are equalized at 32 mV. This is a case in which all echoes result from *equal* reflection coefficients. If reflection coefficients of the various reflectors are different, the resulting echo intensities, even after compensation, will be different. These differences should not be normalized or information about various structure echogenicities would be lost.

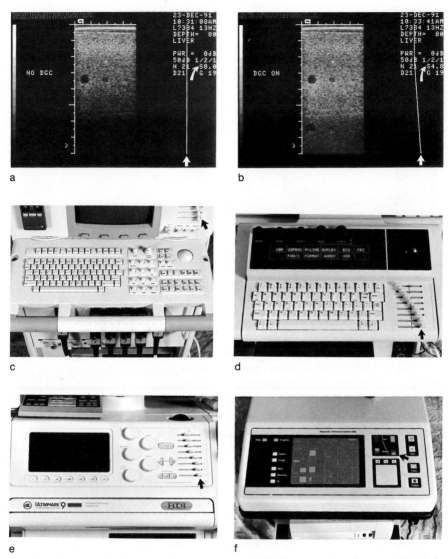

Figure 4.9. Two scans of a tissue-equivalent phantom imaged at 7 MHz without (*a*) and with (*b*) depth gain compensation (DGC). Without DGC, the echo brightness (amplitude, intensity, strength) declines with depth (top to bottom). On the display, DGC settings are shown graphically (*straight arrows*). The slopes (*curved arrows*) are (*a*) 0 dB/cm and (*b*) 4.8 dB/cm. Average tissue attenuation is 0.5 dB/cm/MHz (see Section 2.3). This is calculated per centimeter of sound propagation. Average attenuation, then, is 1 dB/cm/MHz when the centimeter value is the distance from the transducer to the reflector. The sound must travel twice this distance (round trip) so that the attenuation number doubles. Typical DGC slopes will then be about 1 dB/cm/MHz. (*c* through *g*) DGC controls on several instruments (*arrows*).

Illustration continued on following page

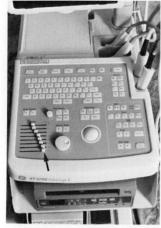

g   **Figure 4.9** *Continued*

sate for the frequency used and the tissues being imaged. DGC is set subjectively by the operator to achieve, on average, uniform brightness throughout the image. Thus, the average attenuation in the tissue cross section at the operating frequency has been compensated for when this is achieved.

Typical DGC amplifiers compensate for about 60 dB of attenuation. At the depth at which maximum gain has been achieved, the echo brightness begins to decrease because the DGC can no longer compensate (the gain is at maximum). Thus, imaging depth has been determined by the attenuation and maximum DGC gain. Table 2.6 indicates that imaging depths occur at the 60-dB attenuation points. For example:

$$1.0 \text{ dB/cm/MHz} \times 5.0 \text{ MHz} \times 12 \text{ cm} = 60 \text{ dB}$$

so that the maximum imaging depth at 5 MHz is about 12 cm. Note that distance (cm) in this instance is one-way, from transducer to the deepest structure imaged. The sound travels twice this distance, so that:

$$0.5 \text{ dB/cm/MHz} \times 5.0 \text{ MHz} \times 24 \text{ cm} = 60 \text{ dB}$$

where distance (cm) refers to that of the sound path (twice the depth above).

Compression is the process of decreasing the differences between the smallest and largest amplitudes (Fig. 4.10). This is accomplished by logarithmic amplifiers (log amps) that amplify weak inputs more than strong ones. The ratio of the largest to the smallest amplitude or power

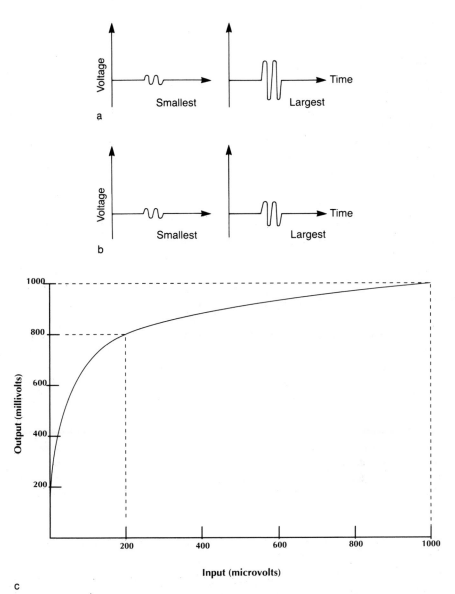

Figure 4.10. Compression decreases the difference between the smallest and largest voltage amplitudes passing through the system. In this example, the ratio of largest to smallest amplitudes before compression is five (*a*). After compression, the ratio is three (*b*). (*c*) A logarithmic amplification curve accomplishes compression. A linear amplifier has a straight-line relationship between input and output, meaning that all input voltages are amplified by the same factor. Here, the relationship is in the shape of a logarithmic curve. This means that weaker voltages are amplified to a greater degree than stronger ones, thereby reducing the differences between them. In this example a 200-μV input voltage is amplified by a factor of nearly 8000 (output is 780 mV). But a 1000-μV input is amplified by a factor of only 1,000 to an output of 1000 mV. Both are amplified, but not by the same amount. The difference between the two is reduced by logarithmic compression: before compression the larger voltage is 5 times the smaller voltage (1000/200 = 5), whereas after compression, the larger voltage is only 1.28 times the smaller one (1000/780 = 1.28).

143

that a system can handle is called the dynamic range. It is expressed in decibels. For example, if an amplifier is insensitive to voltage amplitudes of less than 0.01 mV and cannot properly handle voltage amplitudes of greater than 1000 mV, the ratio of voltages is 1000/0.01, or 100,000. The power ratio is equal to the square of the voltage ratio: $(100,000)^2$, or 10,000,000,000. According to Table 4.2, the dynamic range of the amplifier is 100 dB. Although amplifiers have such a dynamic range (typically 100 to 130 dB), other portions of the electronics might not. Furthermore, our eyes can only handle a dynamic range of about 20 dB.[15] The largest power can be only about 100 times the smallest for our viewing of the display. Thus, the largest voltage amplitude can only be about 10 times the smallest. The dynamic range remaining after compensation is typically 40 to 70 dB. A compressor would have to compress the intensity ratio (100,000) corresponding to 50 dB to an intensity ratio of 100 (acceptable for the display).

Demodulation (sometimes called amplitude detection or envelope detection) is the process of converting the voltages delivered to the receiver from one form (radio frequency [RF]) to another (video) (Fig. 4.11). This is done by rectification and smoothing (filtering) (Fig. 4.12). Because diagnostic ultrasound pulses do not have constant amplitude (see Fig. 2.15), when demodulated, they do not have the blocked appearance shown in Figures 4.11 and 4.12, but rather appear as in Figure 3.39.

Rejection (sometimes called suppression or threshold) eliminates the smaller-amplitude voltage pulses (Figs. 4.13 and 4.4c) produced by weaker echoes or electronic noise . The weaker echoes can come from grating lobes or multiple scattering (see Chapter 6) from within the tissue, thus constituting "acoustic noise." Electronic noise (Fig. 4.14) exists in all electronic circuits. High-quality input amplifier circuit (called

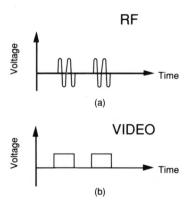

(a)

(b)

Figure 4.11. Echo voltages are produced in a complicated cyclic form (*a*) called radio frequency (RF), which would be difficult to store and display. Furthermore, only the amplitude of each echo is needed for a gray scale display of anatomy. Thus the RF form is converted to video form (*b*), which retains the amplitude of each echo voltage.

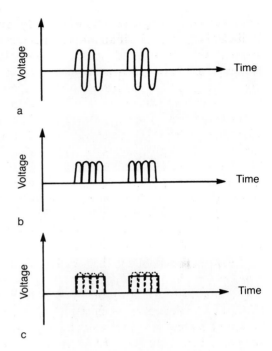

Figure 4.12. Rectification (*b*) and smoothing (filtering) (*c*) of pulses (*a*) results in demodulation.

the preamplifier) noise levels are a few microvolts in amplitude. It is desirable to reduce or eliminate noise, whether electronic or acoustic, from the image, because it contributes no useful information and interferes with the observation of the useful information that *is* presented.

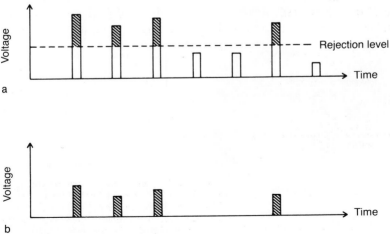

Figure 4.13. Rejection eliminates voltage pulses with amplitudes below the rejection level. (*a*) Before rejection. (*b*) After rejection.

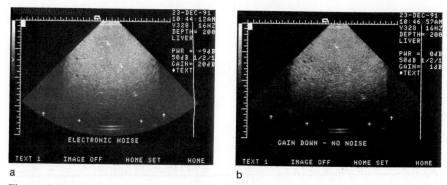

Figure 4.14. (*a*) Near maximum gain conditions, electronic noise can be seen on the display. (*b*) With reduced gain, these weak voltages are not amplified enough to be visualized.

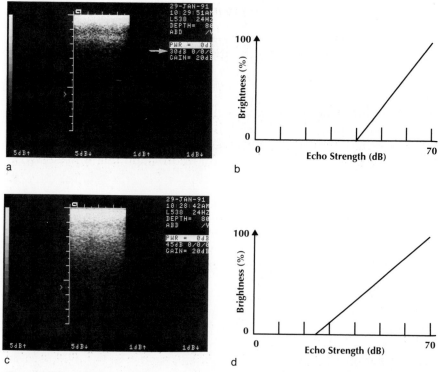

Figure 4.15. (*a*) The dynamic range setting (*arrow*) is 30 dB. The lower 40 dB of echoes returning from a tissue equivalent phantom are set to zero (*black portion*). The remainder have high contrast with brightness progressing from black for 40-dB echoes to white for 70-dB echoes. (*b*) A 30-dB dynamic range setting assigns the weakest 40 dB of echo dynamic range to zero (*black*) and the remaining 30 dB of dynamic range to linearly higher brightnesses. (*c*) A display with a dynamic range of 45 dB. (*d*) Brightness assignment with a 45-dB dynamic range.

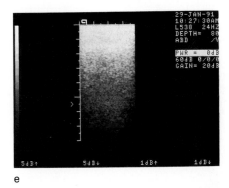

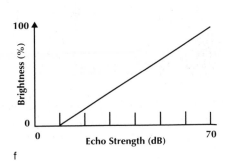

e   f

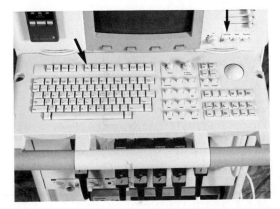

Figure 4.15 *Continued.* (*e*) A display with a dynamic range of 60 dB. (*f*) Brightness assignment with a 60-dB dynamic range. (*g*) Log compression control (*arrows*).

g

Amplification (gain) and compensation (DGC) functions are always operator-adjustable; demodulation is not. Rejection is sometimes an operator-adjustable control (see Fig. 4.4*c*). It can be presented in a different form: a dynamic range or log compression control (Fig. 4.15). Rather than directly controlling the logarithmic compression amplifier, this control reassigns echo amplitude values to a smaller dynamic range by reducing some of the weaker ones to zero. It is, then, something like a threshold control except that, unlike threshold, the remaining echo amplitudes are reassigned new values according to the dynamic range setting. A smaller dynamic range setting eliminates the weaker echoes from the display and presents the remaining ones in a higher-contrast format.

To store echo information in digital memory (see Section 4.3), the demodulated voltage amplitudes representing echoes must pass through an analog-to-digital converter (ADC) (Fig. 4.16). Various instruments perform this conversion at different points in the system ranging all the

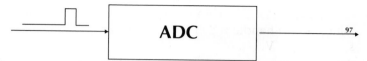

Figure 4.16. The analog-to-digital converter (ADC) converts voltage amplitude to a number. Analog means proportional; digital refers to counting (fingers and toes).

way from before the beam former to after all the receiver functions discussed in this section.

EXERCISES

4.2.1 Five functions performed by the receiver are _____, _____, _____, _____, and _____.

4.2.2 Match the following functions with what they accomplish:

   a. amplification: __2__   1. converts pulses from RF to video form
                                        2. increases all amplitudes
   b. compensation: __5__   3. decreases dynamic range
   c. compression: __3__   4. eliminates weaker voltages
   d. demodulation: __1__   5. corrects for tissue attenuation

   e. rejection: __4__

4.2.3 Input voltage to an amplifier is 1 mV and output voltage is 10 mV. The voltage amplification ratio is _____. The power ratio is _____. The gain is _____ dB.

4.2.4 A receiver with a gain of 60 dB has 1 μW of power applied to the input. The output power is _____ W.

4.2.5 A receiver with a gain of 60 dB has 10 μV of voltage applied to the input. The output voltage is _____ mV.

4.2.6 Compensation is also called (more than one correct answer):
   a. swept beam
   b. swept gain
   c. refraction
   d. diffraction
   e. time gain compensation

4.2.7 Compensation takes into account reflector _depth_ or _distance_.

4.2.8 Compensation amplifies echoes differently, according to their arrival _time_.

4.2.9 Compression decreases the _dynamic_ range to a range that our _eyes_ can handle.

4.2.10 If a display has a dynamic range of 20 dB and the smallest voltage it can handle is 200 mV, the largest voltage it can handle is _2.0_ V.

4.2.11 Demodulation converts voltage pulses from _____ form to _____ form.

4.2.12 Rejection eliminates higher-amplitude echoes. True or false?

4.2.13 Another name for rejection is
a. threshold
b. depth gain compensation
c. swept gain
d. compression
e. demodulation

4.2.14 The log compression or dynamic range control reduces the range of echo amplitudes displayed by reducing the weaker ones to _zero_ and assigning the stronger ones _lower_ to increasing brightness. This produces a _higher_ contrast image with elimination of _weaker_ echoes.

4.2.15 An amplifier has a power output of 100 mW when the input power is 0.1 mW. The amplifier gain is _30_ dB.

4.2.16 If the pulser output to the transducer is reduced by 3, 6, and 9 dB, the ultrasound pulse output intensity is reduced by _50_, _75_, and _87.5_ per cent, respectively.

4.2.17 One watt is _20_ dB below 100 W.

4.2.18 One watt is _10_ dB above 100 mW.

4.2.19 If the input power is 1 mW and the output is 10,000 mW, the gain is _40_ dB.

4.2.20 If an amplifier has a gain of 15 dB, the ratio of output power to input power is _____. (Use Table 4.2.)

4.2.21 If the output of a 22-dB gain amplifier is connected to the input of a 23-dB gain amplifier, the total gain is _45_ dB. The overall power ratio is _____. (Use Table 4.2.)

4.2.22 If a 17-dB electric attenuator is connected to a 15-dB amplifier, the net gain is _-2 dB_ dB. The net attenuation is _2_ dB. For a 1-W input, the output is _____ W. (Use Table 2.3.)

4.3
Memory and Contrast Resolution

Storing each cross-sectional image in memory as the sound beam is scanned through the tissue permits display of a single image (scan) out of the rapid sequence of several images (frames) normally acquired each second in dynamic (real-time) ultrasound instruments. Holding and displaying one scan out of the sequence is called freeze-frame. Some instruments have enough memory to store the last several frames acquired. This is sometimes called cine review, cine-loop (Fig. 4.17*a*), or image review.

Image memories used in diagnostic ultrasound instruments are of the digital type. These memories are sometimes called digital scan converters because they provide a means for displaying, using a television scan format (see Section 4.4), information acquired in a linear or sector

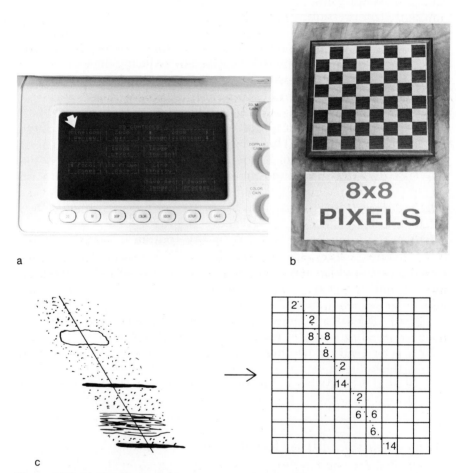

a   b

c

Figure 4.17. (*a*) Cine-loop selection on a control menu. (*b*) A chess or checker board is divided into 8 rows and 8 columns of squares, for a total of 64 "pixels." (*c*) Anatomic cross-section scanned and front view of a portion of the digital scan converter. Numbers are stored in the memory elements according to the intensity of the echoes received from corresponding anatomic locations.

scan line format (see Section 3.3). The image plane is divided into squares called pixels (picture elements), with commonly 512×512 squares on the sides. There are about one quarter million pixels so that they are very tiny and numerous. In each of these spaces in memory, a number is stored that corresponds to the echo intensity received from the point within the body corresponding to that memory position.

A digital scan converter is a computer memory that stores numbers. A matrix (like a checkerboard, Fig. 4.17b) of digital memory elements is used to store echo information. Commonly, a square matrix, with 512 squares on a side (total of 262,144), is used. In each of these elements, a number is stored that corresponds to the echo intensity received from the point within the body corresponding to that memory position (Fig. 4.17c). If the digital memory were made up of a single matrix checkerboard, each pixel could only store one of two numbers, a zero or a one. This is because such memories are binary in nature and can only operate in two conditions—on or off—corresponding to one or zero. This would only allow bistable (black and white) imaging. To image gray scale (several shades of gray or brightness in addition to black and white), it is necessary to store one of several numbers at each location and, therefore, to have more than one checkerboard. These can be thought of as layered back-to-back. In a four-bit (binary digit) memory, there are four checkerboards back to back so that each pixel has four bits associated with it. In the binary numbering system, this allows numbers from 0 to 15 (16-shade system) to be stored.

The use of digital memories in ultrasound imaging instruments necessitates an understanding of the binary numbering system. Digital (computer) memories and data processors use binary numbers in carrying out their functions. This is because they contain electronic components that operate in only two states—off (0) and on (1).

Binary digits (bits) consist of only zeros and ones, represented by their respective numbers (0 and 1). As in the decimal numbering system with which we are so familiar, other numbers must be represented by moving these symbols to different positions (columns). In the decimal system, in which there are 10 symbols (0 through 9), there is no symbol for the number 10 (nine is the largest number for which there is a single symbol). To represent 10 in symbolic form, then, the symbol for one (1) is used, but it is moved to the second (from the right) column. A zero is placed in the right column to clarify this, resulting in the symbol, 10. The symbol for one has been used, but in such a way that it no longer represents one but, rather, ten.

A similar procedure is used in the binary numbering system. The symbol 1 represents the largest number (one) for which there is a symbol in the system. To represent the next number (two), the same thing is done as in the decimal system. That is, the symbol 1 is placed in the next column to represent the number two.

Columns in the two systems represent values as follows.

	Decimal									Binary						
ones	tens	hundreds	thousands	ten-thousands	hundred-thousands	millions	....		ones	twos	fours	eights	sixteens	thirty-twos	sixty-fours	....
									0	1	0	1	0	(		

In the decimal system, each column represents 10 times the column to its right. In the binary system, each column represents two times the column to its right.

The decimal number 1234 represents (reading from right to left) four ones, three tens, two hundreds, and one thousand; that is, $4 + 30 + 200 + 1000 = 1234$. Likewise, the decimal number 10110 represents zero ones, one ten, one hundred, zero thousands, and one ten thousand. The binary number, 10110, represents zero ones, one two, one four, zero eights, and one sixteen, or $0 + 2 + 4 + 0 + 16 = 22$ (in decimal form). This represents a straightforward way of converting a number from the binary system to the decimal system.

EXAMPLE 4.3.1

Convert the binary number 101010 to decimal form. This number represents $0 + 2 + 0 + 8 + 0 + 32$ or 42 in decimal form.

To convert a number from decimal to binary form, one must successively subtract the largest multiples of two (binary) possible from the decimal.

EXAMPLE 4.3.2

Convert the decimal number 60 to binary:

    a. Can 64 be subtracted from 60? no (0)
    b. Can 32 be subtracted from 60? yes (1)
                     $60 - 32 = 28$
    c. Can 16 be subtracted from 28? yes (1)
                     $28 - 16 = 12$

d. Can 8 be subtracted from 12? yes (1)

$$12 - 8 = 4$$

e. Can 4 be subtracted from 4? yes (1)

$$4 - 4 = 0$$

f. Can 2 be subtracted from 0? no (0)

g. Can 1 be subtracted from 0? no (0)

Therefore, decimal 60 equals 0111100 or 111100. To check this answer, convert it back to decimal. This number, 111100, represents $0 + 0 + 4 + 8 + 16 + 32 = 60$ in decimal.

Table 4.3 lists the binary forms of the decimal numbers 0 through 63. Numbers 64 through 127 would have one additional digit, and so forth with higher multiples of 2.

Several examples of digital memories are given in Table 4.4. A 10×10, four-bit (per pixel) memory is shown in Figure 4.18. The total number of memory elements in various digital memories is given in Table 4.5. A group of 8 bits is called a byte and 1024 bytes (8192 bits) are called a kilobyte. Common in ultrasound instruments today are 6-, 7-, and 8-bit memories. Human vision can differentiate approximately 100 gray levels.[15] More than the 256 shades of an 8-bit system could not be appreciated in human vision.

The procedure for storing the information required for display of the two-dimensional cross-sectional image in a digital scan converter is as follows: the beam is scanned through the patient in such a way that it "cuts" through the tissue in cross section. Echoes received from all points on this cross section are converted to numbers that are stored at corresponding places (pixel locations) in the digital memory. All the information necessary for displaying this cross-sectional image is now stored in memory. The information can then be taken out of memory and applied to a two-dimensional display (cathode ray tube [CRT]; see Section 4.4) and displayed in such a way that the numbers coming out of memory are displayed with corresponding brightnesses on the face of the tube (Fig. 4.19). An example of such a display is shown in Figure 4.20. To see the pixels, read magnification (sometimes called zoom) is used. In this presentation, rather than viewing all the pixels in memory, a smaller group of pixels is shown in expanded (magnified) fashion. This increases pixel size, making the square pixel nature of the image more obvious. Write magnification is also available on some instruments. This allows a smaller anatomic field of view to be written into the entire memory, thereby enlarging the image without enlarging pixel size (Fig. 4.21).

Digital (derived from Latin for "finger" or "toe") scan converters are discrete rather than continuous, which means that they can only store

TABLE 4.3
Binary and Decimal
Number Equivalents

Decimal	Binary	Decimal	Binary
0	000000	32	100000
1	000001	33	100001
2	000010	34	100010
3	000011	35	100011
4	000100	36	100100
5	000101	37	100101
6	000110	38	100110
7	000111	39	100111
8	001000	40	101000
9	001001	41	101001
10	001010	42	101010
11	001011	43	101011
12	001100	44	101100
13	001101	45	101101
14	001110	46	101110
15	001111	47	101111
16	010000	48	110000
17	010001	49	110001
18	010010	50	110010
19	010011	51	110011
20	010100	52	110100
21	010101	53	110101
22	010110	54	110110
23	010111	55	110111
24	011000	56	111000
25	011001	57	111001
26	011010	58	111010
27	011011	59	111011
28	011100	60	111100
29	011101	61	111101
30	011110	62	111110
31	011111	63	111111

TABLE 4.4
Characteristics of Digital Memories

Bits per Pixel	Lowest Number Stored		Highest Number Stored		Number of Shades
	Decimal	Binary	Decimal	Binary	
4	0	0000	15	1111	16
5	0	00000	31	11111	32
6	0	000000	63	111111	64
7	0	0000000	127	1111111	128
8	0	00000000	255	11111111	256

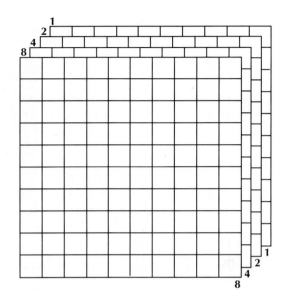

Figure 4.18. A 10 × 10 pixel, 4-bit deep (4 bits per pixel) digital memory.

whole numbers in each pixel location ranging from zero to a maximum that is determined by the number of bits per pixel (see Table 4.4).

For a 512 × 512 matrix in which the represented anatomic depth is 20 cm, each pixel represents an anatomic dimension of 0.4 mm. This represents the spatial resolution of the memory matrix. If the maximum depth represented in memory is 10 cm, then the memory spatial resolution is 0.2 mm.

Preprocessing, in general, includes all that is done to echoes prior to being stored in memory (Fig. 4.22). This includes all the receiver functions and write magnification (Fig. 4.21b). Postprocessing, in general, includes everything done with echoes after they are stored in memory.

TABLE 4.5
Bits (Binary Digits or Memory Elements) in
Digital Memories with 512 × 512
(262,144) Pixels

Bits per Pixel	Total Bits	Total Kilobytes*
4	1,048,576	128
5	1,310,720	160
6	1,572,864	192
7	1,835,008	224
8	2,097,152	256

* 1 byte = 8 bits; 1 kilobyte = 1024 bytes or 8192 bits.

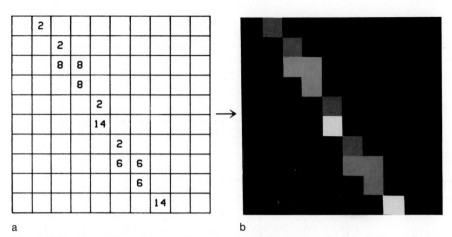

Figure 4.19. For display of scanned anatomic structures, numbers are read out of pixel locations in digital memory (*a*) and applied to the display in such a way that brightness corresponds to those stored numbers (*b*). The display process for the scan line acquired in Figure 4.17*c* is shown.

Read magnification (Fig. 4.21*f*) is an example. Some authors use these terms in a more restricted sense to include only digital processing (those things that occur between the ADC and the digital-to-analog converter [DAC]) functions. An even more specific definition of preprocessing, in digital systems, is the assignment of specific numbers to echo intensities as they are stored in memory (see Figs. 4.15 and 4.23*a*). Postprocessing is the assignment of specific display brightnesses to numbers derived from memory (Fig. 4.24). For most digital systems, the preprocessing scheme is a linear one (see Fig. 4.23). In some, it can be controlled by the operator. For a linear preprocessing assignment, the echo dynamic range is equally divided throughout the gray levels of the system. Tables 4.6 and 4.7 give, for 4- to 8-bit systems, the number of decibels of dynamic range covered by each shade (assuming 40-dB and 60-dB echo dynamic range after attenuation compensation) and the average intensity difference between two echoes for them to be assigned to different shades (numbers in memory) in the system. This is known as contrast resolution. More bits per pixel (more gray shades) improves contrast resolution. For a 4-bit, 40-dB dynamic range system, an echo must have nearly twice the intensity of another one for it to be assigned a different shade. With a 60-dB dynamic range, more than twice the intensity would be required. For a 6-bit, 40-dB system, only a 15 per cent difference is required. For an 8-bit, 60-dB system, a 5 per cent difference is required. Figure 4.23 shows how a larger number of gray shades improves contrast resolution.

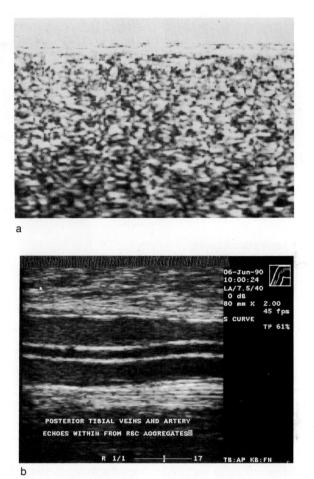

Figure 4.20. Display of pixels of various brightnesses representing various numbers in the corresponding memory locations. The display is magnified (zoom) here to make the square pixels easily seen. Normally they are too small and numerous to be noticed individually. (*a*) Magnified image of tissue-equivalent phantom. (*b*) Magnified image of leg vessels.

It is easy to determine if a function is part of preprocessing or postprocessing. If it cannot be performed on a frozen image, it is a preprocessing function (e.g., write magnification). If it can be performed on a frozen image, it is a postprocessing function. On many instruments, several preprogrammed postprocessing schemes are selectable by the operator. On some, the postprocessing curve may be designed as desired by the operator using panel controls. A linear assignment (see Fig. 4.24) equally divides the display brightness range among the stored gray levels of the system. Other schemes (Fig. 4.25) may be

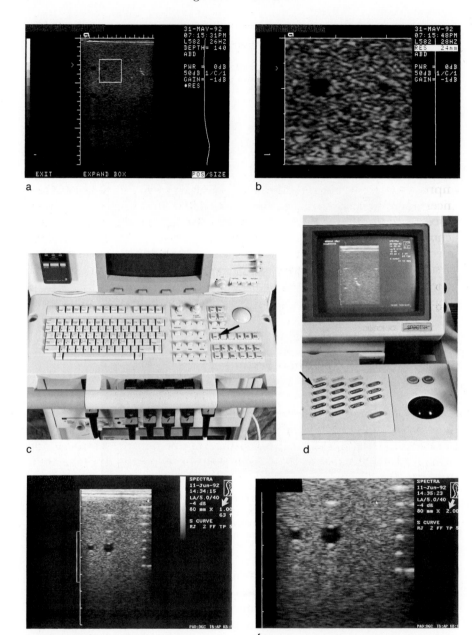

Figure 4.21. (*a*) A scan of a phantom without write magnification. (*b*) A scan using write magnification. Included are 4- and 2-mm simulated cysts. (*c*) (*arrow*) On this control panel, write magnification is indicated by RES, meaning regional expansion selection. (*d*) Read magnification (or zoom), when applied to an "unzoomed" image (*e*), magnifies the stored pixel brightnesses (*f*).

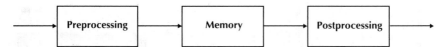

Figure 4.22. Preprocessing includes operations performed on echoes prior to storage in memory. Postprocessing includes operations performed after information is stored in memory.

used that allow assignment of more of the brightness range to certain portions of the stored-number range capability of the system. This can improve the presentation and perception of small echo strength differences stored in memory. Liver metastases (Fig. 4.26) illustrate the importance of contrast resolution, as they can be just slightly more or less echogenic than the surrounding normal liver tissue. The less difference in echogenicity there is, the more difficult it will be to detect the masses. First, more gray shades (more bits per pixel) will be required to store the echoes emanating from metastases with different numbers in memory than those for the surrounding liver. Even then, if a linear postprocessing assignment is used, these small number differences in memory may not be observed in the display. For example, in Figure 4.25a, in which more gray scale range is assigned to the weaker echoes, if normal and abnormal tissue echoes differed by one digit in memory (e.g., normal = 12; abnormal = 13), there would be a 5 per cent difference in brightness (gray level) between the two on the display. This difference would be easily observed. However, with linear postprocessing (see Fig. 4.24a), there would be only a 1.5 per cent brightness difference, which might go unnoticed. In Figure 4.25a, the improvement in contrast resolution for weaker echoes (because of the steeper slope for echoes assigned values 0 through 16 in memory) is accomplished at the cost of reduced contrast

TABLE 4.6
Contrast Resolution of Digital Memories (40-dB Dynamic Range)

Bits per Pixel	Decibels per Shade	Intensity Difference (per cent)*
4	2.5	78
5	1.2	32
6	0.6	15
7	0.3	7
8	0.2	5

* The average difference required between two echoes for them to be assigned different shades.

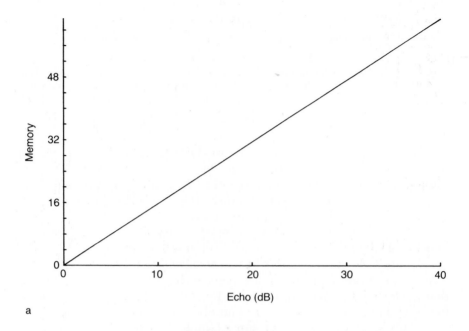

a

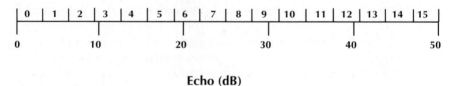

b

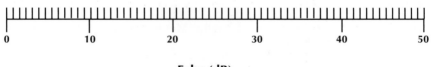

c

Figure 4.23. (*a*) Digital preprocessing is the assignment of numbers (to be stored in memory) to echo intensities. Here, echo intensity is expressed in decibels (relative to the weakest echo, which is represented as 0 dB; 40 dB is the strongest echo, which is 10,000 times the intensity of the weakest) in the form of a straight-line assignment. An instrument dynamic range of 40 dB and a 6-bit (64-shade) memory are assumed. (*b*) With a 4-bit memory, a 50-dB dynamic range is divided into 16 regions (shades). (*c*) With a 6-bit memory, a 50-dB dynamic range is divided into 64 regions, which are numbered 0 through 63.

Memory Shades

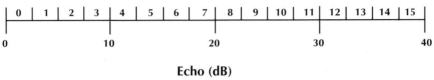

Echo (dB)

d

Memory Shades

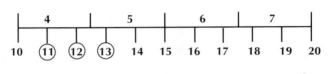

Echo (dB)

e

Memory Shades

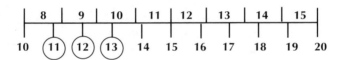

Echo (dB)

f

Figure 4.23 *Continued.* (*d*) With a 4-bit memory, a 40-dB dynamic range is divided into 16 regions. (*e*) The 10- to 20-dB dynamic range portion of (*d*) is expanded here. If normal liver echoes were 12 dB (assigned 4 in memory) and metastases were 13 dB (slightly hyperechoic; assigned 5), the normal and abnormal would be different in memory. If the metastases were 11 dB (slightly hypoechoic), they would be stored as 4s, just as would the normal echoes, and the difference would be lost. (*f*) With a 5-bit (32-shade) memory, both cases in (*e*) would be assigned different numbers and contrast resolution would be maintained.

resolution for the remainder of the dynamic range (shallow slope for echoes assigned values 16 through 63 in memory). Figure 4.27 shows a hemangioma whose presentation is enhanced by using a specially crafted, very steep postprocessing assignment at the echo level corresponding to the hemangioma echogenicity. The contrast between the abnormal and normal tissues is greatly increased. If the mass were not

Text continued on page 166

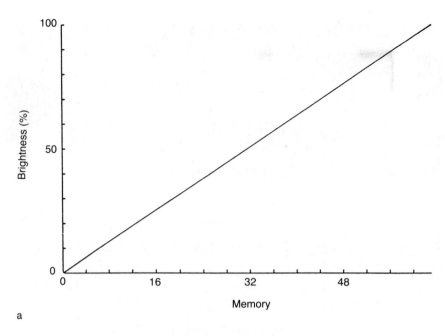

a

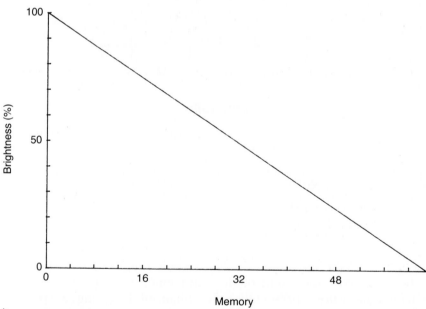

b

Figure 4.24. Digital postprocessing is the assignment of specific display brightnesses to numbers derived from specific pixel locations in memory. (*a*) Brightness increases with increasing echo intensity. This is sometimes called a white-echo display. (*b*) Brightness increases with decreasing echo intensity (black-echo display). Both forms of display were common in the early days of gray-scale imaging. The latter is now seldom used, as the white-echo display has been shown to be superior.[16]

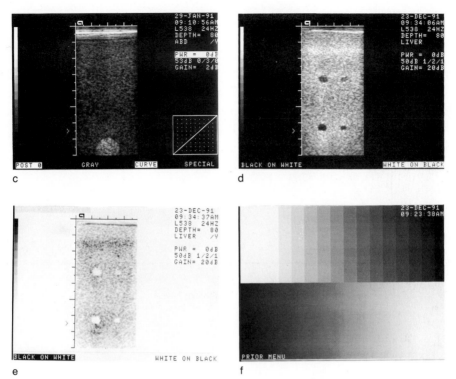

Figure 4.24 *Continued.* (*c* and *d*) Examples of the assignment shown in part *a*. (*e*) Example of the assignment shown in part *b*. (*f*) The upper portion shows 16 shades using an assignment similar to part *b*. The lower portion shows 256 shades using an assignment similar to part *a*.

TABLE 4.7
Contrast Resolution of Digital Memories (60-dB Dynamic Range)

Bits per Pixel	Decibels per Shade	Intensity Difference (per cent)*
4	3.8	140
5	1.9	55
6	0.9	23
7	0.5	12
8	0.2	5

* The average difference required between two echoes for them to be assigned different shades.

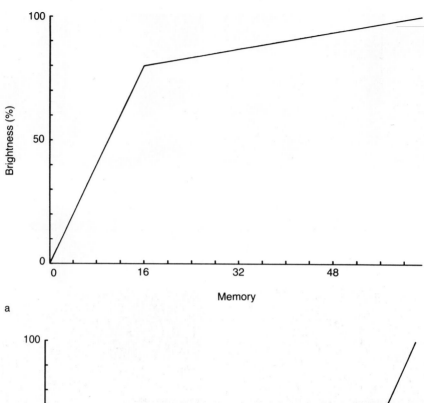

Figure 4.25. Nonlinear postprocessing assignment schemes. A large brightness range is reserved for weak (*a*), strong (*b*), and intermediate (*c*) echoes. These areas have improved contrast resolution.

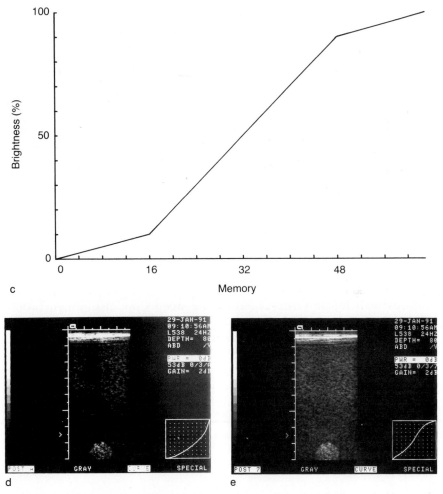

c

Figure 4.25 *Continued.* (*d*) A display using a postprocessing curve similar to that in part *b*. (*e*) A display using a postprocessing curve similar to that in part *c*. Compare parts *d* and *e* with the linear case in Figure 4.24*c*.

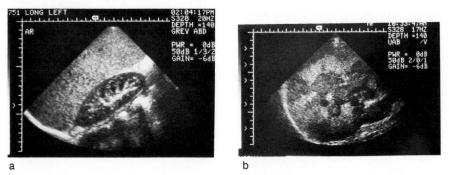

Figure 4.26. (*a*) Normal liver and kidney. (*b*) Liver metastases that are less echogenic (and, therefore, darker) than the surrounding liver tissue.

165

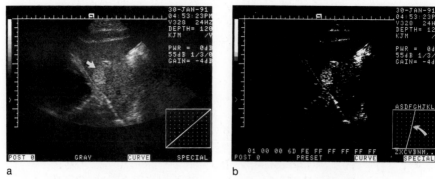

Figure 4.27. (*a*) Ultrasound of a hemangioma (*arrow*) using linear postprocessing. (*b*) Ultrasound of a hemangioma with a very steep postprocessing assignment (*curved arrow*) designed to produce a great contrast between these normal and abnormal tissue echoes.

obvious with linear postprocessing, the steep slope assignment would likely have made it visible.

Some instruments have the ability to present different echo intensities in various colors rather than in gray shades. Because the eye can differentiate more color tints than gray shades,[15] color displays often offer improved contrast resolution capability. This process is called B color or color scale (in comparison to B mode and gray scale). Figure 4.28 (also Plate I) shows examples.

EXERCISES

4.3.1 For the digital memory shown in Figure 4.29, enter the number stored in each pixel location:
   a. lower right: _____
   b. middle right: _____
   c. upper right: _____
   d. upper middle: _____
   e. upper left: _____

4.3.2 The contrast resolution for a digital instrument that has an echo dynamic range of 43 dB and 32 shades is _____ dB per shade.
   a. 1.3
   b. 3.2
   c. 4.3
   d. 32
   e. 43

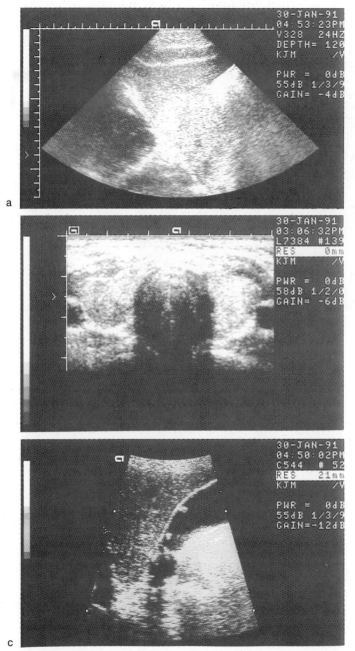

Figure 4.28. Color displays of a hemangioma (*a*) (compare with Fig. 4.27), thyroid (*b*), and gall bladder (*c*). Color assignments, shown in the color bars on the left, are designated as follows: (*a*) temperature (increasing intensity assigned dark orange through yellow to white), (*b*) magenta (dark magenta through light magenta to white), and (*c*) rainbow (dark violet through various colors to white). (See Plate I.)

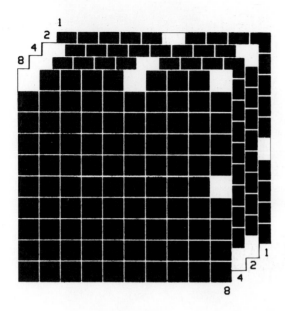

Figure 4.29. Digital memory description for Exercise 4.3.1. White indicates that the memory device is on.

4.3.3 The contrast resolution for a 6-bit digital instrument that has an echo dynamic range of 45 dB is _____ dB/shade.
   a. 0.3
   b. 0.5
   c. 0.7
   d. 0.9
   e. 6

4.3.4 Match the following:
   a. analog: _____   1. picture element
   b. digital: _____   2. assignment of stored
   c. preprocessing: _____   numbers
   d. postprocessing: _____   3. discrete
   e. pixel: _____   4. binary digit
   f. bit: _____   5. continuous
                              6. assignment of displayed
                                 brightnesses

4.3.5 Typical digital pixel matrix dimensions are _____.
   a. 640 x 128
   b. 16 x 64
   c. 100 x 100
   d. 512 x 1540
   e. 512 x 512

4.3.6 Match the number of shades with bits per pixel:

a. 16: _____   1. 1
b. 32: _____   2. 2
c. 64: _____   3. 3
d. 128: _____   4. 4
e. 256: _____   5. 5
               6. 6
               7. 7
               8. 8
               9. 9
               10. 10

4.3.7 _____ total memory elements are required for a 100×100 pixel, 5-bit digital memory.

4.3.8 Memories of _____ bits are common in ultrasound today.

a. 4–8
b. 4–6
c. 6–8
d. 5–7
e. 4–5

4.3.9 Digital scan converters store _____.

a. logarithms
b. electrical magnetism
c. electrical current
d. electrical charge
e. numbers

4.3.10 _____ is commonly controllable by the operator.

a. postprocessing
b. pixel matrix
c. bits per pixel
d. digitization
e. all of the above

4.3.11 In binary numbers, how many symbols are used? _____

4.3.12 The term "binary digit" is commonly shortened into the single word _____.

4.3.13 Each binary digit in a binary number is represented in memory by a memory element, which at any time is in one of _____ states.

4.3.14 Match the following:

Column in an 8-bit binary number hgfedcba: Decimal number represented by a 1 in the column:

a. _____   1. 64
b. _____   2. 32

c. _____   3. 1
d. _____   4. 16
e. _____   5. 8
f. _____   6. 128
g. _____   7. 2
h. _____   8. 4

4.3.15 The binary number 10110 represents zero ones, one two, one four, zero eights, and one sixteen, i.e., $0 + 2 + 4 + 0 + 16 = 22$. What decimal number is represented by the binary number 11001? _____

4.3.16 The decimal number 13 is made up of one one, zero twos, one four, and one eight ($8 + 4 + 0 + 1 = 13$). It is therefore represented by the binary number _____.

4.3.17 Match the following:

Decimal Number	Binary Number
a. 1 _____	1. 0001111
b. 5 _____	2. 0011001
c. 10 _____	3. 0001010
d. 15 _____	4. 0110010
e. 20 _____	5. 0000001
f. 25 _____	6. 1100100
g. 30 _____	7. 0101000
h. 40 _____	8. 0011110
i. 50 _____	9. 0010100
j. 100 _____	10. 0000101

4.3.18 How many binary digits are required in the binary numbers representing the following numbers?

a. 0 _____
b. 1 _____
c. 5 _____
d. 10 _____
e. 25 _____
f. 30 _____
g. 63 _____
h. 64 _____
i. 75 _____
j. 100 _____

4.3.19 Match the following:
How many bits are required to represent each decimal number in binary form?

a. 7 _____   1. 1
b. 15 _____   2. 2
c. 3 _____   3. 3

d. 511 _____   4. 4
e. 1023 _____   5. 5
f. 63 _____   6. 6
g. 255 _____   7. 7
h. 1 _____   8. 8
i. 127 _____   9. 9
j. 31 _____   10. 10

4.3.20 How many bits are required to store numbers representing each number of different gray shades?

a. 2 _____
b. 4 _____
c. 8 _____
d. 15 _____
e. 16 _____4_____
f. 25 _____
g. 32 _____
h. 64 _____
i. 65 _____
j. 128 _____

4.4
Display and Temporal Resolution

There are several ways in which the information delivered to the display may be presented. Those in common use are brightness mode (B mode, B scan, or gray scale) and motion mode (M mode).

The display device used in each case is a CRT. This tube generates a sharply focused beam of electrons that produces a spot of light on the phosphor-coated inner front face (screen) of the tube (Fig. 4.30). The beam (and spot) can be moved across or up and down the face by applying voltages to deflection plates (Fig. 4.31) or, more commonly, by applying electric currents to magnetic deflection coils. If the voltage or current is properly varied, the spot can be made to move across the face in a specific pattern. At the completion of this pattern (i.e., when a frame is completed), the spot jumps rapidly back to the starting point and the next frame is begun.

The brightness of the spot is determined by the strength of the electron beam (which is easily controlled). Because we do not want to display the *numbers* (representing echo amplitude) in memory, but rather pixels of proportional brightness, these numbers must be converted to proportional voltages that control the electron beam strength

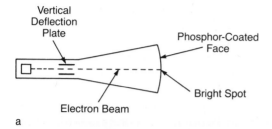

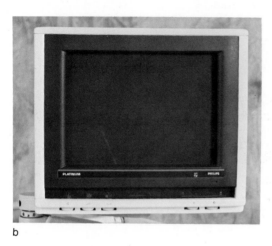

b

Figure 4.30. (*a*) A cathode ray tube (side view). The electron beam produces a spot of light where it strikes the phosphor-coated inner front face of the tube. There is also a set of horizontal deflection plates that is not shown. (*b*) An ultrasound instrument display.

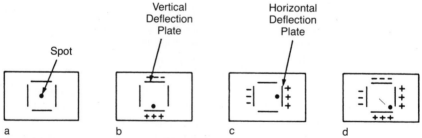

a   b   c   d

Figure 4.31. Spot deflection on the face of a cathode ray tube (front view). (*a*) No voltage is applied to the deflection plates; the spot is centered. (*b*) Voltage is applied to the vertical deflection plates; the spot is deflected down. Increasing the voltage increases the deflection. If the applied voltage were reversed, the spot would be deflected up. (*c*) Voltage is applied to the horizontal deflection plates; the spot is deflected to the right. (*d*) Voltage is applied to both sets of plates; the spot is deflected down and to the right. Magnetic deflection, although more common, is more difficult to illustrate.

in the CRT. Therefore, between the memory and the display, there is a digital-to-analog converter (DAC) (Fig. 4.32).

B mode operation causes a brightening of the spot for each echo in memory. The brightness (gray scale) is proportional to the echo strength. B scan (B mode scan or gray scale) operation depends on entry of echoes (scan lines) into memory, as discussed in Chapter 1. The memory is filled with echoes from many pulses as the beam is scanned through the tissue cross section to be imaged. The B scan is a brightness image that represents a cross section of the object through the scanning plane, as if the sound beam cut a section through the tissue. Each individual image is called a frame. Because several frames can be acquired and presented in each second of time, this is called a real-time display.

Real-time instruments must produce several cross-sectional images per second. This requires the use of mechanical or array automatic scanning transducers (see Section 3.3). The number of images displayed per second is called the frame rate. A rapid sequence yields what appears to be a continuously changing image. When freeze-frame is activated, echo entry into memory is halted and the last frame is shown continuously on the display. Real-time imaging provides rapid and convenient acquisition of the desired image (the display changes continuously as the scan plane is moved through the tissues) and two-dimensional imaging of the motion of moving structures (the display continuously changes as the structures move).

Each frame is made of scan lines. For each focus on each scan line (see Section 3.3) in each frame, a pulse is required. The PRF required is, therefore, determined by the required number of focuses, lines per frame, and the frame rate. Indeed, the PRF is equal to these three quantities multiplied together.

number of focuses ↑	PRF ↑

lines per frame ↑	PRF ↑

frame rate ↑	PRF ↑

However, as discussed in Section 2.4, time is required for echoes to return as a pulse travels into the tissue. The greater the penetration, the

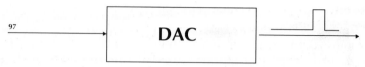

Figure 4.32. The digital-to-analog converter (DAC) converts the numbers (digital) stored in memory to proportional (analog) voltages that control the brightness of the cathode ray tube.

longer it takes for all the echoes to return (remember the 13 μs/cm rule). To avoid range-ambiguity artifact (see Section 6.1), all echoes from one pulse must be received before the next pulse is emitted. Therefore, PRF must decrease as penetration increases.

penetration ↑   PRF ↓

That is, if a lower operating frequency is used, penetration is increased (less attenuation), and PRF must decrease to avoid range ambiguity. This will be experienced as a frame rate reduction (Fig. 4.33) for lower operating frequencies. Likewise, wider images (requiring more scan lines) and multiple focuses also reduce frame rate (Fig. 4.34). The relationship between these competing variables is:

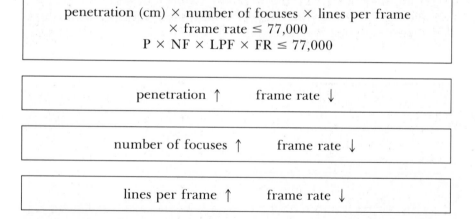

penetration (cm) × number of focuses × lines per frame
× frame rate ≤ 77,000
P × NF × LPF × FR ≤ 77,000

penetration ↑   frame rate ↓

number of focuses ↑   frame rate ↓

lines per frame ↑   frame rate ↓

The 77,000 is one half the average speed of ultrasound in tissues (154,000 cm/s). The one half results because the penetration (expressed in cm) is only half the round-trip distance the sound must travel for the

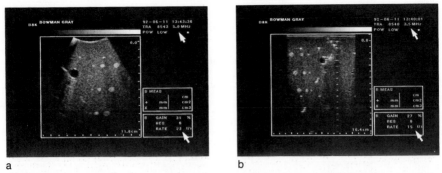

Figure 4.33. A lower operating frequency allows greater penetration, thereby necessitating longer echo arrival time, which slows down the frame rate. (*a*) 5 MHz, penetration of 9 cm, 23 frames per second. (*b*) 3.5 MHz, penetration of 13 cm, 15 frames per second.

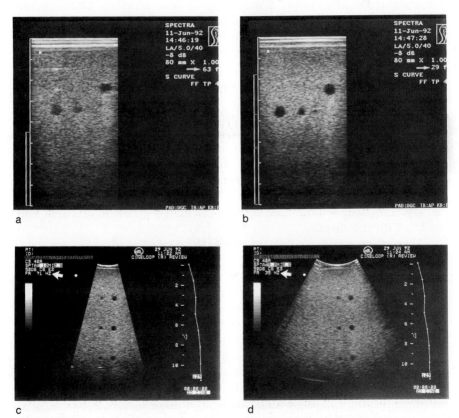

Figure 4.34. (*a*) Frame rate of 63. (*b*) Multiple focuses reduce the frame rate to 29. (*c*) Frame rate of 71. (*d*) An increased frame width reduces the frame rate to 35.

TABLE 4.8
Pulse Repetition Frequencies (PRF) and Frame
Rates (FR) Permitted for Various Single-focus
Imaging Depths (Penetration) and 100 or 200
Scan Lines per Frame

Penetration (cm)	PRF (Hz)	FR 100 Lines	FR 200 Lines
20	3850	38	19
15	5133	51	25
10	7700	77	38
5	15,400	154	77

deepest echoes. The symbol ≤ means less than or equal to. That is, when penetration is multiplied by the number of focuses, the number for scan lines per frame, and the frame rate, the result must not exceed 77,000. Otherwise, the PRF required will not allow return of all echoes prior to emission of the next pulse (resulting in range-ambiguity artifact). Table 4.8 lists the allowable PRFs and frame rates for various penetration and lines-per-frame values. Multiple focuses reduce permitted frame rates inversely (e.g., 2 focuses with a penetration of 20 cm and 100 lines per frame is ½ × 38, or 19 frames per second).

For measurement purposes, most displays include range marker dots or calipers, or both (Fig. 4.35). Marker dots are presented as a series of dots in a line with a given separation (e.g., 1 cm). Calipers are two pluses (or some other symbol), which can be placed anywhere on the display. The distance between them is calculated by the instrument and read out on the display.

The other common display mode (M mode) is used to show the motion of cardiac structures (Fig. 4.36). It is a display form that illustrates depth versus time.

Television monitors are often used as the display devices for ultrasound imaging instruments. A television monitor is a CRT in which a particular electron beam scanning format is utilized. The electron beam current is continually changed as the beam is scanned to provide varying brightness of the spot, thus providing a gray-scale image. The television scanning format consists of a left-to-right and top-to-bottom scanning pattern, which is similar to the way in which this page of text is read. The resulting display consists of 525 horizontal display scan lines that produce one frame of a dynamic image (Fig. 4.37a). Each horizontal line

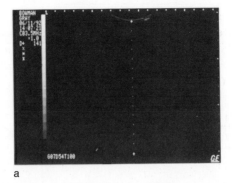

a

b

Figure 4.35. (*a*) Range marker dots. (*b*) Calipers with 5.7-mm (×) and 5.9-mm (+) separations.

corresponds to a row of echo information in memory. This picture is updated (real-time imaging) 30 times each second. This compares to motion picture film, in which 24 frames per second are used. The 30-frame-per-second television picture is scanned in alternate odd and even line fields to reduce flicker. The field rate is 60 per second (two fields make up one frame). External monitors (Fig. 4.37*b*) connected to the ultrasound instrument use the television scan format described here. By comparison, some internal monitors (see Fig. 4.30*b*) in instruments use more horizontal scan lines to improve resolution and higher frame rates for improved imaging of rapidly moving structures. In all cases, though, the images consist of horizontal scan lines on the display.

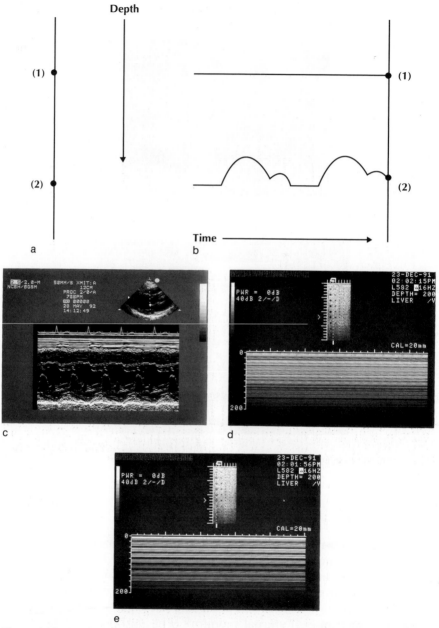

Figure 4.36. (*a*) B-mode presentation of echo depth with echoes from both a stationary structure (*1*) and a moving one (*2*). (*b*) If pulses are sent down the same path repeatedly and vertical scan lines are placed next to each other, a display of depth versus time results. The pattern of motion of moving structures (*2*) is traced out on the display for evaluation. This is called an M-mode display. (*c*) M-mode presentation of a moving structure (mitral valve) in the adult heart. Time increases to the right. The two-dimensional real-time anatomic cross-sectional image is shown also. (*d*) Stationary structures appear on M-mode display as straight horizontal lines because there is no motion. (*e*) The echo-free regions in the cyst phantom are seen as stationary horizontal dark regions on the M-mode display.

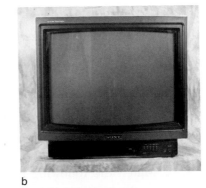

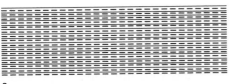

a b

Figure 4.37. (*a*) The television display format has 525 horizontal display scan lines, which are written out in ⅟₃₀th of a second. Half of these (*alternate odd solid lines*) are written first, followed by the remaining (*alternate even dashed*) ones. Each of these sets of lines (solid and dashed on this illustration) makes up a "field." Two fields make a frame. Writing each frame in the format of an odd and an even field reduces flicker. (*b*) A television monitor.

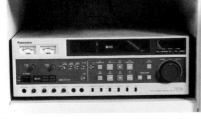

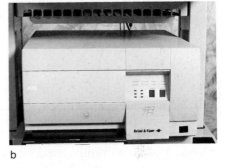

a b

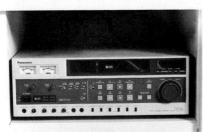

Figure 4.38. Videocassette recording of real-time scanning (*a*). Film (*b*) and print recording (*c*) of frozen images.

c

Recording devices (Fig. 4.38) are often provided to allow videotaping of real-time scanning or hard copy of frozen images.

EXERCISES

4.4.1 The common methods of image presentation are called _____ mode and _____ mode.

4.4.2 Match the following display modes with the appropriate statements (answers may be used more than once):

    a. B mode: _____, _____, _____

    b. M mode: _____, _____, _____

        1. cross-sectional display (two spatial dimensions)
        2. dot is brightened by echo
        3. a depth versus time display
        4. requires the beam to be scanned to develop the image
        5. not a cross-sectional display

4.4.3 The display device used in each mode is a _____ _____ tube.

4.4.4 The spot on a cathode ray tube may be moved by applying voltage to the _____ plates.

4.4.5 Most commonly, electron-beam scanning is accomplished with _____ coils.

4.4.6 The _____ mode is used for studying the motion of a reflector.

4.4.7 The B scan presents a cross section through the _____ plane.

4.4.8 A display that shows various echo strengths as different brightnesses is called a _____ or _____ display.

4.4.9 The _____ _____ stores the gray-scale image and allows it to be displayed on a television monitor.

4.4.10 Television monitors produce _____ images per second.

    a. 10
    b. 15
    c. 30
    d. 60
    e. 100

4.4.11 How many horizontal lines are used to produce a picture on a television monitor?
   a. 60
   b. 100
   c. 256
   d. 525
   e. 1024

4.4.12 It takes _____ ms to produce a single frame on a television monitor using the television scan format.

4.4.13 It takes _____ μs of time to write one horizontal line of brightness information on a television monitor.

4.4.14 Match the following:

Real-time transducer   Display
   a. linear array _____   1. rectangular
   b. oscillating mechanical   2. sector

   _____

   c. convex array _____
   d. annular array _____
   e. phased array _____
   f. vector array _____

4.4.15 If the pulse repetition frequency of an instrument is 1 kHz and it displays (single focus) 25 frames per second, there are _____ lines per frame.

4.4.16 The pulse repetition frequency is _____ Hz if there are 30 frames (40 lines each) per second (single focus).

4.4.17 Imaging involving 10-cm penetration, a single focus, 100 scan lines per frame, and 30 frames per second can be accomplished without range ambiguity. True or false?

4.4.18 The maximum frame rate permitted for 15-cm penetration, three focuses, and 200 scan lines per frame is:
   a. 3.0
   b. 5.5
   c. 8.5
   d. 15
   e. 30

4.5
Review

Diagnostic ultrasound imaging systems are of the pulse-echo type. They use the direction, strength, and arrival time of received echoes to generate B mode and M mode displays. Imaging systems consist of a pulser, beam former, transducer, receiver, memory, and display. Receivers amplify, compensate, compress, demodulate, and reject echoes. Compensation equalizes the differences in received echo amplitudes caused by attenuation. B and M modes use a brightness display. M mode shows reflector motion in time. The B scan shows a cross section through the scanning plane. Digital scan converters store gray-scale image information and permit display on television monitors. Digital scan converters are computer memories that store echo amplitude information as numbers in memory elements. Contrast resolution improves with increasing bits per pixel. Real-time imaging is the rapid sequential display of ultrasound images resulting in a moving presentation. Such imaging requires rapid, repeatable, sequential scanning of the sound beam through the tissue. This is accomplished by mechanical transducers and electronic transducer arrays. Rectangular or sector display formats result from such scanning techniques.

The definitions for terms discussed in this chapter are listed below:

Amplification. The process of increasing small voltages to larger ones.

Amplifier. A device that accomplishes amplification.

Analog. Related to a procedure or system in which data are represented by continuously variable physical quantities (e.g., electric voltage).

Analog-to-digital converter (ADC). A device that converts voltage amplitude to a digital number.

B mode. Mode of operation in which the display records a spot brightening for each echo pulse delivered from the receiver.

B scan. A brightness image that represents a cross section of the object through the scanning plane.

Beam former. The part of an instrument that accomplishes electronic beam scanning, apodization, steering, focusing, and aperture with arrays.

Bit. Binary digit.

Burst. A cycle or two of voltage.

Cathode ray tube. A display device that produces an image by scanning an electron beam over a phosphor-coated screen.

Compensation. Equalization of received reflection amplitude differences caused by different attenuations for different reflector depths. Also called DGC or TGC.

Compression. A decrease in the differences between small and large amplitudes.

Contrast resolution. Ability of a gray-scale display to distinguish between echoes of slightly different amplitude or intensity.

CRT. Cathode ray tube.

Demodulation. Conversion of voltage pulses from RF to video form.

DGC. Depth gain compensation. See Compensation.

Digital. Related to a procedure or system in which data are represented by discrete units (numerical digits).

Digital scan converter. Computer memory that stores echo information.

Digital-to-analog converter (DAC). A device that converts a digital number to a proportional voltage amplitude.

Dynamic focusing. Continuously variable receiving focus that follows the changing position of the transmitted pulse.

Dynamic imaging. Rapid-frame-sequence imaging.

Dynamic range. Ratio (in decibels) of largest power to smallest power that a system can handle; ratio of the largest to the smallest intensity of a group of echoes.

Frame. Display image produced by one complete scan of the sound beam.

Frame rate. Number of frames displayed per second.

Freeze frame. Constant image of the last frame entered into memory.

Gain. Ratio of output to input of electric power.

Gray scale. Continuous range of brightnesses between white and black.

Gray-scale display. Display in which several values of spot brightness may be displayed.

Impulse. A brief excursion of voltage.

M mode. Mode of operation in which the display presents a spot brightening for each pulse delivered from the receiver, producing a two-dimensional recording of reflector position (motion) versus time.

Noise. Thermally generated random variations in a voltage signal.

Pixel. Picture element; the unit into which imaging information is divided for storage and display in a digital instrument.

Postprocessing. Signal processing done after the memory process.

Preprocessing. Signal processing (gain, compensation, etc.) done before the memory process.

Radio frequency. Voltages representing echoes in cyclic form.

Real-time. Imaging with a real-time display.

Real-time display. A display that continuously images moving structures.

Rectification. Conversion from an alternating (reversing) to a direct (one-way) form of voltage.

Rejection. Elimination of smaller-amplitude voltage pulses.

RF. Radio frequency.

Scan converter. A device that stores imaging information in one scanning format and reads it out for display in another.

Scan line. A line produced on a display that represents the echoes from a pulse.

Scanning. Sweeping a sound beam to produce an image.

Temporal resolution. The ability of a display to distinguish closely spaced events in time (it improves with an increased frame rate).

TGC. Time gain compensation. See Compensation.

Time gain compensation. Compensation.

Variable focusing. Transmit focus with various focal lengths.

Video. Demodulated amplitude voltages representing echoes.

Exercises

4.5.1 The six primary components of a diagnostic ultrasound imaging system are the _____, _____ _____, _____, _____, _____, and _____.

4.5.2 Match each component with its function:

a. pulser: _____
b. transducer: _____
c. receiver: _____
d. memory: _____
e. display: _____

1. produces ultrasound pulses
2. processes voltages received from the transducer
3. receives electric information from the memory
4. produces electric pulses that drive the transducer
5. provides electric information to the display

4.5.3 Match the following ultrasound parameters with the instrument components that determine them (answers may be used more than once):

a. frequency: _____

b. period: _____

c. wavelength: _____, _____

d. propagation speed: _____

e. pulse repetition frequency: _____

f. pulse repetition period: _____

g. pulse duration: _____

h. duty factor: _____, _____

i. spatial pulse length: _____, _____

j. axial resolution: _____, _____

k. amplitude: _____, _____

l. intensity: _____, _____

m. attenuation: _____, _____

n. imaging depth: _____, _____

o. beam width: _____, _____

p. lateral resolution: _____, _____

1. pulser
2. transducer
3. tissue

4.5.4 The information that can be obtained from an M mode display includes

a. distance and motion pattern

b. transducer frequency, reflection coefficient, and distance

c. acoustic impedances, attenuation, and motion pattern

d. none of the above

4.5.5 The compensation (swept gain, DGC, and so forth) control serves to

a. compensate for machine instability in the warm-up time

b. compensate for attenuation

c. compensate for transducer aging and the ambient light in the examining area

d. decrease patient examination time

4.5.6 A gray-scale display shows

a. gray color on a white background

b. reflections with one brightness level

c. a white color on a gray background

d. a range of echo amplitudes

4.5.7 The dynamic range of an ultrasound system is defined as

a. the speed with which ultrasound examination can be performed

b. the range over which the transducer can be manipulated while performing an examination

    c. the ratio of the maximum amplitude to the minimum ampli-
       tude or power that can be displayed
    d. the range of pulser voltages applied to the transducer

4.5.8 A digital scan converter is a _____.
    a. compressor
    b. receiver
    c. display
    d. computer memory
    e. none of the above

4.5.9 Which of the following is not performed in a receiver?
    a. rejection
    b. amplification
    c. digital-to-analog conversion
    d. RF to video conversion
    e. compression
    f. compensation

4.5.10 Television displays produce _____ frames per second with _____ lines in each.
    a. 30, 60
    b. 30, 525
    c. 60, 512
    d. 512, 512
    e. 60,120

4.5.11 In a digital instrument, echo intensity is represented by
    a. positive charge distribution
    b. a number stored in memory
    c. electron density of the scan converter writing beam
    d. a and c
    e. all of the above

4.5.12 If there were no attenuation in tissue, _____ would not be needed.
    a. rejection
    b. compression
    c. demodulation
    d. compensation

4.5.13 The television scanning format uses _____ fields per frame so that there are _____ fields presented on the monitor per second.

4.5.14 Which of the following are capable of displaying gray-scale information?
    a. storage cathode ray tube
    b. television monitor
    c. demodulator

d. a and b

e. none of the above

4.5.15 Echo imaging includes ultrasound generation, propagation and reflection in tissues, and reception of returning _____.

4.5.16 The diagnostic ultrasound systems in common clinical use today are of the _____ type.

4.5.17 Gray-scale instruments show echo amplitude as _____ on the display.

4.5.18 Pulse-echo instruments look for three things: the _____, _____, and arrival _____ of echoes emanating from tissues.

4.5.19 A digital scan converter stores image information in the form of _____ numbers.

a. electric charge

b. binary

c. decimal

d. impedance

e. none of the above

4.5.20 Imaging systems produce a visual _____ from the electrical _____ received from the transducer.

4.5.21 The transducer is connected to the memory through the _____.

4.5.22 The transducer receives voltages from the _____ in pulse-echo systems.

4.5.23 The _____ receives voltages from the transducer.

4.5.24 Increasing gain generally produces the same effect as

a. decreasing attenuation

b. increasing attenuation

c. increasing compression

d. increasing rectification

e. both b and c

4.5.25 Voltages occur at the output of the

a. pulser

b. transducer

c. receiver

d. display

e. both a and b

f. both c and e

4.5.26 Ultrasound pulses from the pulser are applied to the _____.

4.5.27 Rectification and smoothing are parts of

a. amplipression

b. rejection

c. a and b

    d. compression

    e. demodulation

4.5.28 If gain is reduced by one half and if input power is unchanged, the output power is _____ what it was before.

    a. equal to

    b. twice

    c. one half

    d. none of the above

4.5.29 If gain is 30 dB and output power is reduced by one half, the new gain is _____ dB.

    a. 15

    b. 60

    c. 33

    d. 27

    e. none of the above

4.5.30 If four shades of gray are shown on a display, each twice the brightness of the preceding one, the brightest shade is _____ times the brightness of the dimmest shade.

    a. 2

    b. 4

    c. 8

    d. 16

    e. 32

4.5.31 The dynamic range displayed in Exercise 4.5.30 is _____ dB.

    a. 10

    b. 9

    c. 5

    d. 2

    e. 0

4.5.32 Gain and attenuation are usually expressed in which unit(s)?

    a. dB

    b. dB/cm

    c. cm

    d. cm/3 dB

    e. none of the above

4.5.33 Compensation (swept gain) makes up for the fact that reflections from deeper reflectors arrive at the transducer with greater amplitude. True or false?

4.5.34 The mode that shows one-dimensional (depth) real-time images is _____ mode.

4.5.35 The mode that shows two-dimensional real-time images is _____ mode.

4.5.36 A real-time B mode display may be produced by rapid _____ transducer scanning or by _____ scanning of a transducer array.

4.5.37 Each complete scan of the sound beam produces an image on the display that is called a _____.

4.5.38 For a single focus, the number of lines in each frame is equal to the number of times the transducer is _____ while the frame is produced (while the sound beam is scanned).

4.5.39 In real-time scanning, the pulse repetition frequency depends upon the number of _____ per frame and the _____ rate.

4.5.40 Increasing the number of focuses reduces _____ _____.

4.5.41 To correct for attenuation, the TGC must (increase or decrease) _____ the amplification (gain) for increasing depth.

4.5.42 If a higher frequency is used, resolution is (improved or worsened), imaging depth (increases or decreases), and the TGC slope must be (increased or decreased)?

4.5.43 Images are typically divided into 512 pixels on each side (512 × 512). This means that an image typically contains how many pixels?

4.5.44 Which type of real-time transducer gives a wide view close to the transducer? Which of the following produce(s) a sector format image?
   a. mechanical real-time
   b. linear array
   c. phased array
   d. all of the above

4.5.45 If a single-focus ultrasound instrument produces 1000 pulses per second and 20 frames per second, how many scan lines make up each frame?

CHAPTER 5

Doppler Instruments

One item of information not used by the instruments described in Chapter 4 is the Doppler shift of the received echoes. Doppler instruments respond to moving reflectors or scatterers (usually blood cells in circulation) by detecting Doppler shift. This information is converted to audible sound and to visual displays. Doppler instruments are of three types:

1. Continuous-wave (CW) spectral
2. Pulsed-wave (PW) spectral
3. Color-flow (CF)

Doppler ultrasound has been used for many years in medicine as a tool for monitoring fetal heart rate during labor and for detecting and quantifying blood flow in the heart and a variety of vessels throughout the body. This flow information is presented as an audible sound and visually as a flow-versus-time plot or as a color-coded two-dimensional presentation. Any of these presentations can be evaluated and used for diagnostic purposes. In most applications, the visual presentation of the flow information is combined with the two-dimensional anatomic presentation of sonography. Broader and more detailed presentation of Doppler principles can be found elsewhere.[1,8–10,17–20]

In this chapter, we consider the following questions: How does ultrasound detect and measure flow? In what ways is flow information presented? How is flow detection localized to a specific site in tissue? How is two-dimensional flow determined and presented in real-time? The following terms are discussed in this chapter:

autocorrelation	Doppler angle
bidirectional	Doppler effect
color flow (CF)	Doppler shift
cosine (cos)	duplex
disturbed flow	fast Fourier transform (FFT)

fluid
frequency spectrum
generator gate
laminar flow
parabolic flow
plug flow
pulsatile flow
receiver gate

sample volume
spectral analysis
spectral broadening
turbulence
turbulent flow
variance
viscosity

5.1
Hemodynamics

Blood flows from the heart through arteries, capillaries, and veins to supply the cells of the body with oxygen and nutrients. Blood is a fluid—that is, it is a material that flows and conforms to the shape of its container. Flow is classified as normal, disturbed, or turbulent. Two types of normal flow are plug flow and laminar flow. At the entrance to a tube, the speed of the fluid is essentially constant across the tube (Fig. 5.1a). This is called plug flow. Further down the tube, laminar flow develops. This occurs as the layers (laminae) of the fluid slide over each other, with the central portion moving at maximum speed and portions next to the vessel wall hardly moving at all (see Fig. 5.1a). Laminar flow is also called parabolic flow because a curve connecting the arrowheads describing laminar flow has the shape of a parabola. Disturbed flow occurs when the parallel stream lines that characterize normal flow are disturbed (i.e., not straight) (Fig. 5.1, b and c). Particles of fluid still flow generally in a forward direction. Turbulent flow is random and chaotic, with individual particles moving in all directions while still maintaining a net forward flow (Fig. 5.1, d and e). Turbulent flow can easily occur beyond an obstruction, such as an atherosclerotic plaque (Fig. 5.1e).

Pressure is the driving force behind fluid flow. A pressure difference at the ends of a fluid-filled pipe, tube, or vessel causes the fluid to flow from the high-pressure to the low-pressure end. The greater the pressure difference, the greater the volume flow rate (expressed in liters per minute or milliliters per second). The greater the resistance to flow, the less the volume flow rate will be. Viscosity, vessel length, and vessel diameter contribute to resistance. Viscosity is the resistance of a fluid to flow (e.g., water has low viscosity, whereas molasses has high viscosity). The longer the vessel, the greater the resistance. The larger the diame-

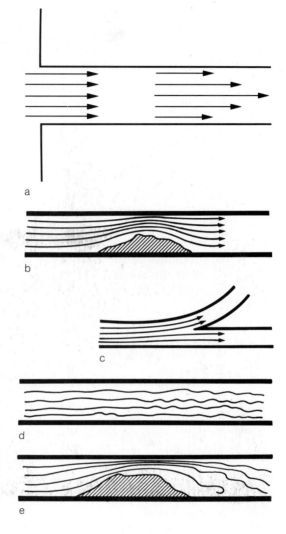

Figure 5.1. (*a*) At the entrance to a tube or vessel, plug flow (*1*) exists. After some distance, laminar flow (*2*) develops. (*b*) Disturbed flow at a stenosis. (*c*) Disturbed flow at a bifurcation. (*d*) Turbulent flow in a vessel resulting from too great a flow speed. (*e*) Turbulent flow resulting from an obstruction.

ter, the less the resistance. Diameter is the variable of interest in most vascular disease studies. With constant pressure difference, flow is steady. Flow in many veins is like this. With pulsatile pressure variations from the beating heart, flow is pulsatile in arteries. In the case of a stenosis, flow speed increases to maintain volume flow rate through the narrowed lumen. Beyond a significant stenosis, turbulent flow is likely to develop.

EXERCISES

5.1.1 The characteristic of a fluid that offers resistance to flow is called
   a. resistance
   b. viscosity
   c. kinematic viscosity
   d. impedance
   e. density
5.1.2 Flow is a response to pressure _difference_.
5.1.3 If the pressure is greater at one end than it is at the other, the liquid will flow from the _____ pressure end to the _____ pressure end.
   a. higher, lower
   b. lower, higher
   c. (depends on the liquid)
   d. all of the above
   e. none of the above
5.1.4 The flow in a tube is determined by _pressure_ difference and _resistance_.
5.1.5 If the following is increased, flow increases.
   a. pressure difference
   b. pressure
   c. resistance
   d. a and b
   e. all of the above
5.1.6 As flow resistance increases, volume flow _decreases_.
5.1.7 Tubes that carry blood in the circulatory system are called _vessels_.
5.1.8 Flow resistance in a vessel depends upon
   a. vessel length
   b. vessel radius
   c. blood viscosity
   d. all of the above
   e. none of the above
5.1.9 Flow resistance decreases with an increase in which of the following?
   a. vessel length
   b. vessel radius
   c. blood viscosity
   d. all of the above
   e. none of the above

5.1.10 Volume flow decreases with an increase in which of the following?
   a. pressure difference
   b. vessel radius
   c. vessel length
   d. blood viscosity
   e. c and d

5.1.11 When the speed of a fluid is essentially constant across a vessel, the flow is called _____ flow.
   a. volume
   b. parabolic
   c. laminar
   d. viscous
   e. plug

5.1.12 disturbed flow occurs when the parallel stream lines describing the flow are altered.

5.1.13 turbulent flow involves random and chaotic flow patterns, with particles moving in all directions.

5.1.14 A narrowing of a tube is called a stenosis.

5.1.15 Proximal to, at, and distal to a stenosis _____ must be constant.
   a. laminar flow
   b. disturbed flow
   c. turbulent flow
   d. volume flow rate
   e. none of the above

5.1.16 For the answer to Exercise 5.1.15 to be true, flow speed at the stenosis must be _____ that proximal and distal to it.
   a. greater than
   b. less than
   c. less turbulent than
   d. less disturbed than
   e. none of the above

5.1.17 Which of the following flows are the same?
   a. steady
   b. pulsatile
   c. plug
   d. laminar
   e. disturbed
   f. turbulent
   g. parabolic

5.1.18 Which flows in 5.1.17 relate to temporal characteristics?
5.1.19 Which flows in 5.1.17 relate to spatial characteristics?

5.2
Doppler Effect

Doppler ultrasonography is useful in detecting and quantifying the presence, direction, speed, and character of blood flow in vessels. Various Doppler patterns are characteristic of plug, laminar, disturbed, and turbulent flows. The Doppler effect is a change in the frequency or wavelength of a wave as a result of motion (Fig. 5.2). The wave can be of light, sound, or any other type. The motion may be that of the wave source, the observer (receiver), or a reflector. An example of the Doppler effect with a moving source of sound is the higher pitch of a siren as an ambulance approaches an observer (compared with the lower pitch the observer hears after the ambulance has passed and is receding in the distance). The same effect could be observed if the ambulance were stationary and the observer were approaching or moving away from it in a moving vehicle. Ultrasonic Doppler effect is used in home alarm systems (Fig. 5.2c). Microwave Doppler effect is used in police radar speed detectors. In medical applications of Doppler ultrasonography, a moving reflector or scatterer of sound is used. In blood flow measurements, the dominant scatterer of sound is the erythrocyte (Fig. 5.2, *a* and *b*), which is the dominant cell in blood. The change in frequency secondary to scatterer motion (blood flow) is called the Doppler shift frequency or, more simply, the Doppler shift. It is the difference between the frequency of the emitted ultrasound and that of the returning echoes. Subtraction of transmitted frequency from echo frequency is equal to Doppler shift. It is proportional to the emitted frequency (operating frequency of the transducer) and to the speed of flow. These quantities are related to each other through the Doppler equation:

Doppler shift (MHz) = echo frequency (MHz)
$$- \text{operating frequency (MHz)}$$

$$= \frac{\begin{array}{c}2 \times \text{operating frequency (MHz)} \\ \times \text{ reflector speed (m/s)} \times \cos \theta\end{array}}{\text{propagation speed (m/s)}}$$

$$f_D = f_e - f_o = \frac{2f_o \times v \times \cos \theta}{c}$$

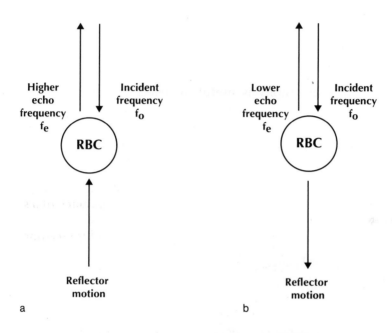

a   b

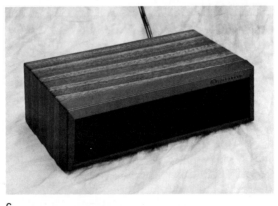

c

Figure 5.2. Doppler effect. (*a*) If the reflector (red blood cell [RBC], erythrocyte) moves toward the ultrasound source, the reflected (echo) frequency is higher than the incident frequency. (*b*) If the reflector moves away from the ultrasound source, the reflected frequency is lower than the incident frequency. (*c*) Ultrasonic motion detection "burglar" alarm.

reflector speed ↑   shift ↑

operating frequency ↑   shift ↑

Doppler angle ↑   shift ↓

The shift is positive when the reflector is moving toward the transducer and it is negative when the reflector is moving away from the transducer. The Doppler equation can be rearranged and the average speed of sound in tissue incorporated to yield the following form of the equation:

$$\text{reflector speed} = \frac{\text{propagation speed} \times \text{Doppler shift}}{2 \times \text{operating frequency} \times \cos\theta}$$

$$v\ (\text{cm/s}) = \frac{77\ f_D(\text{kHz})}{f_o(\text{MHz})\cos\theta}$$

The 77 is valid when v, f_D, and f_o are given in the units shown. The Doppler angle is the angle between the sound propagation and blood flow directions (Fig. 5.3a). The larger the angle is, the smaller the Doppler shift will be for a given flow speed (Fig. 5.3b). Doppler instruments determine the Doppler shifts of the returning echoes. It is important to realize that, as shown by the Doppler equation, a calculated flow speed v depends on the Doppler angle θ. Therefore, values of v calculated from the observed f_D are only as accurate as the estimated Doppler angle θ. This is one reason why sonography is combined with Doppler techniques. With a cross-sectional image of the vessel walls, the sonographer can adjust a flow direction indicator which, when combined with an indication of the beam direction, can yield the Doppler angle. The instrument uses this value of angle to convert Doppler shift to flow speed (Fig. 5.3c). Table 5.1 lists Doppler frequency shifts for several reflector or scatterer speeds, Doppler angles, and operating frequencies.

If the sides and angles of a right triangle (a triangle in which one of the angles equals 90 degrees) are labeled as in Figure 5.4, the cosine of angle A (cos A) is defined as the length of side b divided by the length of side c.

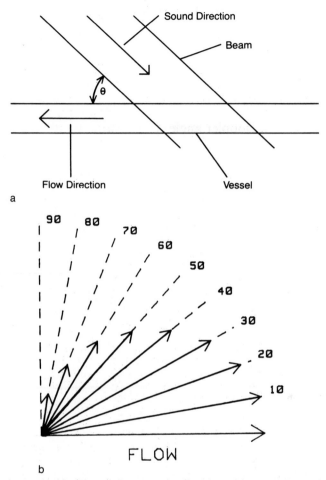

a

b

FLOW

Figure 5.3. (*a*) Angle θ is the angle between the direction of flow and the sound propagation direction. (*b*) As Doppler angle increases, echo Doppler shift frequency decreases.

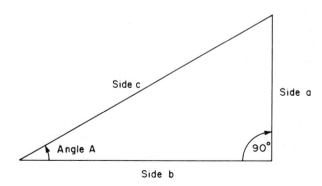

Figure 5.4. Sides and angles of a right triangle.

TABLE 5.1
Doppler Shifts for Various Frequencies, Angles, and Speeds

Frequency (MHz)	Angle (Degrees)	Speed (cm/s)	Shift (kHz)
2	0	10	0.26
2	0	50	1.30
2	0	100	2.60
2	30	10	0.22
2	30	50	1.12
2	30	100	2.25
2	45	10	0.18
2	45	50	0.92
2	45	100	1.84
2	60	10	0.13
2	60	50	0.65
2	60	100	1.30
5	0	10	0.65
5	0	50	3.25
5	0	100	6.49
5	30	10	0.56
5	30	50	2.81
5	30	100	5.62
5	45	10	0.46
5	45	50	2.30
5	45	100	4.59
5	60	10	0.32
5	60	50	1.62
5	60	100	3.25
10	0	10	1.30
10	0	50	6.49
10	0	100	13.0
10	30	10	1.12
10	30	50	5.62
10	30	100	11.2
10	45	10	0.92
10	45	50	4.59
10	45	100	9.18
10	60	10	0.65
10	60	50	3.25
10	60	100	6.49

EXAMPLE 5.2.1

If the lengths of sides a, b, and c are 1, $\sqrt{3}$, and 2, respectively, what is cos A?

$$\cos A = \frac{\sqrt{3}}{2} = 0.87$$

If the cosine is known, angle A may be found using a calculator or a table, such as Table 5.2.

EXAMPLE 5.2.2

If cos A is 0.87, what is A? From Table 5.2, it can be determined that A = 30 degrees.

If angle A is known, cos A may be found using a calculator or a table, such as Table 5.2.

TABLE 5.2
Cosines for Various Angles

Angle A (degrees)	cos A
0	1.00
1	1.00
2	1.00
3	1.00
4	1.00
5	1.00
6	0.99
7	0.99
8	0.99
9	0.99
10	0.98
20	0.94
30	0.87
40	0.77
50	0.64
60	0.50
70	0.34
80	0.17
90	0.00

EXAMPLE 5.2.3

If A = 40 degrees, what is cos A? From Table 5.2, it can be determined that cos A = 0.77.

For a 90-degree Doppler angle, the Doppler shift is zero. In practice, there is some Doppler shift observed even at a 90-degree angle because beams are not cylindrical in shape (see Section 3.2). Thus, even when the beam axis (center line) is perpendicular to the flow, portions of the beam encounter the flow at other (nonperpendicular) angles. An instrument designed to measure the difference between the incident and reflected frequencies can yield information on reflector motion. The moving reflector could be a tissue boundary (e.g., a blood vessel wall or heart wall) or blood cells in circulation. Commonly used operating frequencies are within the 2- to 10-MHz range.

The optimum angle range for most vascular studies is approximately 30 to 60 degrees. With greater angles, the Doppler shift becomes too small (except for extremely high flow speeds), whereas with smaller angles, refraction and critical-angle effects inhibit successful signal acquisition. In cardiac studies, most views of the heart result in reasonably small Doppler angles so that angle correction is seldom used.

In all Doppler techniques, the Doppler angle is important. In Doppler echocardiography, it is commonly assumed to be zero because the views used allow the beam to be approximately parallel to the measured flow. Here, a 5-degree error in Doppler angle produces less than 1 per cent error in calculated flow speed. In peripheral vascular work, because many vessels run approximately parallel to the skin surface, the Doppler angles encountered vary over a range of about 30 to 60 degrees. A 5-degree error in Doppler angle can produce a calculated flow speed error of 5 per cent to 12 per cent in this range. Beyond 60 degrees, the error rapidly increases. Therefore, it is not wise to operate at a Doppler angle of greater than 60 degrees. Initially, it might seem that calibrating spectral displays in Doppler shift frequency, rather than flow speed, would avoid the problem. However, this is not true. Rather, is it the dependence of Doppler shift frequency on the Doppler angle that causes the problem. That is, as the Doppler angle increases, frequency shift decreases. Therefore, Doppler shift information from various instruments or laboratories can only be compared with each other or against a standard, either by using a constant angle or by correcting for angle. However, two advantages of using flow speed information rather than Doppler shift frequencies are (1) the operating frequency of the transducer is accounted for (and therefore eliminated) and (2) the information is physiologically relevant. After all, it is information regarding blood flow that we desire, not some acoustic frequency.

EXERCISES

5.2.1 The Doppler effect is a change in reflected _____ caused by reflector _____.

5.2.2 If the reflector is moving toward the source, the reflected frequency is _____ than the incident frequency.

5.2.3 If the reflector is moving away from the source, the reflected frequency is _____ than the incident frequency.

5.2.4 If the reflector is stationary with respect to the source, the reflected frequency is _____ _____ the incident frequency.

5.2.5 Measurement of Doppler shift yields information about reflector _____.

5.2.6 If the incident frequency is 1 MHz, the propagation speed is 1600 m/s, and the reflector speed is 16 m/s toward the source, the Doppler shift is _0.02_ MHz and the reflected frequency is _1.02_ MHz.

5.2.7 If 2-MHz ultrasound is reflected from a soft tissue boundary moving at 10 m/s toward the source, the Doppler shift is _.026_ MHz.

5.2.8 If 2-MHz ultrasound is reflected from a soft tissue boundary moving at 10 m/s away from the source, the Doppler shift is _____ MHz.

5.2.9 Doppler shift is the difference between _____ and _____ frequencies.

5.2.10 When incident sound direction and reflector motion are not parallel, calculation of the reflected frequency involves the _____ of the angle between these directions.

5.2.11 If the angle between incident sound direction and reflector motion is 60 degrees, the Doppler shift and reflected frequency, given the parameters in Exercise 5.2.6, are _____ MHz and _____ MHz, respectively.

5.2.12 If the angle between incident sound direction and reflector motion is 90 degrees, the cosine of the angle is _____ and the reflected frequency, given the parameters in Exercise 5.2.6, is _____ MHz.

5.2.13 A policeman in a (Doppler) radar-equipped patrol car detects the speed of an automobile to be 55 mph. If the angle between the radar beam and the direction of the automobile is 60 degrees, the actual speed of the automobile is _____ mph.

5.2.14 If side a, b, and c in Figure 5.4 have lengths of 3, 4, and 5, respectively, cos A is _____.

5.2.15 If angle A is 90 degrees, cos A is _____.

5.2.16 If cos A is 0.94, angle A is _____ degrees.

5.2.17 Doppler ultrasonography is good for detecting and quantifying the presence , direction, speed , and character of blood flow in vessels.

5.3
Spectral Instruments

The three types of instruments that implement the Doppler effect medically include CW, PW, and color-flow (CF) instruments. The CW Doppler instrument (Fig. 5.5) uses a continuously transmitted sound beam. Echoes are thus continuously received by the transducer. Therefore, a

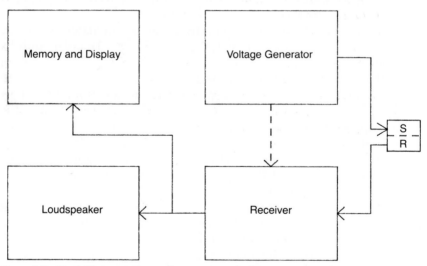

Figure 5.5. Block diagram of a continuous-wave Doppler instrument. The voltage generator produces a continuously alternating voltage that drives the source transducer (S). The receiving transducer (R) produces continuous voltage in response to the reflections it continuously receives. The receiver detects any difference in frequency between the voltages produced by the continuous-wave generator and those produced by the receiving transducer. The Doppler shift produces a voltage that drives a loudspeaker in the audible range and a visual display. The frequency of the audible sound is equal to the Doppler shift. It is proportional to the reflector speed and to the cosine of the angle between the sound propagation direction and the reflector motion (see Section 5.2).

dual-element transducer—one element for transmitting and one for receiving—is required. The receiver compares the frequency of the returning echoes with the frequency of the transmitted sound, yielding the Doppler shift. This is applied to a loudspeaker, which produces audible sounds because Doppler shifts for typical operating frequencies and physiologic flow speeds are in the audible range (see Table 5.1). The system is sensitive to Doppler-shifted echoes returning from moving scatterers within the overlapping region of the beams of the transmit and receive elements of the dual-element transducer. Any Doppler-shifted echoes from within this region will be detected by the system and presented audibly or visually. The Doppler demodulator in the receiver is generally a phase-quadrature detector[1,8] that has two output channels representing forward and reverse flow (positive and negative Doppler shifts). These two channels can be presented on separate loudspeakers, or can be displayed visually as positive and negative Doppler shifts above and below a zero baseline on the display (see Figs. 5.3c and 5.6).

To eliminate the high-intensity, low-frequency Doppler shift echoes resulting from vessel or heart wall motion during pulsatile flow, a high-pass filter (a filter that rejects frequencies below an adjustable value) is used. Sometimes called a wall filter, it rejects the strong echoes that would overwhelm the weaker echoes from the blood.

To separate flow information from two vessels or to localize it within a vessel, range selectivity or resolution must be provided. This is the principle feature of the PW Doppler instrument (Fig. 5.7). The voltage generator provides voltage bursts of several cycles in length to the transducer. Thus, this is a pulse-echo system, similar to those used for sonography except that longer pulses are used. The receiver detects and presents Doppler shift information audibly and visually, as in a CW doppler instrument. However, the receiver includes a gate which, when

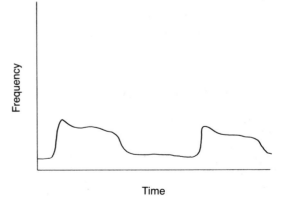

Figure 5.6. A display of spectrum as a function of time (cardiac cycle). The amplitude of each frequency component at each instant of time is represented by gray level or color. A thin line presentation like this would result if pulsatile plug flow (see Fig. 5.1a) were encountered.

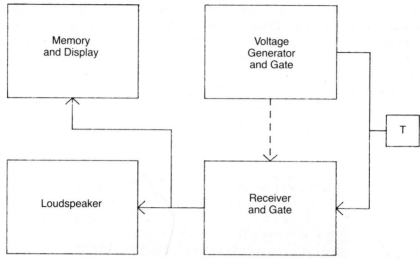

Figure 5.7. Block diagram of a pulsed Doppler instrument. The voltage generator produces a continuously alternating voltage. The generator gate converts this continuous voltage to voltage bursts that drive the transducer (*T*). Received pulses are delivered to the receiver, where their frequency is compared with the frequency of the generator. The difference (Doppler shift) is sent to the loudspeaker and display. The receiver also contains a gate that selects reflections from a given depth according to arrival time, thus providing motion information as a function of depth.

open, allows the passage of voltages representing echoes and, when closed, prevents the passage of voltages. Because echo arrival time (see Table 2.7) corresponds to echo generation depth (13 μs/cm), the receiver gate can control the location (depth) from which Doppler information is received. Indicators are included on the display (see Figs. 5.3*c* and 5.8) to indicate the points at which the gate opens and closes and the included region (Table 5.3) from which Doppler-shifted echoes are being received (the sample volume). While searching for the desired Doppler signal, a longer gate length (i.e., 10 mm) is used. When the signal is localized, a smaller gate length (i.e., 2 mm) is used to improve the signal-to-noise ratio. Because pure plug flow is not found in blood vessels, flow in vessels is not perfectly uniform. That is, not all of the cells are moving at the same speed within a sample volume. Furthermore, with disturbed and turbulent flow, cells are moving in different directions. A parabolic flow profile is common for smaller vessels, whereas a profile approximating plug flow is characteristic for larger vessels, particularly in systole. Thus, it is apparent that, even for normal flow, a range of Doppler shift frequencies will return to the transducer at any instant throughout the cardiac cycle, even from a small sample volume. This occurs because echoes are returning from scatterers that are moving at different speeds and/or directions (i.e., different velocities). Abnormal and turbulent flows increase the range of the Doppler shift frequencies received (this is called spectral broadening) and sometimes include both positive and negative Doppler shifts (above and below the baseline). Because, even in normal flow, many Doppler shift frequencies are received simultaneously, the sound representing these Doppler shifts is a combination of several frequencies. The human auditory system is able to analyze this complex signal and recognize normal and abnormal flow sounds. In

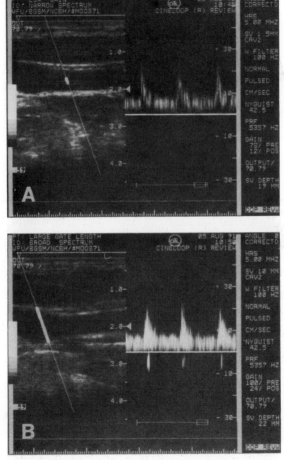

Figure 5.8. (*a*) Narrow spectrum from a common carotid artery using a small (1.5-mm) sample gate. (*b*) Spectral broadening resulting from the inclusion of all the flow across the vessel with a large (10-mm) gate. (Reproduced from Kremkau, F.W.: Doppler principles. Sem. Roentg. 27:6–16, 1992, with permission.)

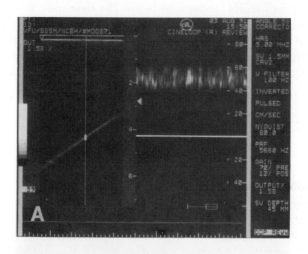

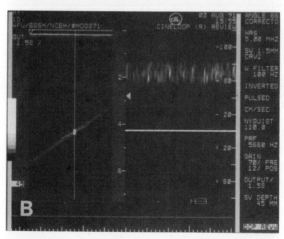

Figure 5.9. A moving string test object is imaged and the Doppler spectrum shown. (*a*) With proper angle correction (56°), the 50 cm/s string speed is shown correctly. (*b*) With improper angle correction (66°), an incorrect string speed of 70 cm/s is shown, representing 40 per cent error. (Reproduced from Kremkau, F.W.: Doppler principles. Sem. Roentg. 27:6–16, 1992, with permission.)

TABLE 5.3
Spatial Gate Length for Various
Temporal Gate Lengths*

Time (μs)	Length (mm)
1.3	1
2.6	2
3.9	3
5.2	4
6.5	5
13.0	10
19.5	15
26.0	20
39.0	30

* Time is from gate turn-on to turn-off. Pulse
duration adds to the time and effective gate length.

addition to audible presentation, the component frequencies of the complex received signal can be separated through a process called spectral analysis.[1] This is accomplished digitally by the fast fourier transform (FFT). This spectral analysis is analogous to the spreading out of white light by a prism into its component colors, called a color spectrum (hence, the term spectral analysis, for "to analyze" is to take apart). FFTs can be calculated rapidly enough to be presented in real-time, allowing Doppler shift spectra to be presented as a function of time on the display (see Fig. 5.8). In arterial flow, as shown in Figure 5.8, it is observed that Doppler shift frequency (and calculated flow speed) increases and decreases over the cardiac cycle. Although the calculated flow speed values at any point and time are dependent on Doppler angle, the relationship between peak-systolic and end-diastolic values (i.e., their ratio) is independent of angle. Thus, measures of these parameters (pulsatility indices) are useful descriptors of flow characteristics.[1]

Duplex instruments that combine imaging with Doppler technology allow more intelligent use of the Doppler effect in that they provide information regarding the location of the source of the Doppler signal. Thus, the observer knows the vessel (and for small gates, the location within the vessel) from which the Doppler information is being obtained. The display generated from such duplex systems present anatomic cross sections along with the Doppler spectral information (see Fig. 5.8).

Spectral broadening is an indicator of flow disturbance and turbulence. However, technique is important in its use because it is affected by gain settings and gate length (see Fig. 5.8).

Angle correction is important on spectral displays. Even small angle errors can produce large speed errors (Fig. 5.9).

EXERCISES

5.3.1 All Doppler instruments distinguish between positive and negative Doppler shifts. True or false?

5.3.2 Instruments that distinguish between positive and negative Doppler shifts yield motion _____ information and are called _____.

5.3.3 Continuous-wave Doppler instruments use single-element transducers similar to those used in imaging. True or false?

5.3.4 The components of a continuous-wave Doppler system include a _____ _____, _____ _____, _____ _____, _____, _____, _____, and _____.

5.3.5 Quantitative information about the frequencies contained in returning Doppler-shifted echoes can be obtained using the _____ _____ _____ (FFT) mathematical technique.

5.3.6 To display the pattern of time change of a Doppler frequency spectrum, a display of _____ _____ versus _____ can be used.

5.3.7 In Exercise 5.3.6, the amplitude of each frequency component is represented by _____ level or _____.

5.3.8 The received frequency spectrum exists (rather than a single frequency) because of the distribution of _____ _____ encountered by the pulse.

5.3.9 Because velocity is speed *and* direction, variations in either of these in the flow region monitored by the Doppler instrument may contribute to the received frequency spectrum. True or false?

5.3.10 The components of a pulsed Doppler instrument are the same as those for a continuous-wave instrument except for the addition of two _____ and the combining of two _____ _____ into one.

5.3.11 The purpose of the generator gate is to convert a _____ voltage to a voltage _____.

5.3.12 The purpose of the receiver gate is to allow selection of Doppler-shifted echoes from specific _____ according to their _____ _____.

5.3.13 Pulsed Doppler instruments require a two-element transducer assembly. True or false?

5.3.14 If the receiver gate opens later, the gate location moves deeper. True or false?

5.4
Color-Flow Instruments

CW and PW Doppler instruments provide one-dimensional Doppler information. That is, the flow information originates somewhere along a stationary Doppler beam. CF instruments provide real-time two-dimensional flow information.[18–20] The process is analogous to pulse-echo sonography (see Chapter 1), where echo information from a two-dimensional section of tissue is stored in a memory and displayed. In sonography, echo location and amplitude are the essential parameters. In Doppler CF instruments, echo location and Doppler shift are the essential parameters. In time-shift CF instruments, the Doppler effect is not used. Rather, echo arrival time shifts are used to determine reflector motion.[21] In CF instruments, the two-dimensional Doppler shift or time shift information is color-coded and superimposed on the two-dimensional gray-scale real-time anatomic display. Color is used primarily to indicate direction of flow. However, it is also an indicator of the speed of flow and, sometimes, of the flow disturbance or turbulence (spectral broadening). The colors red, blue, yellow (red + green), cyan (blue + green), and white are used; for example, red indicates a positive shift (flow toward the transducer), whereas blue indicates a negative shift (away from the transducer). The beam is automatically scanned electronically using an array, as in real-time imaging (see Section 3.3). When shifted echoes are received, the shift is stored in corresponding memory locations. The combined color and gray-scale image is derived from the stored shifted and nonshifted echoes, which represent flow and anatomy, respectively. Imaging frame rates are decreased because of the added time required to acquire the Doppler information. Typically, 7 to 20 pulses along a scan line are required to determine Doppler shift. In gray-scale anatomic imaging, only one pulse is required per scan line (unless multiple transmit focuses are used, in which case each additional focus requires another pulse).

Because there is no way a Doppler spectrum from an FFT (which requires a two-dimensional display) can be shown at each of many pixel locations on the display, an autocorrelation technique is commonly used.[8,18] Each echo is correlated with the corresponding one from the previous pulse, thus determining the motion that has occurred during each pulse. The autocorrelation yields the sign, the mean, and spread (variance) around the mean Doppler shift. Thus, it is possible to present on the display real-time, color-coded, two-dimensional information on flow direction, speed, and character. The CF display does not provide all of the details of the Doppler spectrum that a spectral display does.

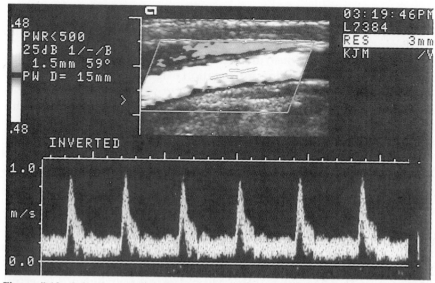

Figure 5.10. Color-flow display of a common carotid artery, including a color-coded pulsed-Doppler spectrum. Colors are assigned to the spectrum according to Doppler shift amplitudes. (See Plate II.) (Reproduced from Kremkau, F.W.: Doppler principles. Sem. Roentg. *27*:6–16, 1992, with permission.)

However, the spectral display can only provide this information from one sample volume, whereas the CF display provides limited information (direction, mean, and variance) from hundreds of locations in the anatomic cross section (Fig. 5.10; also Plate II).

Because only flow direction, mean speed, and sometimes, an indication of variance are presented, the Doppler information is quite restricted compared with the conventional spectral display. However, two-dimensional CF instruments are useful in identifying regions of

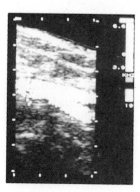

Figure 5.11. Superficial femoral artery and profunda branch flow are shown in color; a wedge was used to avoid 90-degree Doppler angle. (See Plate II.)

abnormal flow at which the gate of a PW instrument can be located for further analysis.

Peripheral vascular work with CF instruments using linear arrays would often result in no color because the ultrasound pulses would be directed at the flow at close to a 90-degree Doppler angle. To avoid this and to allow detection of Doppler shifts and, therefore, presentation of color information, the Doppler angle is reduced from 90 degrees by two

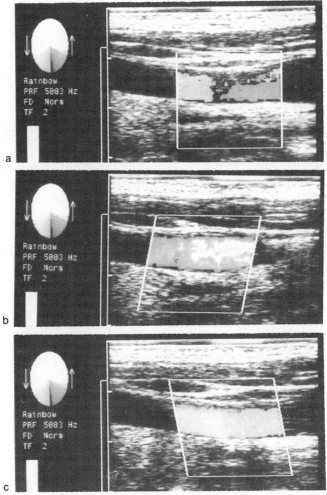

Figure 5.12. Color scan lines are directed (*a*) vertically, (*b*) to the left of vertical, and (*c*) to the right of vertical. Flow is from left to right, producing positive and negative Doppler shifts depending on the relationship between scan lines and flow. (See Plate III.) (Reproduced from Kremkau, F.W.: Doppler principles. Sem. Roentg. 27:6–16, 1992, with permission.)

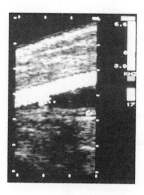

Figure 5.13. The profunda branch off the femoral artery appears to have no flow (no color within it) because of the 90-degree Doppler angle between the scan lines and the flow. Compare this with Figure 5.11, in which the wedge has been reversed. (See Plate II.)

methods; standoff wedge and phase-steered beams (Figs. 5.11, also Plate II, and 5.12, also Plate III). If the wedge were not used in Figure 5.11, the upper vessel (superficial femoral artery) would probably not contain color because it would be parallel to the transducer face, resulting in a 90-degree Doppler angle. Indeed, the profunda branch in Figure 5.13 (also Plate II) contains no color and might be thought to be occluded. However, Figure 5.11 shows that, with the wedge reversed (thereby eliminating the perpendicularity), color fills the profunda, confirming that it is patent. In CF instruments as in all color instruments, 90-degree Doppler angles must be avoided to detect flow. Figure 5.12a reveals the difficulty that may be encountered in obtaining color in a vessel whose flow is perpendicular to the scan lines. Angling the scan lines to the left or right of perpendicular yields positive (Fig. 5.12b) and negative (Fig. 5.12c) Doppler shifts in the vessel, respectively (flow is from left to right).

Spectral Doppler presents the entire range of Doppler shift frequencies received as they change over cardiac cycle. Color Doppler displays can only present statistical representations of the complete spectrum at each pixel location on the display. The sign, mean value, and possibly, the variance of the spectrum, are color-coded into the hue, saturation, and luminance presented at each display pixel location. Some instruments provide a readout of the quantitative digital values for mean Doppler shift at chosen pixel locations. It is important to realize that these are mean values that cannot be compared with the peak-systolic values that are commonly used in evaluating spectral displays. In the case of detection of a stenosis in the presence of turbulence, the implication of this is that the turbulence causes increased weighting of lower Doppler shifts, thus reducing the mean Doppler shift. The peak is unchanged in the presence of turbulence, as observed on a spectral display. However, in the CF display, the mean would be reduced in the presence of turbulence.

EXERCISES

5.4.1 Color-flow instruments present two-dimensional color-coded images representing _____ that are superimposed on gray-scale images representing _____.

5.4.2 The following colors are commonly used in color-flow maps.
a. red, blue
b. yellow, cyan
c. white
d. magenta, green
e. a, b, and c
f. all of the above

5.4.3 Non-Doppler color-flow instruments detect echo arrival _____ shifts to determine flow speeds.

5.4.4 Doppler color-flow instruments commonly use an _____ technique to yield _____ flow speed in real-time.

5.4.5 The autocorrelation technique yields
a. mean Doppler shift
b. sign of Doppler shift
c. spread around the mean (variance)
d. all of the above
e. none of the above

5.4.6 In color-flow instruments, color is used only to represent flow direction. True or false?

5.4.7 Approximately _____ pulses are required to obtain one line of color-flow information.
a. 1
b. 10
c. 100
d. 1000
e. 1,000,000

5.4.8 There are approximately _____ samples per line on a color-flow display.
a. 2
b. 20
c. 200
d. 2000
e. 2,000,000

5.4.9 Color-flow displays are not dependent on the Doppler angle. True or false?

5.4.10 If two colors are shown in the same vessel using a color-flow instrument, it always means flow is occurring in opposite directions in the vessel. True or false?

5.5
Review

Flow in vessels depends on pressure difference and resistance. Viscosity, vessel length, and vessel diameter contribute to resistance. Flow types include steady, pulsatile, plug, laminar (parabolic), disturbed, and turbulent. The Doppler effect is a change in frequency resulting from reflector or scatterer motion toward or away from the ultrasound source. Doppler instruments make use of this frequency shift to yield information regarding motion and flow. CW systems provide motion and flow information without depth information or selection capability. Pulsed Doppler systems provide depth information and the ability to select the depth at which Doppler information is generated. Spectral analysis provides information on the distribution of received frequencies resulting from the distribution of scatterer velocities (speeds and directions) encountered. In addition to audible output, imaging of vessel flow spectra is accomplished in Doppler systems. Combined systems utilizing dynamic B-scan imaging and CW and PW Doppler technology are available commercially. CF systems provide displays of two-dimensional, real-time flow superimposed on gray-scale anatomic scans.

Definitions of the terms used in this chapter are listed below:

Autocorrelation. A rapid technique (used in color-flow instruments) for obtaining mean Doppler shift frequency.

Bidirectional. Indicates Doppler instruments that are capable of distinguishing between positive and negative Doppler shifts (forward and reverse flow).

Color flow. The presentation of two-dimensional, real-time Doppler or time-shift information superimposed on a real-time, gray-scale anatomic cross-sectional image. Flow directions toward and away from the transducer (i.e., positive and negative Doppler or time shifts) are presented as different colors on the display.

Cos. Abbreviation for cosine.

Cosine. The cosine of angle A in Figure 5.4 is the length of side b divided by the length of side c.

Disturbed flow. Flow that cannot be described by straight, parallel stream lines.

Doppler angle. The angle between the sound beam and flow direction.

Doppler effect. Frequency change of a reflected sound wave as a result of reflector motion relative to the transducer.

Doppler shift. Reflected frequency minus incident frequency.

Duplex. Combination of B-mode imaging and PW Doppler technology.

Fast Fourier transform. Rapid digital implentation of Fourier transform.

Fluid. A material that flows and conforms to the shape of its container; a gas or a liquid.

FFT. Fast Fourier transform.

Fourier transform. A mathematical technique for obtaining a Doppler frequency spectrum.

Frequency spectrum. The range of frequencies present. In a Doppler instrument, the range of Doppler shift frequencies present in the returning echoes.

Generator gate. The electronic portion of a pulsed Doppler system that converts the continuous voltage of the voltage generator to a pulsed voltage.

Laminar flow. Flow in which fluid layers slide over each other to produce a parabolic flow speed profile.

Parabolic flow. Laminar flow.

Plug flow. Flow with all fluid portions traveling with nearly the same flow speed and direction.

Pulsatile flow. Flow that accelerates and decelerates with each cardiac cycle.

Receiver gate. A device that allows only echoes from a selected depth (arrival time) to pass.

Sample volume. Region of tissue from which pulsed Doppler echoes are accepted.

Spectral analysis. Use of fast Fourier transform to determine Doppler shift frequency range several times each second.

Spectral broadening. The widening of the Doppler shift spectrum; that is, the increase of the range of Doppler shift frequencies present as a result of a broader range of flow velocities encountered by the sound beam. This occurs for normal flow in smaller vessels and for turbulent flow in any vessel.

Turbulence. Random, chaotic, multidirectional flow of a fluid.

Turbulent flow. See turbulence.

Variance. Spread around a mean value.

Viscosity. Resistance of a fluid to flow.

EXERCISES

5.5.1 Doppler systems convert _____ _____ information to audible sound and visual display.

5.5.2 Pulses similar to those used in gray-scale imaging systems are used in Doppler systems. True or false?

5.5.3 Continuous-wave Doppler system transducers require _____ elements.

5.5.4 The receiver in a Doppler system compares the _____ of the voltage generator and the voltage from the receiving transducer.

5.5.5 The Doppler shift usually is not in the audible frequency range and must be converted by the receiver to a frequency that can be heard. True or false?

5.5.6 Doppler shift is determined by reflector _____ and by the _____ of an angle.

5.5.7 A component that pulsed Doppler systems have but continuous-wave Doppler systems do not have is the _____.

5.5.8 A Doppler system may have as an output a visual _____.

5.5.9 In a pulsed Doppler system, the pulse repetition frequency is determined by the generator _____, and the source ultrasound frequency is determined by the _____ _____.

5.5.10 Pulsed Doppler systems can give motion information for a specific _____.

5.5.11 Spectral analysis is accomplished by _____ _____ transform analysis.

5.5.12 The sound received by the transducer in a Doppler instrument is in the audible frequency range. True or false?

5.5.13 Frequencies used in Doppler ultrasound are in approximately the same range as those for pulse-echo imaging. True or false?

5.5.14 If the incident frequency is 4 MHz, the reflector speed is 100 cm/s, and the angle between beam and motion directions is 60 degrees, the Doppler shift is _____ kHz.

5.5.15 Color-flow instruments use

   a. continuous-wave Doppler

   b. pulsed Doppler

   c. compressed Doppler

d. all of the above

e. none of the above

5.5.16 The _____ effect is used to detect and measure blood ____ in vessels.

5.5.17 Motion of an echo-generating structure causes an echo to have a different _____ than the emitted pulse.

5.5.18 Why are multiple transmit focus and color Doppler flow imaging normally not combined?

a. the two are incompatible

b. resolution is not important in color-flow imaging

c. the Doppler shifts interfere with the phased arrays

d. frame rate too low

e. all of the above

CHAPTER 6

Artifacts

In imaging, an artifact is anything that is not properly indicative of the structures or flow imaged. It is caused by some characteristic of the imaging technique. Because some artifacts are useful (e.g., shadowing and enhancement), imaging can, at times, reveal more than direct viewing of the anatomy (if it were possible). This is because some ultrasound imaging artifacts, though considered to be errors from an anatomic imaging standpoint, provide valuable information on the nature of objects or lesions that might not be apparent with other imaging methods or even with direct viewing. In addition to helpful artifacts, there are several that hinder proper interpretation and diagnosis. These must be avoided or properly handled when encountered.

Artifacts in sonography occur as structures that are either:

1. not real
2. missing
3. improperly located
4. of improper brightness, shape, or size

Some artifacts are produced by improper equipment operation or settings (e.g., incorrect receiver gain and compensation settings). Others are inherent in the pulse-echo ultrasound imaging method and can occur even with proper equipment and technique.

Artifacts that occur in sonography[22,23] are listed in Table 6.1, where they are grouped as they are considered in the next two sections.

The assumptions in the design of ultrasound imaging instruments are that sound travels in straight lines, that echoes originate only from objects located on the beam axis, that the amplitude or intensity of returning echoes is directly related to the reflecting or scattering properties of distant objects, and that the distance to reflecting or scattering objects is proportional to the round trip travel time (13 μs per cm of depth).

TABLE 6.1
Sonographic Artifacts

Propagation Group	Attenuation Group
Axial resolution	Shadowing
Lateral resolution	Enhancement
Section thickness	Refraction (edge) shadowing
Speckle	Focal enhancement
Reverberation	
Refraction	
Multipath	
Mirror image	
Side lobe	
Grating lobe	
Comet tail	
Ring-down	
Speed error	
Range ambiguity	

Several artifacts may be encountered in Doppler ultrasound, including incorrect presentations of Doppler-flow information, either in spectral or color-flow (CF) form. The most common of these is aliasing. Others do occur, however, including range ambiguity, spectrum mirror image, location mirror image, and speckle.

In this chapter, the following questions are considered: What causes ultrasound images to appear incorrectly? How can specific artifacts be recognized? How can they be handled properly to avoid the pitfalls and misdiagnoses that they can cause? The following terms are discussed in this chapter:

aliasing	range ambiguity
comet-tail	refraction
enhancement	reverberation
grating lobes	section thickness
mirror image	shadowing
multipath	side lobes
multiple reflections	speckle
Nyquist limit	speed error

6.1
Propagation

Axial and lateral resolution limitations are artifactual because a failure to resolve means a loss of detail, and two adjacent structures may be visualized as one. Detail resolution is discussed in Section 3.4.

The beam width perpendicular to the scan plane (the third dimension) (Fig. 6.1) results in section-thickness artifacts—for example, the appearance of false debris in echo-free areas (Fig. 6.2a) and the presentation of cystic objects as echogenic (Fig. 6.2, b through e). This is because the interrogating beam has finite thickness as it scans through the patient. Echoes are received that originate not only from the center of the beam but also from off axis. These are all collapsed into a thin two-dimensional image that is composed of echoes that have come from a not-so-thin tissue volume scanned by the beam. Figure 3.31b shows an anechoic vessel lumen resulting from a thin section thickness from an annular array (see Section 3.3).

Apparent image resolution can be deceiving. This is sometimes not directly related to the scattering properties of tissue (texture), but is a result of interference effects of the scattered sound from the distribution of scatterers in the tissue. This phenomenon is called acoustic speckle (see Section 2.4) (Fig. 6.3).

Multiple reflections (reverberations) can occur between the transducer and a strong reflector. These may be sufficiently strong to be detected by the instrument and to cause confusion on the display. The process by which they are produced is shown in Figure 6.4a. This results in the display of reflectors that are not real (Fig. 6.4, b and c). The

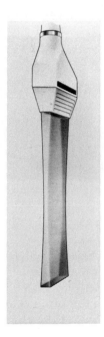

Figure 6.1. The scan "plane" through the tissue is really a three dimensional volume. Two dimensions (axial and lateral) are in the scan plane, but there is a third dimension (called section thickness, z-axis, or elevational axis). The third dimension is collapsed to zero thickness when the image is displayed in two-dimensional format.

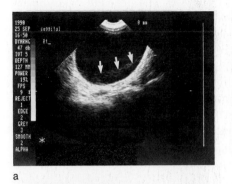

a

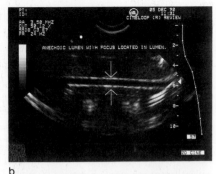

b

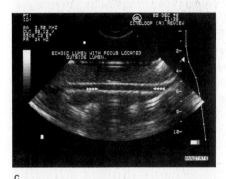

c

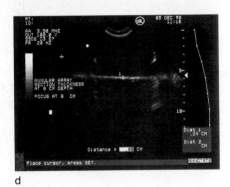

d

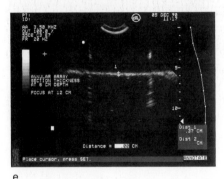

e

Figure 6.2. (*a*). An ovarian cyst that should be echo-free has an echogenic region (arrows). These off-axis echoes are a result of scan plane section thickness. Using an annular array, the section-thickness focus can be located (*b*) at the position of a vessel (correctly appearing anechoic) or away from the vessel (*c*), causing it to contain off-axis echoes because of the increased section thickness. Using a section-thickness test object (see Section 7.1), section thickness is seen to increase from 2.4 mm to 3.7 mm as the section-thickness focus is moved from the reflector location (*d*) to well beyond it (*e*). (Parts *b*, *c*, *d*, and *e* reprinted from J. Diag. Med. Sonography, 7:85–90, 1991, with permission.)

multiple reflections are placed beneath the real reflector at separation intervals equal to the separation between the transducer and the real reflector. Each subsequent reflection is weaker than prior ones, but this diminution is at least partially counteracted by the compensation function of the receiver.

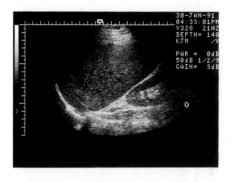

Figure 6.3. The typically grainy appearance of ultrasound images is not primarily the result of detail resolution limitations, but rather of speckle, which is the interference pattern resulting from constructive and destructive interference of echoes returning simultaneously from many scatterers within the propagating ultrasound pulse at any particular time.

Refraction (see Section 2.4) can cause a reflector to be positioned improperly (laterally) on the display (Fig. 6.5). This is likely to occur, for example, when the transducer is placed on the abdominal midline (Figs. 6.5c and 6.6). Beneath are the rectus abdominis muscles, which are surrounded by fat. These tissues represent a refracting boundary because of their different propagation speeds.

The term multipath describes a situation in which the paths to and from a reflector are different (Fig. 6.7). Multipath results in improper positioning of the reflector image (increased range). Because multiple reflections are involved, these echoes are quite weak and probably "muddy" the image somewhat. Like speckle, this contributes to acoustic noise in the image (see Fig. 6.3).

The mirror image artifact presents structures that are on one side of a strong reflector on the other side as well (Fig. 6.8). This commonly occurs around the diaphragm and pleura because of the total reflection from air-filled lung. Sometimes, the mirrored structure is not in the unmirrored scan plane (Fig. 6.8c).

Side lobes (see Section 3.2) are beams that propagate from a single-element transducer in directions different from the primary beam. Grating lobes (see Section 3.3) are extra beams emitted from an array transducer (Fig. 6.9). Side and grating lobes are weaker than the primary beam and do not normally produce echoes that are imaged, particularly if they fall on a normally echogenic region of the scan. However, if these lobes encounter a strong reflector (e.g., bone or gas), their echoes may well be imaged, particularly if they fall within an anechoic region. If so, they will appear in incorrect locations (Figs. 6.10 and 6.11).

An artifact that has been termed a comet tail is shown in Figure 6.12. It is a series of closely spaced, discrete echoes (i.e., a particular form of reverberation). Figure 6.13 appears to be similar, but is fundamentally different from this type of artifact. Discrete echoes cannot be identified because a continuous emission of sound from the origin may be occur-

Text continued on page 230

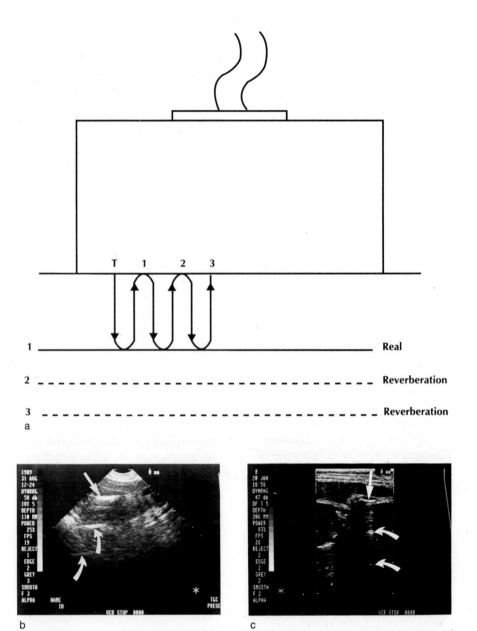

Figure 6.4. (*a*) A pulse (*T*) is transmitted from the transducer. A strong echo is generated at the real reflector and is received (*1*) at the transducer, allowing correct imaging of the reflector. However, the echo is partially reflected by the transducer so that a second echo (*2*) is received, as well as a third (*3*). These later echoes appear deeper on the display, where there are no reflectors. (*b*) A chorionic villi sampling catheter (*straight arrow*) and two reverberations (*curved arrows*). (*c*) A fetal scapula (*straight arrow*) and two reverberations (*curved arrows*).

226

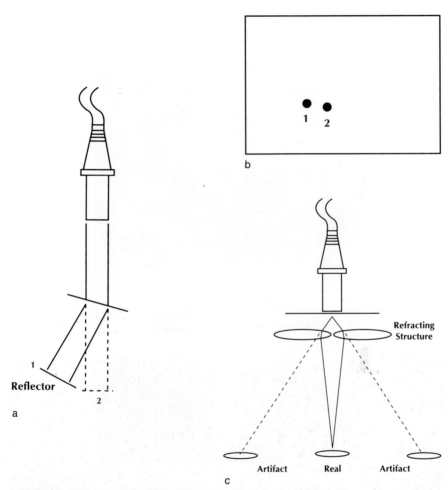

Figure 6.5. Refraction (*a*) results in improper positioning of the reflector on the display (*b*). The system thinks the reflector is at position 2 because that is the direction from which the echo was received when, in fact, the reflector is actually at position 1. (*c*) One real structure is imaged as two artifactual objects because of the refracting structure close to the transducer. If unrefracted pulses can propagate to the real structure, a triple presentation (one correct, two artifactual) can result.

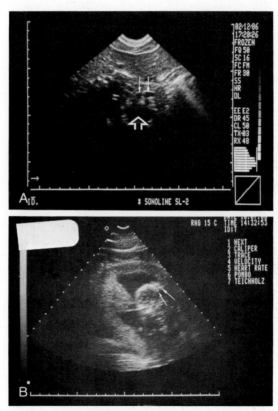

Figure 6.6. (*a*) Refraction (probably through the rectus abdominis muscle) has widened the aorta (*open arrow*) and produced a double image of the celiac trunk (*arrows*). (*b*) Refraction has produced a double image of a fetal skull (*arrows*).

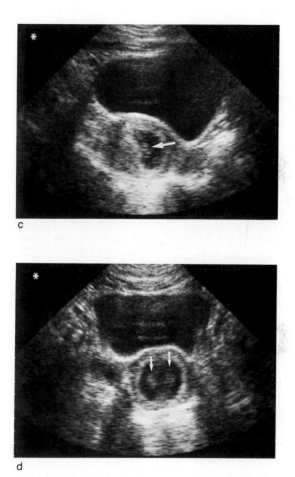

Figure 6.6 *Continued.* Refraction may also cause a single gestation (*c*) to appear as a double gestational sac (*d*).

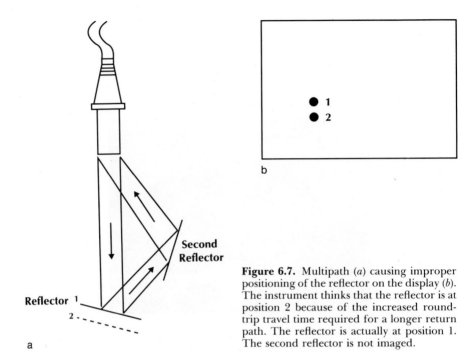

Figure 6.7. Multipath (*a*) causing improper positioning of the reflector on the display (*b*). The instrument thinks that the reflector is at position 2 because of the increased round-trip travel time required for a longer return path. The reflector is actually at position 1. The second reflector is not imaged.

ring. The mechanism for such a continuous effect (termed ring-down artifact) is not well understood, but it may be caused by a resonance phenomenon associated with gas bubbles.

Propagation speed error occurs when the assumed value for propagation speed (1.54 mm/μs leading to the 13 μs/cm rule) is incorrect. If the propagation speed that exists over a path traveled is greater than 1.54 mm/μs, the calculated distance to the reflector is too small, and the display will place the reflector too close to the transducer (Fig. 6.14). This is because the higher speed causes the echoes to arrive sooner. If the actual speed is less than 1.54 mm/μs, the reflector will be displayed too far from the transducer (Fig. 6.15). Refraction and propagation speed error can also cause a structure to be displayed with incorrect shape.

In two-dimensional gray-scale and M-mode imaging, it is assumed that, for each pulse, all echoes are received before the next pulse is emitted. If this were not the case, ambiguity could result (Figs. 6.16 and 6.17). The maximum depth imaged unambiguously by an instrument is determined by its pulse repetition frequency (PRF) (discussed in Sec-

Text continued on page 238

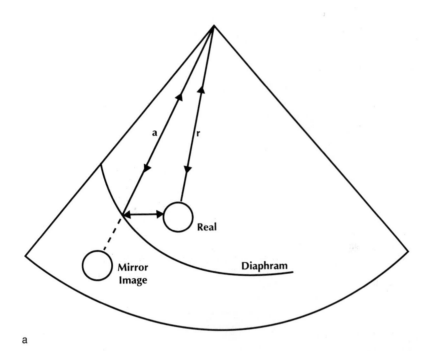

a

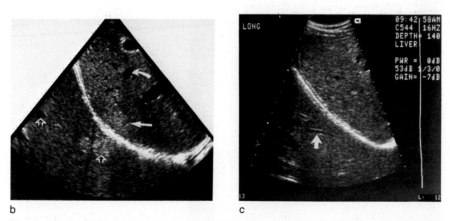

b   c

Figure 6.8. (*a*) When pulses encounter a (real) structure directly (scan line *r*), the structure is imaged correctly. If the pulse first reflects off the diaphragm (also the returning echo) (scan line *a*), the structure is imaged on the other side of the diaphragm. (*b*) A hemangioma (*straight arrow*) and vessel (*curved arrow*) with their mirror images (*open arrows*). (*c*) A vessel is mirror-imaged (*arrow*) superior to the diaphragm, but does not appear inferior because it is outside the unmirrored scan plane.

Illustration continued on following page

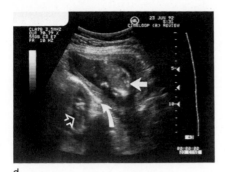

d

Figure 6.8 *Continued.* (*d*) A fetus (*straight arrow*) also appears as a mirror image (*open arrow*). The mirror (*curved arrow*) is probably echogenic muscle.

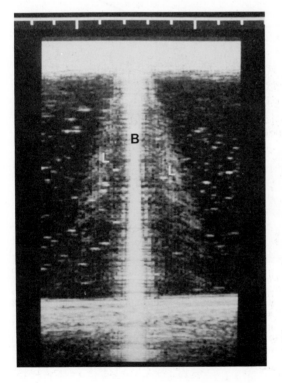

Figure 6.9. Primary beam (*B*) and grating lobes (*L*) from a linear-array transducer.

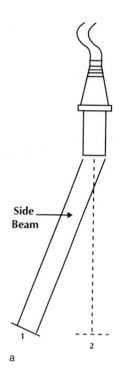

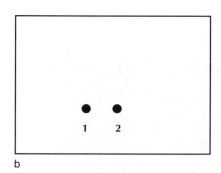

Figure 6.10. (*a*) A side lobe or grating lobe can produce and receive a reflection from a "side view." (*b*) This will be placed on the display at the proper distance from the transducer but in the wrong location (direction). This is because the instrument assumes that echoes originate from points along the main beam axis. The instrument thinks that the reflector is at position 2 because that is the direction in which the main beam travels. The reflector is actually in position 1.

Figure 6.11. Side and grating lobes in obstetrical scans can produce the appearance of amniotic sheets or bands. (*a*) A real amniotic sheet (*arrow*). (*b*) and (*c*) Grating lobe (*open arrow*) duplication of fetal bones (*curved arrow*) appearing like amniotic bands or sheets.

Illustration continued on following page

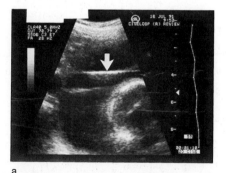

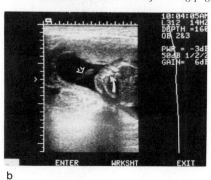

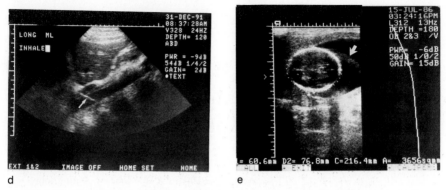

d   e

Figure 6.11 *Continued.* (*d*) Artifactual grating lobe echoes (*arrow*) cross the aorta. (*e*) Grating lobe (*arrow*) duplication of a fetal skull.

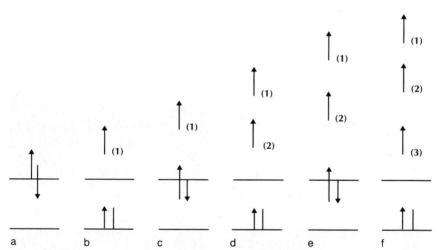

a   b   c   d   e   f

Figure 6.12. The generation of comet tail (closely spaced reverberations). Action progresses in time from left to right. (*a*) An ultrasound pulse encounters the first reflector and is partially reflected and partially transmitted. (*b*) Reflection and transmission at the first reflector are complete. Reflection at the second reflector is occurring. (*c*) Reflection at the second reflector is complete. Partial transmission and partial reflection are again occurring at the first reflector. (*d*) The echoes from the first (*1*) and second (2) reflectors are traveling toward the transducer. A second reflection (repeat of *b*) is occurring at the second reflector. (*e*) Partial transmission and reflection are again occurring at the first reflector. (*f*) Three echoes are now returning: the echo from the first reflector (*1*); the echo from the second reflector (*2*); and the echo from the second reflector (*3*), reflected from the back side of the first reflector (*c*) and reflected again from the second reflector (*d*). A fourth echo is being generated at the second reflector (*f*).

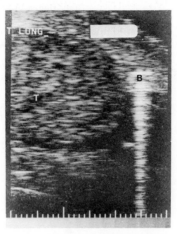

g

Figure 6.12 *Continued.* (*g*) Comet tail from an air rifle BB shot pellet (*B*) adjacent to the testicle (*T*). The front and rear surface of the BB are the two reflecting surfaces involved in this example. (Part *g* from Kremkau, F.W., and Taylor, K.J.: Artifacts in ultrasound imaging. J. Ultrasound Med., 5:227, 1986. Reprinted with permission.)

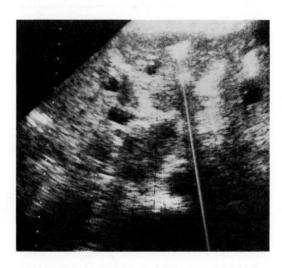

Figure 6.13. Ring-down from air in the bile duct. (From Kremkau, F.W., and Taylor, K.J.: Artifacts in ultrasound imaging. J. Ultrasound Med., 5:227, 1986. Reprinted with permission.)

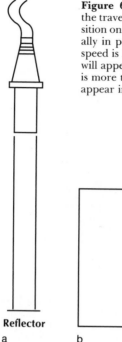

Reflector

a   b

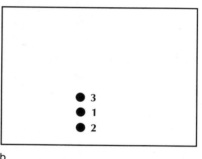

Figure 6.14. The propagation speed over the traveled path (*a*) determines reflector position on the display (*b*). The reflector is actually in position 1. If the actual propagation speed is less than that assumed, the reflector will appear in position 2. If the actual speed is more than that assumed, the reflector will appear in position 3.

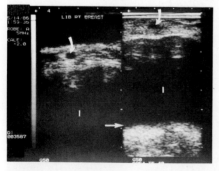

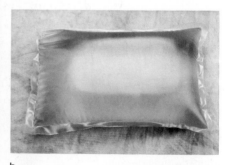

a   b

Figure 6.15. (*a*) The low propagation speed in a silicone breast implant (*I*) causes the chest wall (*straight arrow*) to appear deeper than it should. Note that a cyst (*curved arrow*) is shown more clearly on the left image than on the right. That is because a gel standoff pad (*b*) has been placed between the transducer and the breast, moving the beam focus closer to the cyst.

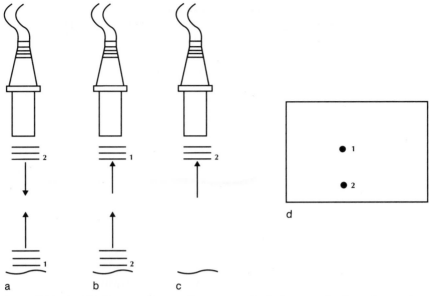

Figure 6.16. Ambiguity caused by sending out a pulse before an echo from the previous pulse is received. (*a*) A pulse (*2*) is sent out just as a previous pulse (*1*) is reflected. (*b*) The first echo arrives at the transducer when the second pulse reflects. (*c*) The second echo arrives at the transducer. (*d*) The spot (*1*) in the center of the display resulting from the arrival of the earlier pulse indicates a reflector at a location where there is none. The spot below (*2*) is in the correct reflector location.

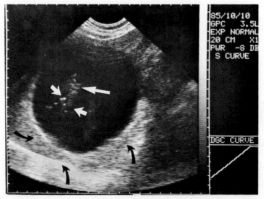

Figure 6.17. A large renal cyst (having a diameter of about 10 cm) has artifactual range-ambiguity echoes within it (*white arrows*). These came from structure(s) below the display. These deep echoes arrived after the next pulse was emitted, so they were thought to have arrived earlier and were placed closer to the transducer than they should have been. Echoes arrived from much deeper (later) than usual in this case because the sound passed through the long, low-attenuation paths in the cyst. These echoes may have come from bone or a far body wall. Low attenuation in the cyst is indicated by the strong echoes (enhancement) below it (*curved black arrows*).

tions 2.2 and 4.4). To avoid range ambiguity, PRF is automatically reduced in deeper imaging situations. This usually causes a reduction in frame rate.

6.2
Attenuation

Shadowing is the reduction in echo amplitude from reflectors that lie behind a strongly reflecting or attenuating structure, such as a bone (Fig. 6.18) or a stone (Fig. 6.19). Enhancement is the increase in echo amplitude from reflectors that lie behind a weakly attenuating structure (see Figs. 6.17, 6.18, and 6.19). Shadowing and enhancement result in reflectors being placed on the image with amplitudes that are too low and too high, respectively. Brightening of echoes can also be attributable to the increased intensity in the focal region of a beam. This is called focal enhancement or focal banding (Fig. 6.20). Shadowing can also occur behind the edges of objects that are not necessarily strong or weak attenuators (Figs. 6.21). In this case, the cause may be the defocusing action of a refracting curved surface (Fig. 6.22). Alternatively, it may be attributable to destructive interference caused by sound passing through different speeds and getting out of phase. Either cause decreases the intensity of the beam beyond the surface, causing echoes to be weakened. Shadowing and enhancement are often useful artifacts for determining the nature of masses.[22,23]

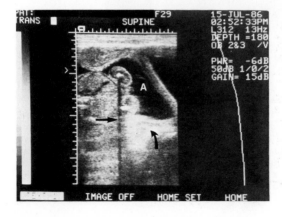

Figure 6.18. Shadowing (*straight arrow*) from a fetal limb bone and enhancement (*curved arrow*) caused by the low attenuation of amniotic fluid (*A*) through which the ultrasound travels.

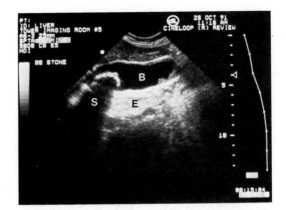

Figure 6.19. Shadowing (*S*) from a gallstone and enhancement (*E*) caused by the low attenuation of bile (*B*).

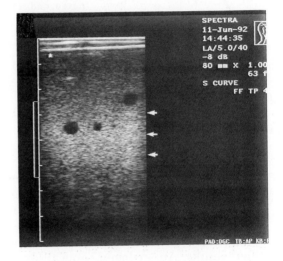

Figure 6.20. Focal banding (*arrows*) is the brightening of echoes around the focus where intensity is increased by the narrowing of the beam.

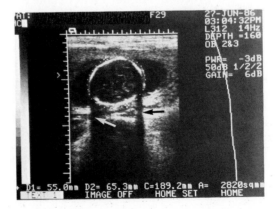

Figure 6.21. Edge shadows (*arrows*) from a fetal skull.

239

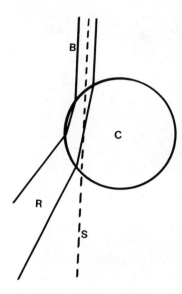

Figure 6.22. As a sound beam (*B*) enters a circular region (*C*) of higher propagation speed, it is refracted, and refraction occurs again as it leaves. This causes spreading of the beam with decreased intensity. The echoes from region *R* are presented deep to the circular region in the neighborhood of the dashed line. They are weak owing to the beam spread, thus giving the shadow in the region *S*.

6.3
Spectral Doppler

Aliasing is the most common artifact encountered in Doppler ultrasound. There is an upper limit to Doppler shift that can be detected by pulsed instruments. If the Doppler shift frequency exceeds one half the PRF (normally in the 5- to 30-kHz range), aliasing occurs (Fig. 6.23).[1] Improper Doppler shift information (improper direction and improper value) results. An analogous optical form of aliasing occurs in motion pictures when wagon wheels appear to rotate at various speeds and in reverse direction. Higher PRFs (Table 6.2) permit higher Doppler shifts to be detected, but also increase the likelihood of range-ambiguity artifact (discussed in Section 6.1 and later in this section). Continuous-wave (CW) Doppler instruments do not have this limitation (but neither do they provide depth selectivity).

Aliasing is a result of the sampling character of pulsed-wave (PW) instruments. Because they use pulses of ultrasound, they acquire portions of the Doppler shift that is to be detected. These samples must be connected together to yield the resulting Doppler shift frequency. In any sampling system, if sampling occurs often enough, the correct result will be found. If sampling does not occur often enough (under sampling), an incorrect result will be obtained (Fig. 6.24). For a single-frequency, sinusoidal wave, there must be at least two samples per cycle to

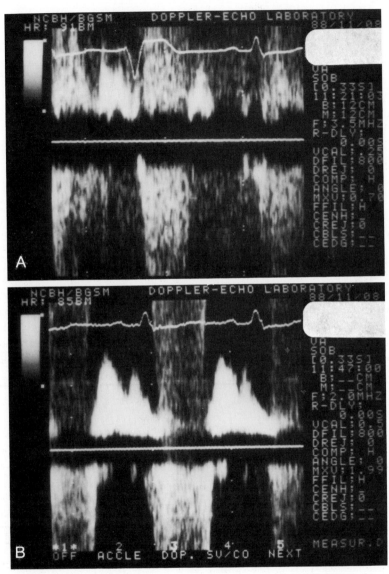

Figure 6.23. Two examples of aliasing in Doppler echocardiography.

avoid aliasing. For a complex signal containing many frequencies, the sampling frequency must be at least double the highest frequency present to avoid aliasing. Stated in another way, the highest Doppler shift frequency encountered in the signal must not exceed one half of the PRF of the PW instrument (this is called the Nyquist limit fre-

TABLE 6.2
Aliasing and Range-Ambiguity
Artifact Values

Pulse Repetition Frequency (kHz)	Doppler Shift Above Which Aliasing Occurs (kHz)	Range Beyond Which Ambiguity Occurs (cm)
2.5	1.2	30
5.0	2.5	15
7.5	3.7	10
10.0	5.0	7
12.5	6.2	6
15.0	7.5	5
17.5	8.7	4
20.0	10.0	3
25.0	12.5	3
30.0	15.0	2

quency). If it does, aliasing will result. When aliasing occurs, incorrect flow information is presented (Fig. 6.25). Generally, peak flow information appears incorrectly on the opposite side of the baseline (i.e., a high positive flow appears as a negative flow). There are several approaches to avoiding this problem, including increasing PRF, increasing Doppler

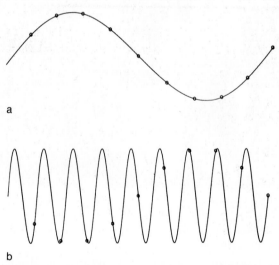

a

b

Figure 6.24. Doppler shift signal sampled at 10 points (*open circles*). (*a*) One cycle. (*b*) Nine cycles. As signal frequency is increased, aliasing occurs when the Nyquist limit is exceeded. It can be seen that connection of the open circles with a smooth curve in (*b*) would yield a 1-cycle representation of what is actually a 9-cycle Doppler shift.

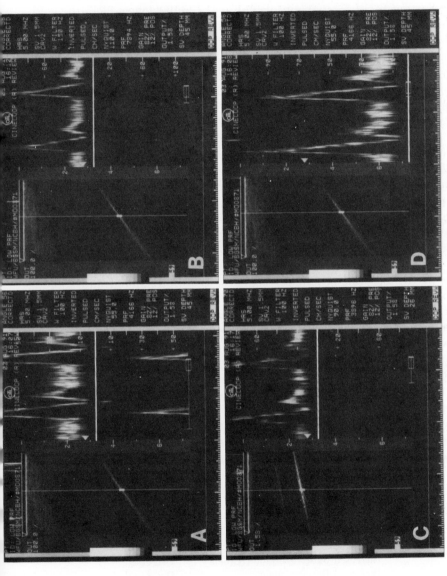

Figure 6.25. A moving string test object (see Section 7.1) simulating a common carotid artery spectrum. (*a*) Aliasing is occurring because peak systolic flow exceeds the Nyquist limit (55 cm/s). (*b*) Increasing the pulse repetition frequency (and therefore the Nyquist limit) removes the aliasing. (*c*) Increasing the Doppler angle reduces the Doppler shift so that it does not exceed the Nyquist limit and there is no aliasing. (*d*) Baseline shifting scrolls the aliased portions below the baseline to their proper position in peak systole. (Reproduced from Kremkau, F.W.: Doppler principles. Sem. Roentg. 27:6–16, 1992, with permission.)

angle, baseline shifting, lowering transducer frequency, and switching to CW techniques. The first three of these are illustrated in Figure 6.25. Increasing the PRF increases the likelihood of range-ambiguity artifact (see Section 6.1).[1] Deeper sample volumes require lower PRFs to avoid range ambiguity and, therefore, are associated with an increased likelihood of aliasing for higher flow rates. Baseline shifting, essentially a cosmetic rearrangement of information on the display (electronic cutting and pasting), moves the aliased information back to its proper place. However, when this is done, legitimate Doppler information in the region of the display that has been rearranged appears in an incorrect location. Table 6.3 summarizes various influences on aliasing.

The mirror image artifact described in Section 6.1 can also occur with Doppler systems. This means that an image of a vessel and a source of Doppler-shifted echoes can be duplicated on the opposite side of a strong reflector (such as bone). The duplicated vessel containing flow could, therefore, be misinterpreted as an additional vessel. It would have a spectrum similar to that for the real vessel. Figure 6.26 shows an example of image and spectrum duplication of the subclavian artery. The strong reflector in this case is the pleura.

A mirror image of a Doppler spectrum can appear on the opposite side of the baseline when, in fact, flow is unidirectional and should appear on only one side of the baseline. This is an electronic duplication of the spectral information. It can occur when receiver gain is set too high (causing overloading in the receiver and cross talk between the two flow channels). It can also occur when the Doppler angle is near 90 degrees (Fig. 6.27). In this case, the duplication is usually legitimate. This is because beams are focused and not cylindrical in shape. Thus, portions of the beam can experience approaching flow, whereas other portions can experience receding flow.

Doppler spectra have a speckle quality to them that is similar to that observed in sonography. Speckle (see Section 6.1) is a result of interference effects of scattered sound from the distribution of scatterers (eryth-

TABLE 6.3
Aliasing Influences

Influence	Aliasing
Increased pulse repetition frequency	Decreased
Increased Doppler angle	Decreased
Proper baseline shift	Decreased
Decreased transducer frequency	Decreased
Switch to continuous wave	Eliminated
Increased sample volume depth	Increased

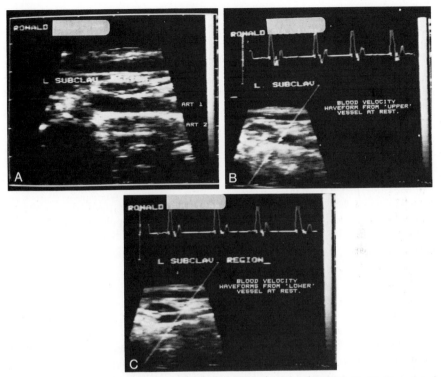

Figure 6.26. (*a*) Subclavian artery (*ART 1*) and its mirror image (*ART 2*). (*b*) Flow signal from the artery. (*c*) Flow signal from the mirror image.

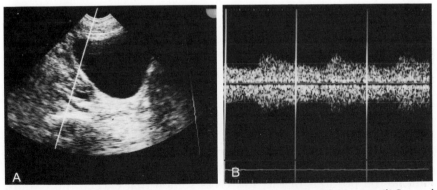

Figure 6.27. (*a*) The Doppler angle is nearly 90 degrees at the ovarian artery. (*b*) Spectral mirror image with low-impedance flow on both sides of the baseline.

Illustration continued on following page

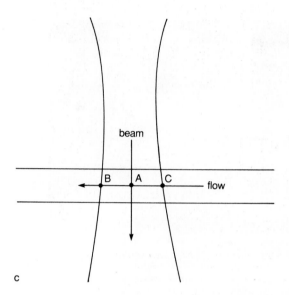

Figure 6.27 *Continued.* (*c*) Because beams are focused and not cylindrical in shape, portions of the beam (*C*) can experience flow toward, while other portions (*B*) can experience flow away, when the beam axis intersects (*A*) the flow at 90 degrees. (Parts *a* and *b* from Taylor K.J.W., and Holland S.: Doppler ultrasound. I. Basic principles, instrumentation and pitfalls. Radiology, *174*:297–307, 1990; reprinted with permission.)

rocytes) in the blood. Because the ultrasound pulse encounters several scatterers at any point in its travel, several echoes are generated simultaneously. These may arrive at the transducer in such a way that they reinforce (constructive interference) or partially or totally cancel (destructive interference) each other. This results in a displayed dot pattern that does not directly represent individual scatterers, but instead represents an interference pattern of the scatterer distribution scanned. This phenomenon is called acoustic speckle. It is analogous to the speckle phenomenon observed when a laser is shone on a wall.

6.4
Color-Flow Imaging

The aliasing artifact appears in color-flow displays as a region of different color (apparent opposite flow) wherein the Doppler shift exceeds half the PRF (Nyquist limit). The maximum Doppler shift on the color map (the nyquist limit) is set at the lowest value that generally does not produce aliasing (although aliasing is not always "bad") so that slower flows will not go undetected. Aliasing can be used as a quantitative tool to indicate the portions of the flow cross section that exceed the Nyquist limit. It can easily be distinguished from true flow reversal, as shown in Figure 6.28 (also Plate IV). An aliased color change must pass through

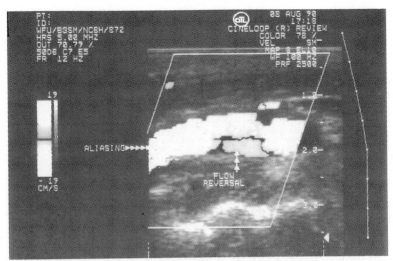

Figure 6.28. Color-flow presentation of common carotid artery flow, including flow reversal and aliasing. The two can be distinguished because the boundary between the different directions with flow reversal passes through the baseline (*black*), whereas the aliasing boundary passes through the upper and lower extremes of the color bar (*white*). In this particular color bar assignment, the maximum positive Doppler shifts are assigned the color green so that there is a thin green region showing the exact boundary where aliasing occurs. The aliasing occurs in the distal portion of the vessel because it is curving down, reducing the Doppler angle between the flow and the scan lines. (See Plate IV.) (Reproduced from Kremkau, F.W.: Doppler principles. Sem. Roentg. 27:6–16, 1992, with permission.)

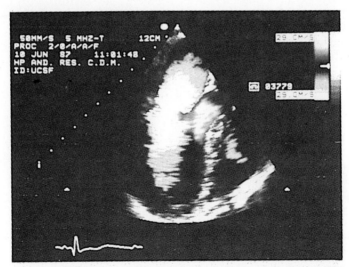

Figure 6.29. Transesophageal cardiac color-flow image of the long axis in diastole. The blue colors between the left atrium and left ventricle represent blood traveling away from the transducer. However, because of high flow speeds through the mitral valve, aliasing has occurred and the yellow and orange colors have replaced the blue colors. (See Plate IV.)

247

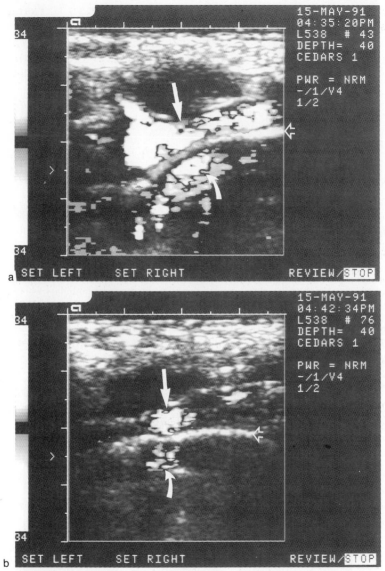

Figure 6.30. Color-flow imaging of the subclavian artery (*straight arrow*) in longitudinal (*a*) and cross-sectional (*b*) views. The pleura (*open arrow*) causes the mirror image (*curved arrow*). (See Plate V.)

the extremes of the color map, whereas true flow reversal passes through the zero baseline and black wall filter region of the color map. Thus, the region between the two different colors with flow reversal is black, whereas with aliasing, it is bright, with the colors assigned at the color map extremes. Figure 6.29 (also Plate IV) shows an example of aliasing in the heart.

Range ambiguity in color-flow Doppler, as in sonography, places echoes (color Doppler shifts in this case) that have come from deep locations (after a subsequent pulse was emitted) in shallow locations where they do not belong.

Other artifacts discussed in Sections 6.1 and 6.2 occur with color-flow imaging also. These include speckle, refraction, mirror image (Fig. 6.30, also Plate V), grating lobe,[19] and shadowing.[19] Color-flow information will often not be acquired at Doppler angles close to 90 degrees (see Fig. 5.13, also Plate II).

6.5
Review

Axial resolution is determined by spatial pulse length, whereas lateral resolution is determined by beam width. The beam width perpendicular to the scan plane causes section-thickness artifacts. Apparent resolution close to the transducer is not directly related to tissue texture, but is a result of interference effects from a distribution of scatterers in the tissue (speckle). Reverberation produces a set of equally spaced artifactual echoes distal to the real reflector. Refraction displaces echoes laterally. In a mirror-image artifact, objects that are present on one side of a strong reflector are displayed on the other side as well. Shadowing is caused by high-attenuation objects in the sound path. Enhancement results from low-attenuation objects in the sound path. Propagation speed error and refraction can cause objects to be displayed in improper locations or incorrect sizes, or both. Refraction can also cause edge shadowing.

Artifacts that can occur with Doppler ultrasound include aliasing, range ambiguity, color-flow image and Doppler signal mirroring, and spectral trace mirroring. Aliasing is the most common artifact. It occurs when the Doppler shift frequency exceeds one half the PRF. It can be reduced or eliminated by increasing the PRF or Doppler angle, using baseline shift, reducing operating frequency, or using a CW instrument.

In this chapter, several ultrasound imaging and Doppler-flow artifacts have been discussed, all of which are listed in Table 6.4 along with their causes. In some cases, artifact names are identical to their causes. Some artifacts are useful in interpretation and diagnosis (e.g., shadowing and enhancement), whereas some can cause confusion and error (e.g., aliasing and reverberation). A proper understanding of artifacts

TABLE 6.4
Artifacts and Their Causes

Artifact	Cause
Axial resolution	Pulse length
Lateral resolution	Pulse width
Section thickness	Pulse width
Speckle	Interference
Reverberation	Multiple reflection
Refraction	Refraction
Multipath	Multiple reflection
Mirror image	Multiple reflection
Side lobe	Side lobe
Grating lobe	Grating lobe
Comet tail	Reverberation
Ring down	Resonance
Speed error	Speed error
Range ambiguity	High pulse repetition frequency
Shadowing	High attenuation
Enhancement	Low attenuation
Edge shadowing	Refraction or interference
Focal enhancement	Focusing
Aliasing	Low pulse repetition frequency
Spectrum mirror	High Doppler gain

and how to deal with them when encountered enables sonographers and sonologists to use them in diagnosis while avoiding the pitfalls that they can cause.

The definitions of terms discussed in this chapter are as follows:

Aliasing. Improper Doppler shift information from a pulsed Doppler or color-flow instrument when true Doppler shift exceeds one half the pulse repetition frequency.

Comet tail. A series of closely spaced reverberation echoes.

Enhancement. Increase in echo amplitude from reflectors that lie behind a weakly attenuating structure.

Grating lobes. Additional minor beams of sound traveling out in directions different from the primary beam. These result from the multielement structure of transducer arrays.

Mirror image. An artifactual gray-scale, color-flow, or Doppler signal appearing on the opposite side (from the real structure or flow) of a strong reflector.

Multipath. Paths to and from a reflector that are not the same.

Multiple reflections. Several reflections produced by a pulse encountering a pair of reflectors.

Nyquist limit. The Doppler-shift frequency above which aliasing occurs; one half the pulse repetition frequency.

Range ambiguity. Echoes placed too close to the transducer because a second pulse was emitted before they were received.

Refraction. Change of sound direction occurring when sound passes from one medium to another.

Reverberation. Multiple reflections.

Section thickness. Thickness of the scanned tissue volume perpendicular to the scan plane.

Shadowing. Reduction in echo amplitude from reflectors that lie behind a strongly reflecting or attenuating structure.

Side lobes. Minor beams of sound traveling out from a single-element transducer in directions different from the primary beam.

Speckle. The granular appearance of images caused by the interference of echoes from the distribution of scatterers in tissue.

Speed error. Propagation speed that is different than its assumed value (1.54 mm/μs).

EXERCISES

6.1 The maximum pulse repetition frequency that will unambiguously image to a maximum depth of 15 cm is _____ kHz.

6.2 The maximum depth for unambiguous imaging with an instrument having a pulse repetition frequency of 1 kHz is _____ cm.

6.3 If the propagation speed in a soft tissue path is 1.60 mm/μs, a diagnostic instrument assumes a propagation speed too _____ and will show reflectors too _____ the transducer.
   a. high, close to
   b. high, far from
   c. low, close to
   d. low, far from

6.4 Multipath can occur with only one reflector. True or false?

6.5 The most common artifact encountered in Doppler ultrasound is
   a. aliasing
   b. range ambiguity

    c. spectrum mirror image

    d. location mirror image

    e. electromagnetic interference

6.6 Which of the following can reduce or eliminate aliasing?

    a. increased pulse repetition frequency

    b. increased Doppler angle

    c. increased operating frequency

    d. use of continuous-wave mode

    e. more than one of the above

6.7 The fine texture in the region near the transducer indicates the extremely excellent resolution that actually exists in that region. True or false?

6.8 The fact that a beam, as it scans through tissue, has some finite width results in the _____ artifact.

6.9 Which of the following can cause improper location of objects on a display? (More than one correct answer)

    a. shadowing

    b. enhancement

    c. speed error

    d. mirror image

    e. refraction

    f. side lobe

6.10 Refraction can cause shadowing. True or false?

6.11 The transducer face is one of the reflectors involved in reverberations in which illustration—Fig. 6.4*b* or 6.12*g*?

6.12 Match these artifact causes with their result:

    a. reverberation: _____

    b. shadowing: _____, _____

    c. enhancement: _____

    d. propagation speed error:

    _____, _____

    e. refraction: _____, _____

    f. multipath: _____

    1. unreal structure displayed

    2. structure missing on the display

    3. structure displayed with improper brightness

    4. improperly positioned structure

    5. improperly shaped structure

    6. structure of improper size

6.13 Reverberation results in added reflectors being imaged with equal _____.

6.14 In reverberation, subsequent reflections are _____ than previous ones.

6.15 Enhancement is caused by a
    a. strongly reflecting structure
    b. weakly attenuating structure
    c. strongly attenuating structure
    d. refracting boundary
    e. propagation speed error
6.16 Which of the following can decrease or eliminate aliasing?
    a. decreased pulse repetition frequency
    b. decreased Doppler angle
    c. increased operating frequency
    d. baseline shifting
    e. more than one of the above
6.17 Shadowing results in decreased echo amplitudes. True or false?
6.18 Propagation speed error results in improper _____ position of a reflector on the display.
    a. lateral
    b. axial
6.19 To avoid aliasing, a signal voltage must be sampled at least _____ times per cycle.
    a. 1
    b. 2
    c. 3
    d. 4
    e. 5
6.20 If the highest Doppler shift frequency present in a signal exceeds _____ the pulse repetition frequency, aliasing will occur.
    a. one tenth
    b. one half
    c. 2 times
    d. 5 times
    e. 10 times
6.21 When receiver gain is set too high, which artifact is likely to occur?
    a. aliasing
    b. range ambiguity
    c. spectrum mirror image
    d. location mirror image
    e. speckle
6.22 Which artifact should be suspected if one observes twin gestational sacs when scanning through the rectus abdominis muscle?
6.23 Range ambiguity can occur in which of the following?
    a. imaging instruments

    b. duplex instruments

    c. pulsed Doppler instruments

    d. color-flow instruments

    e. all of the above

6.24 If the pulse repetition frequency is 4 kHz, which of the following Doppler shifts will cause aliasing?

    a. 1 kHz

    b. 2 kHz

    c. 3 kHz

    d. 4 kHz

    e. more than one of the above

6.25 If the pulse repetition frequency is 10 kHz, which of the following Doppler shifts will cause aliasing?

    a. 1 kHz

    b. 2 kHz

    c. 3 kHz

    d. 4 kHz

    e. none of the above

6.26 There is no problem with aliasing as long as the Doppler shifts are _____ half the pulse repetition frequency.

    a. less than

    b. equal to

    c. greater than

    d. all of the above

    e. none of the above

6.27 If Doppler shift is 2.6 kHz, there is no problem with aliasing with a pulse repetition frequency of 10 kHz. True or false?

6.28 If there were a problem in Exercise 6.27, _____ Doppler ultrasound could be used to avoid it.

6.29 If red represents a positive Doppler shift and blue represents a negative one, what color would be seen for normal flow toward the transducer? What color would be seen for aliasing flow toward the transducer? What colors would be seen for normal flow away and for aliasing flow away?

CHAPTER 7

Performance and Safety

Several devices are used to determine whether diagnostic ultrasound imaging instruments are operating correctly and consistently. These devices are considered in two groups: (1) those that test the operation of the instrument (imaging performance) and (2) those that measure the acoustic output of the instrument. Group 1 takes into account the operation of all the components shown in Figure 4.1. Group 2 considers the pulser and the transducer acting as a source. Imaging performance is important for evaluating the instrument as a diagnostic tool. The acoustic output of an instrument is important when considering bioeffects and safety, which are also topics presented in this chapter.

Bioeffects are useful in therapeutic applications of ultrasound, a subject not considered in this book. Of concern is what the bioeffects of ultrasound tell us about the safety or risk of diagnostic ultrasound. We desire knowledge of the probability of damage or injury and under what conditions this probability is maximized (to avoid those conditions) and minimized (to seek those conditions).

In this chapter, we consider the following questions: How do we determine whether or not an imaging or Doppler instrument is working properly? What devices are available for testing various performance characteristics of instruments? What is the difference between a test object and a phantom? How is instrument output measured? What are typical instrument output values? Are there any known risks in the use of imaging or Doppler ultrasound? How can an operator of an ultrasound instrument minimize exposure of the patient to ultrasound? The following terms are discussed in this chapter:

cavitation

dynamic range

hydrophone

phantom

polyvinylidene fluoride (PVDF)

sensitivity

test object

7.1
Performance Measurements

Imaging performance[24–26] is determined by measuring primarily the following parameters, which have been discussed in previous chapters:

1. detail resolution
2. contrast resolution
3. penetration and dynamic range
4. compensation (swept gain) operation
5. range (depth or distance) accuracy

Several devices are available commercially for testing imaging performance. These fall into two categories: tissue-equivalent or tissue-mimicking phantoms and test objects. Tissue-equivalent phantoms have some characteristics representative of tissues (such as scattering and attenuation properties); test objects do not. Some devices are combinations of the two (e.g., tissue-equivalent phantoms containing resolution targets). Phantoms and test objects can be used not only by service personnel, but also by instrument operators.

Tissue-equivalent phantoms are made of graphite-filled aqueous gels or urethane rubber materials. The graphite particles act as the ultrasound scatterers (echo producers) in the materials (graphite is the soft carbon that is used in pencils and as a lubricant). Attenuation in these materials is typically 0.5 to 0.7 dB/cm-MHz, and propagation speed is 1.54 mm/μs in the gels and 1.45 mm/μs in the rubber. The latter speed error is compensated for by physically shifting targets in the rubber material to closer locations. Tissue-equivalent phantoms typically contain echo-free (cystic) regions of various diameters and thin nylon lines (about 0.2 mm in diameter) for measuring detail resolution and distance accuracy. Some contain cones or cylinders containing material of various scattering strengths (various graphite concentrations) that are hyperechoic or hypoechoic compared to the surrounding material. Examples of several phantoms are given in Figures 7.1–7.6.

Test objects do not simulate tissue characteristics, but do provide some specific measure of instrument performance. The beam-profile slice-thickness test object (Fig. 7.7) contains a thin scattering layer in an echo-free (anechoic) material. It can be used to show beam width either in the scan plane or perpendicular to the scan plane (section thickness).

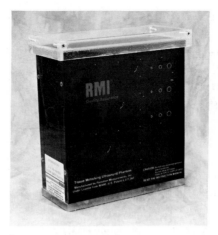

a

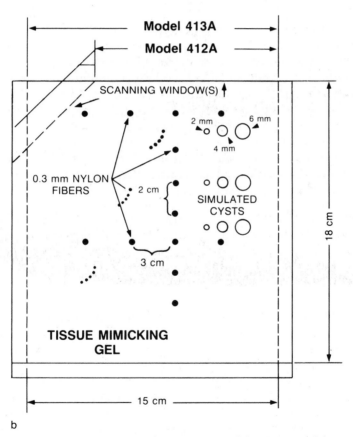

b

Figure 7.1. (*a*) A tissue-equivalent phantom (RMI Model 413A) containing groups of nylon lines and cystic regions of various sizes. (*b*) Diagram detailing the construction of such a phantom.

Illustration continued on following page

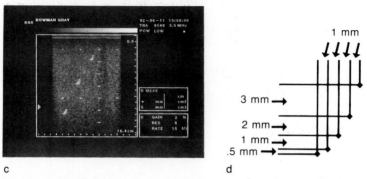

c   d

Figure 7.1 *Continued.* (*c*) Scan of phantom. (*d*) Arrangement of the axial resolution line set in this phantom and in that pictured in Figure 7.2.

The particle image resolution test object (PIRTO) (Fig. 7.8) is filled with small polystyrene spheres that are randomly distributed in a low-attenuation, low-scatter gel. These spheres scatter the ultrasound independently. Their smeared appearance is an indication of detail resolution throughout the image. The speckle pattern (see Sections 2.4 and 6.1) generated by graphite dispersions masks the detail resolution in phantoms, giving the appearance of better resolution than is actually achieved. Nylon lines are added to provide an indication of detail resolution. The polystyrene sphere dispersion in a PIRTO provides detail resolution throughout the image, rather than at localized spots where lines are positioned.

In addition to test objects and phantoms designed for anatomic imaging performance evaluation, devices are also available for Doppler system evaluation. These are of two types: (1) string test objects (Fig. 7.9) and (2) flow phantoms (Fig. 7.10, also Plate VI). The string test object is useful in checking the accuracy of calculated flow speeds on spectral displays. However, the Doppler-shifted echoes are stronger than those encountered with blood, and there is no flow profile. Flow phantoms provide a more physiological model of flow in a tissue-equivalent environment. However, flow profiles and speeds are not accurately known, and bubbles are often a problem in these phantoms. Thus, each type of test device has its strengths and weaknesses. The two together provide a good approach to flow evaluation. There is presently no generally accepted method for measuring Doppler sensitivity.

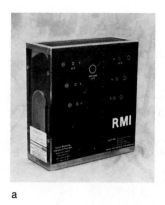

a

Model 415

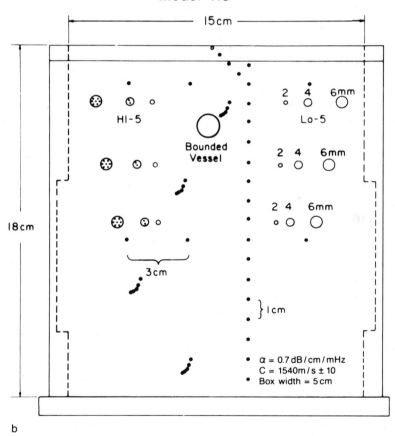

b

Figure 7.2. (*a*) A tissue-equivalent phantom (RMI Model 415) containing nylon lines, simulated cysts, a cystic region with an echogenic rim (simulated bounded vessel) and hyperechoic simulated lesions of various sizes. (*b*) Diagram detailing the construction of such a phantom.

Illustration continued on following page

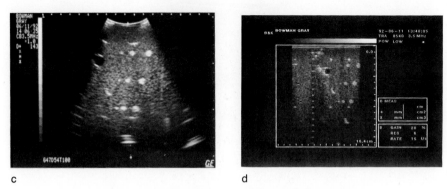

c   d

Figure 7.2 *Continued. (c* and *d)* Scans of phantom.

7.2
Output Measurements

Several devices can measure the acoustic output of ultrasound imaging instruments. They are normally used by engineers and physicists, rather than the instrument operators. Only one, the hydrophone, will be discussed here. It is sometimes called a microprobe. The hydrophone is used in two forms (Fig. 7.11): (1) a small transducer element (1 mm in diameter or less) mounted on the end of a hollow needle, or (2) a large piezoelectric membrane with small metallic electrodes on both sides. The membrane is made of polyvinylidene fluoride (PVDF). PVDF is used in both types of hydrophone because of its wide bandwidth. Various construction approaches are used for hydrophones,[27–30] but these will not be considered here. Hydrophones receive sound reasonably well from all directions without altering the sound by their presence. In response to the varying pressure of the sound, they produce a varying voltage that can be displayed on an oscilloscope. A picture similar to that in Figure 2.15c is produced, from which period, pulse repetition period, and pulse duration can be determined. From these quantities, frequency, pulse repetition frequency, and duty factor can be calculated. Using the hydrophone calibration (relationship between voltage produced and pressure applied), pressure amplitude may also be determined. Wavelength, spatial pulse length, and intensities can also be calculated. Figure 7.12 shows an array hydrophone system.

Using hydrophones and other devices with careful techniques, acoustic output levels (pressures, powers, and intensities) have been measured for various diagnostic ultrasound instruments and transducers.[31–36] Figure 7.13 and Table 7.1 provide summaries of the data from

Text continued on page 271

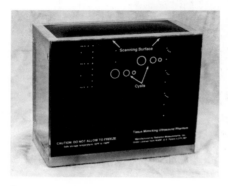

a

Model 414B

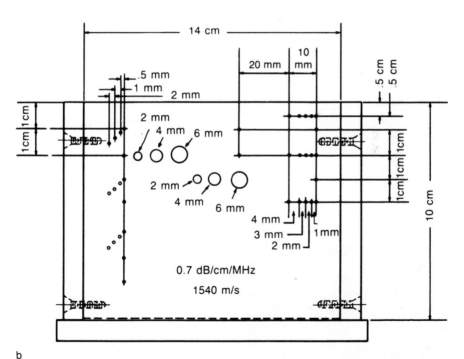

b

Figure 7.3. (*a*) A smaller phantom for higher-frequency "small parts" applications (RMI Model 414B). (*b*) Diagram detailing the construction of such a phantom.

Illustration continued on following page

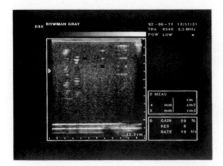

c

Figure 7.3 *Continued.* (*c*) Scan of phantom.

Sector Scan Phantom

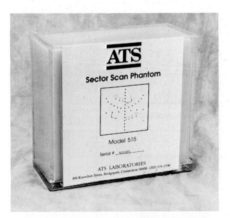

a

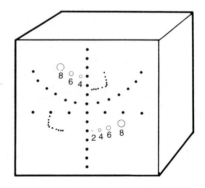

Model 515

b

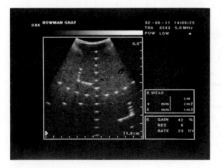

c

Figure 7.4. (*a*) A phantom designed for sector scan applications (ATS Model 515). (*b*) Diagram detailing the construction of such a phantom. (*c*) Scan of phantom.

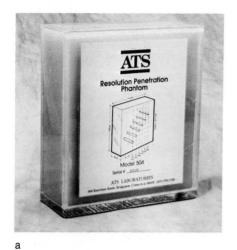

a

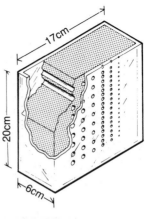

Model 504 & 534

b

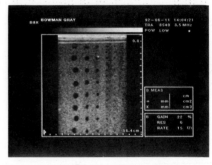

c

Figure 7.5. (*a*) A resolution–penetration phantom that contains columns of simulated cysts of various sizes (ATS Model 504). (*b*) Diagram detailing the construction of such a phantom. (*c*) Scan of phantom.

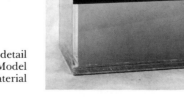

a

Figure 7.6. (*a*) A contrast–detail phantom (Nuclear Associates Model 84-319) containing cones of material of various echogenicities.
Illustration continued on following page

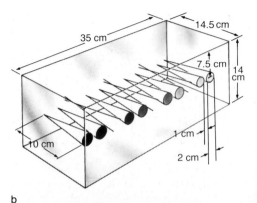

Figure 7.6 *Continued.* (*b*) Diagram detailing the construction of such a phantom. (*c*) Scan of hyperechoic sections of phantom. (*d*) Scan of hypoechoic sections of phantom.

b

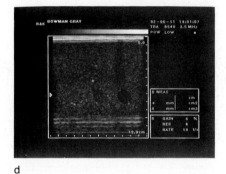

c

d

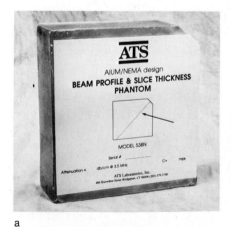

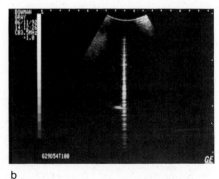

a

b

Figure 7.7. (*a*) A beam-profile and section-thickness test object (ATS Model 538N). It contains a thin scattering layer (*arrow*) in an anechoic material. (*b* and *c*) Scans of beam profiles. Figures 6.2*d* and 6.2*e* show section-thickness images for an annular array using this test object.

Illustration continued on following page

264

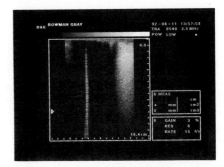

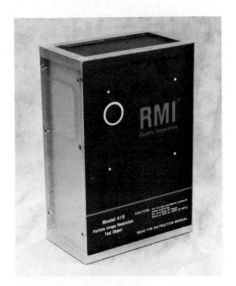

Figure 7.7 *Continued*

c

Figure 7.8. (*a*) A particle image resolution test object (PIRTO) (RMI Model 419). (*b* and *c*) Scans of PIRTO.

a

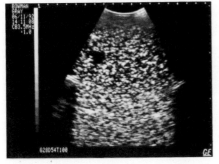

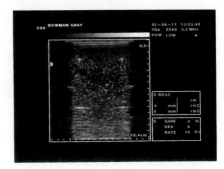

b

c

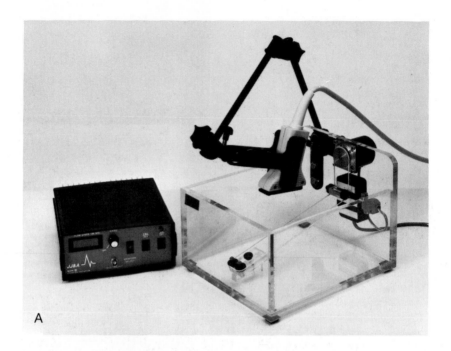

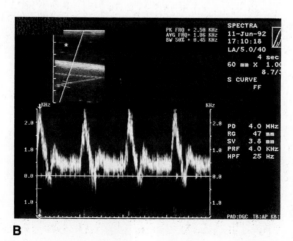

Figure 7.9. (*a*) Moving string test object and controller (JJ&A Mark 4). (*b*) Spectral display of moving string operating in pulsatile mode.

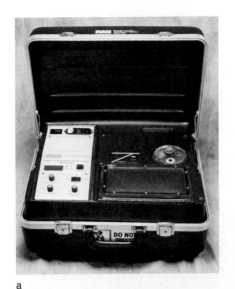

a

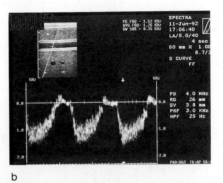

b

c

Figure 7.10. (*a*) Doppler flow phantom (RMI Model 425). (*b*) Spectral display from flow phantom. (*c*) Color-flow image from flow phantom. (See Plate VI.)

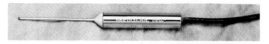

a

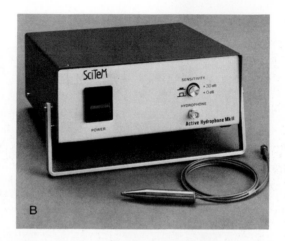

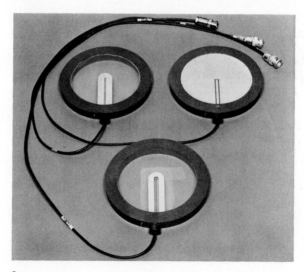

c

Figure 7.11. A hydrophone consists of a small transducer element mounted on the end of a needle (*a* and *b*) or a thin membrane with metal electrodes (*c*). (Part *c* reproduced by permission of Crown Copyright—The National Physical Laboratory, United Kingdom.)

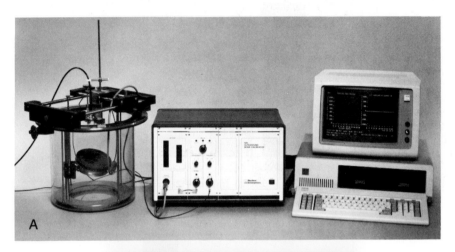

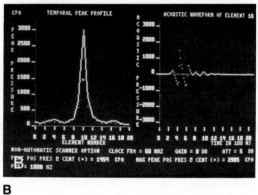

Figure 7.12. Linear array membrane hydrophone system (*a*) for measuring pulse waveform and bandwidth (*b*).

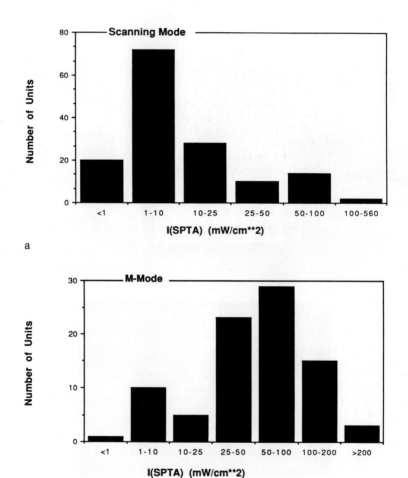

Figure 7.13. Histograms showing the spatial peak–temporal average (SPTA) intensities reported by manufacturers participating in the American Institute of Ultrasound in Medicine commendation process[32,33] for (*a*) imaging mode, (*b*) M-mode, and (*c*) pulsed Doppler. (Reprinted with permission from Ide, M., Zagzebski, J.A., and Duck, F.A.: Acoustic output of diagnostic equipment. Ultrasound Med. Biol. *15*(Suppl. 1): 47–65. Copyright 1989, Pergamon Press, Ltd.)

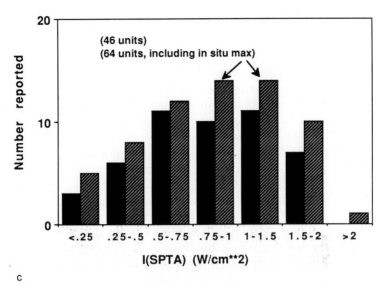

c

Figure 7.13 *Continued*

several sources. Generally, anatomic imaging outputs are lowest and pulsed spectral Doppler outputs are highest, with M-mode and color-flow imaging outputs falling between the two. These data will be compared with bioeffects data in Section 7.4.

TABLE 7.1
Spatial Peak–Temporal Average (SPTA) Output Intensities

Type of Instrument	SPTA Output Intensity (mW/cm²)
All Instruments	0.01–2500
Imaging Instruments	0.01–680
Scanning	0.01–440
Linear array	0.01–48
Phased array	0.1–85
Mechanical	0.1–440
Stopped	0.5–680
Linear array	3.8–332
Phased array	10.1–240
Mechanical	1.6–680
Static	0.5–200
Doppler Instruments	0.6–2500
Continuous wave (CW) obstetrics	0.6–80
CW cardiac/PV (peripheral vascular)	20–2500
Pulsed	40–1945

7.3
Bioeffects

The biological effects and safety of diagnostic ultrasound have received considerable attention during the past few years. Several review articles, textbooks, and institutional documents have been published on this subject.[35-44] In this section, we review current knowledge regarding bioeffects in cells, plants, and experimental animals, as well as the mechanisms of interaction between ultrasound and biological cells and tissues. Regulatory activities, epidemiology, risk and safety considerations, and elements of prudent practice are discussed in Section 7.4.

As with any diagnostic test, there may be some risk (some probability of damage or injury) with the use of diagnostic ultrasound. This risk, if known, must be weighed against the test's benefit to determine the appropriateness of the diagnostic procedure. Knowledge of how to minimize the risk (even if it is unidentified) is useful to everyone involved in diagnostic ultrasound. Sources of information utilized in developing a policy regarding the use of diagnostic ultrasound (whether it be an individual, departmental, institutional, national, or world policy) are diagrammed in Figure 7.14. Included are bioeffects data from experimental systems, output data from diagnostic instruments, and knowledge and experience regarding how the diagnostic information obtained is of benefit in patient management. Comparison of the first two components allows an assessment of risk, whereas the combination of the latter two components yields awareness of benefit. It seems reasonable to assume

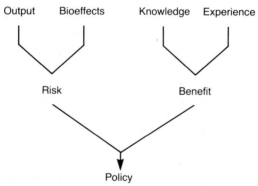

Figure 7.14. Ultrasound risk and benefit information. Risk information comes from experimental bioeffects, epidemiology, and instrument output data. Benefit information comes from knowledge and experience in the use and efficacy of ultrasound imaging. Together, they lead to policy on the prudent use of ultrasound imaging in medicine.

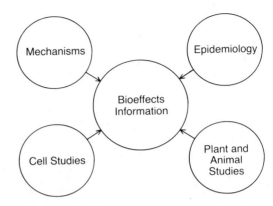

Figure 7.15. Bioeffects information sources.

that there is some risk (however small) in the use of diagnostic ultrasound because ultrasound is a form of energy and has, at least, the potential to produce a biological effect that could constitute risk. Even if this risk is so minimal that it is difficult to identify, prudent practice dictates that routine measures be implemented to minimize the risk while obtaining the necessary information to achieve the benefit.

Our knowledge of bioeffects resulting from ultrasound exposure comes from several sources (Fig. 7.15), including experimental observations in cell suspensions and cultures, plants, and experimental animals; epidemiologic studies with humans; and an understanding of interaction mechanisms, such as heating and cavitation. These categories will be discussed separately in the following sections.

Cells

Several endpoints have been used in studies to evaluate the effects of ultrasound on cells in suspension or in culture. Ultrastructural changes and altered motility patterns in fibroblasts have been reported. These results have not been independently confirmed. Single-strand breaks in the DNA of human leukocytes after exposure to ultrasound have been observed. Various continuous and pulsed exposure frequencies and intensities were used, some involving cavitation and some not. Only one (94 W/cm^2 spatial peak–temporal average [SPTA] at 8 MHz continuous wave [CW]) yielded a significantly increased frequency of breaks which may have resulted from the chemical activity associated with transient cavitation. It appears that, for virtually all bioeffects found in cell suspensions, cavitation is involved.

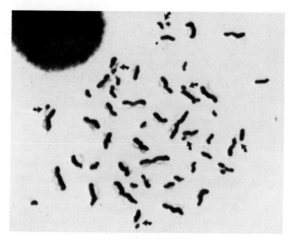

Figure 7.16. Sister-chromatid exchange indicated by arrows. Bromodeoxyuridine (BUdR)-substituted, Giemsa-stained human lymphocyte metaphase. (Reprinted from Kremkau, F. W.: Biologic effects and safety. *In* Rumack, C. M., Wilson, S. R., and Charboneau, J. W. (eds.): Diagnostic Ultrasound. St. Louis, Mosby Year Book, 1991, pp. 19–29, by permission.)

The most extensively studied endpoint with ultrasound exposure of cells is sister chromatid exchange (Fig. 7.16). Over a 10-year period, about two dozen reports have been published on this subject. Most studies have yielded negative results, whereas a few have reported positive results. Of importance is the fact that there is no independent confirmation of a published positive effect. Attempts to do so have lead to the conclusion that the cause of small but statistically significant effects is unknown; however, it seems clear that the ultrasound exposure either does not produce increased exchanges or the effect is not reproducible and is too small to be consistently produced.[35] Even if ultrasound had been shown to produce consistently increased exchanges with all this activity, sister-chromatid exchanges usually have no genetic effect and therefore do not constitute a risk.[35]

Because cells in suspension or in culture are so different from those in the intact patient in a clinical environment, restraint must be exercised in extrapolating clinical significance from *in vitro* results. Cellular studies are useful in determining mechanisms of interaction and in guiding the design of experimental animal studies and epidemiologic studies. The official statement on *in vitro* biological effects published by the American Institute of Ultrasound in Medicine (AIUM)[36] is as follows:

It is difficult to evaluate reports of ultrasonically induced *in vitro* biological effects with respect to their clinical significance. The predominant physical and biological interactions and mechanisms involved in an *in vitro* effect may not pertain to the *in vivo* situation. Nevertheless, an *in vitro* effect must be regarded as a real biological effect. Results from *in vitro* experiments suggest new endpoints and serve as a basis for design of *in vivo* experiments. *In vitro* studies provide the capability to control experimental variables and thus offer a means to explore and evaluate specific mechanisms. Although they may have limited applicability to *in vivo* biological effects, such studies can disclose fundamental intercellular or intracellular interactions. While it is valid for authors to place their results in context and to suggest further relevant investigations, reports of *in vitro* studies which claim direct clinical significance should be viewed with caution.

Plants

The primary components of plant tissues—stems, leaves, and roots—contain gas-filled channels between the cell walls. Plants have thus served as useful biological models for studying the effects of cavitation. Through this mechanism, normal cellular organization and function can be disturbed. Irreversible effects appear to be limited to cell death. Reversible effects include chromosomal abnormalities, reductions in mitotic index, and growth-rate reduction. Membrane damage induced by microstreaming shear stress appears to be the cause of cell death in leaves. Intensity thresholds for lysis of leaf cells are much higher with pulsed ultrasound than they are with CW. Apparently, the response of bubbles within the tissues to CW and pulsed fields is different.

Animals

With experimental animals (mostly mice and rats), reported *in vivo* effects include fetal weight reduction, postpartum fetal mortality, fetal abnormalities, tissue lesions, hind limb paralysis, blood flow stasis, wound repair enhancement, and tumor regression. Recent negative studies include B-cell development, ovulatory response, and teratogenicity, all studied in mice.[35]

Many studies on fetal weight reduction in mice and rats have been performed. All rat and several mouse studies have yielded negative results. A linear dose-effect dependence of exposure condition versus average fetal weight has been reported in which the dose parameter was defined as I^2t, where I is the spatial average exposure intensity and t is the exposure time. This exposure dependence has not been independently confirmed. In one attempt, no effect on fetal weight was found at dose parameter values large enough to produce measurable heating in the fetal and maternal tissues.

Focal lesion production is a well-documented bioeffect reported by at least three laboratories. It has been observed over a wide range of intensity and exposure duration conditions (Fig. 7.17).

The AIUM has summarized the conditions under which mammalian bioeffects have been reported in its statement on conclusions regarding *in vivo* mammalian bioeffects[36]:

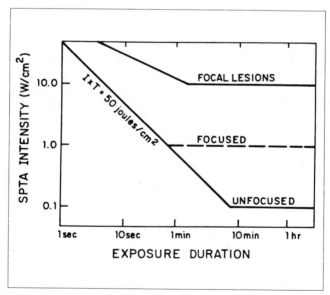

Figure 7.17. Comparison of the minimum spatial peak–temporal average (SPTA) intensities required for ultrasonic bioeffects specified in the *AIUM Statement on Mammalian Bioeffects*. The minimum levels required for focal lesions are also shown on the figure for comparison. Note that logarithmic scaling has been used for the axes of this figure so that the horizontal lines are separated by factors of 10 in intensity. (Reprinted from Bioeffects Committee: Safety Considerations for Diagnostic Ultrasound. Rockville, MD, American Institute of Ultrasound in Medicine, 1991, by permission.)

A review of bioeffects data supports the following statement as an update of the AIUM Statement on *In Vivo* Mammalian Bioeffects: In the low megahertz frequency range there have been (as of this date) no independently confirmed significant biological effects in mammalian tissues exposed *in vivo* to unfocused ultrasound with intensities* below 100 mW/cm, or to focused† ultrasound with intensities below 1 W/cm. Furthermore, for exposure times‡ greater than 1 second and less than 500 seconds (for unfocused ultrasound) or 50 seconds (for focused ultrasound), such effects have not been demonstrated even at higher intensities, when the product of intensity and exposure time is less than 50 joules/cm.

---

* Free-field spatial peak, temporal average (SPTA) for continuous-wave exposures and for pulsed-mode exposures with pulses repeated at a frequency greater than 100 Hz.
† Quarter-power (−6 dB) beam width smaller than four wavelengths or 4 mm, whichever is less at the exposure frequency.
‡ Total time includes off-time as well as on-time for repeated pulse exposures.

A graphic presentation of the statement is given in Figure 7.17. In the latest revision of this statement, the sentence on focused beams was added to indicate their importance and current knowledge relevant to them. The difference between the unfocused and focused levels for bioeffects is consistent with a thermal mechanism whereby, for a given intensity, a more focused beam produces a smaller temperature rise. In summary, no independently confirmed significant biological effects have been observed below 100 mW/cm². For focused beams, the value is 1 W/cm². Focal lesions occur at intensities greater than 10 W/cm². Over this two-decade range of intensities, mammalian bioeffects have been observed for values depending on exposure duration and beam focusing.

Mechanisms

The mechanisms of action by which ultrasound could produce biological effects can be characterized into two groups: heating and mechanical. Attenuation in tissue is primarily attributable to absorption—that is, conversion of ultrasound to heat. Thus, ultrasound produces a temperature rise as it propagates through tissues. The heating produced depends on the applied intensity and frequency of sound (as the absorption coefficient is approximately proportional to frequency) and on the beam focusing and tissue perfusion. Heating increases as intensity or frequency is increased. For a given transducer output intensity, at greater tissue depths, heating is decreased at higher frequencies because of the increased attenuation, which reduces the intensity arriving at depth. Temperature rises of greater than 1°C are considered to be significant.[37] Intensities greater than a few hundred milliwatts per squared centimeter can produce such temperature increases. Absorption coefficients are higher in bone than they are in soft tissues. Bone heating, particularly in the fetus, should, therefore, receive special consideration.

Heating has been shown to be an important consideration in some bioeffects reports. Mathematical models have been developed for calculating temperature rises in tissues.[37–39] These have been used, for example, to calculate the estimated intensities required for a given temperature rise (e.g., 1°C). The AIUM has summarized these calculations in its conclusions regarding a thermal bioeffects mechanism,[37] as follows:

1. A thermal criterion is one reasonable approach to specifying potentially hazardous exposures for diagnostic ultrasound.

2. Based solely on a thermal criterion, a diagnostic exposure that produces a maximum temperature rise of 1°C above normal physiologic levels may be used in clinical examinations without reservation.

3. An *in situ* temperature rise to or above 41°C is considered hazardous in fetal exposures; the longer this temperature elevation is maintained, the greater the likelihood for damage to occur is.

4. Analytic models of ultrasonically induced heating have been applied successfully to *in vivo* mammalian situations. In those clinical situations in which local tissue temperatures are not measured, estimates of temperature elevations can be made by employing such analytic models.

5. Calculations of ultrasonically induced temperature elevation, based on a simplified tissue model and a simplified model of stationary beams, suggest the following: For examinations in soft fetal tissues with typical perfusion rates, employing center frequencies between 2 and 10 MHz and beam widths* less than 11 wavelengths, the computed temperature rise will not be significantly above 1°C if the *in situ* SATA [spatial average–temporal average] intensity† does not exceed 200 mW/cm. If the beam width does not exceed eight wavelengths, the corresponding intensity is 300 mW/cm. However, if the same beam impinges on fetal bone, the local temperature rise may be much higher.

Experimental measurements have been performed that have shown reasonable confirmation of the mathematical calculations. Bone heating has not been found to be significantly greater than that calculated for

---

* Beam width of −6 dB, according to AIUM/National Electrical Manufacturers Association definition.

† SATA = average over focal area.

soft tissues. Biological consequences of hyperthermia include fetal absorption or abortion, growth retardation, microphthalmia, cataract production, abdominal wall defects, renal agenesis, palate defects, brain wave reduction, microencephaly, anencephaly, spinal cord defects, amyoplasia, forefoot hypoplasia, tibial and fibular deformations, and abnormal tooth genesis. There are about 80 known biological effects secondary to hyperthermia. None have occurred at temperatures less than 39°C. Above that, the occurrence of a biological effect depends on temperature and exposure time, as shown in Figure 7.18.

Cavitation is the production and dynamics of bubbles in a liquid medium.[38,40,42] A propagating sound wave is one means by which cavitation can occur. Two types of cavitation are recognized to occur. Stable cavitation is the term used to describe bubbles that oscillate in diameter with the passing pressure variations accompanying the sound wave. Streaming of surrounding liquid can occur in this situation, resulting in shear stresses on suspended cells or intracellular organelles. Cavitation in tissues has been reported to occur with CW high-intensity conditions.

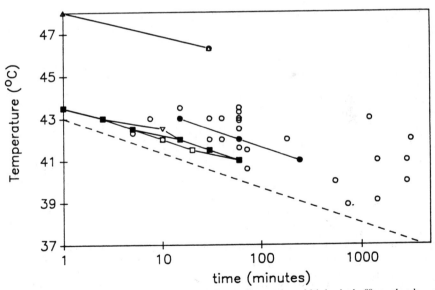

Figure 7.18. Thermal bioeffects. A plot of thermally produced biological effects that have been reported in the literature in which the temperature elevation and exposure durations are provided. Each data point represents either the lowest temperature reported for any duration or the shortest duration for any temperature reported for a given effect. The solid lines represent multiple data points relating to a single effect. The dashed line represents a lower boundary ($t_{43} = 1$) for observed thermally induced biological effects. (Reprinted with permission from Miller, M.W., Ziskin, M.C.: Biological consequences of hyperthermia. Ultrasound Med Biol 15:707–722. Copyright 1989, Pergamon Press, Ltd.)

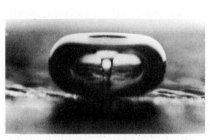

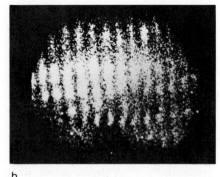

a   b

Figure 7.19. (*a*) Photograph of a liquid jet produced by a collapsing cavitation bubble. The width of the bubble is approximately 1 mm. (*b*) Photograph taken from a TV monitor of an image intensifier system showing light emission from an acoustic standing wave produced in amniotic fluid at 37°C. The vertical bands are separated by approximately 0.75 mm, or half the wavelength for the applied acoustic frequency of 1.0 MHz. The light emission is caused by transient cavitation in the standing wave. (Reprinted from Kremkau, F. W.: Biologic effects and safety. *In* Rumack, C. M., Wilson, S. R., and Charboneau, J. W. (eds.): Diagnostic Ultrasound. St. Louis, Mosby Year Book, 1991, pp. 19–29, by permission.)

Transient (collapse) cavitation occurs when bubble oscillations are so large that the bubble collapses (Fig. 7.19*a*), producing pressure discontinuities (shock waves), localized extremely high temperatures, and light emission in clear liquids (Fig. 7.19*b*). Transient cavitation has the potential for significant destructive effects. It is the means by which laboratory cell disruptors operate. A theory has been developed that predicts that ultrasound could produce transient cavitation under diagnostically relevant conditions in water. Also, a theory has been developed incorporating a range of bubble sizes that yields a predicted dependence of the cavitation threshold on pressure and frequency. Experimental verification of this dependence has been carried out with stabilized microbubbles in water. Thresholds for cavitation in soft tissue and body liquids have not been determined. The AIUM has summarized information on the cavitation mechanism[37] as follows:

1. Acoustic cavitation may occur with short pulses and has the potential for producing deleterious biologic effects.

2. Currently available information indicates that pulses with peak pressures greater than 10 MPa (3300 W/cm) can induce cavitation in mammals.*

---

* Evidence from observations with lithotripters.

3. With the limited data available, it is not possible to specify *threshold* pressure amplitudes at which acoustic cavitation will occur, in mammals, with diagnostically relevant pulse lengths and repetition rates.

7.4
Safety

Information from *in vitro* and *in vivo* experimental studies has yielded no known risks in the use of diagnostic ultrasound. Thermal and mechanical mechanisms have been considered, but do not appear to be operating significantly at diagnostic intensities. Currently, there is no known risk associated with the use of diagnostic ultrasound. Experimental animal data have helped to define the intensity-exposure time region in which bioeffects can occur. However, differences, both physical and biological, between the two situations make it difficult to apply results from one to risk assessment in the other. In the absence of known risk, but recognizing the possibility that bioeffects could be occurring that are subtle, of low incidence, or delayed, a conservative approach to the medical use of ultrasound is recommended. This approach will be described in more detail later in this section.

Instrument Outputs

Intensities cited in Section 7.3 include 100 mW/cm^2 SPTA and 1 W/cm^2 SPTA from the AIUM's statement on *in vivo* mammalian bioeffects, 200 and 300 mW/cm^2 SATA from AIUM's conclusions regarding a thermal bioeffects mechanism, and 3300 W/cm^2 SPTP from the AIUM's conclusions regarding cavitation. We now consider measurements of output intensities from commercial diagnostic instruments (see Section 7.2). Several reports and compilations of output data have been published. Instrument output may be expressed in many ways. Intensity has been the most popular quantity presented to describe instrument output. There are several intensities that may be used. SPTA intensity is used in the AIUM's statement on mammalian bioeffects, and it relates well to a thermal mechanism of interaction. It is also the output intensity that is most commonly presented. Table 7.1 gives a compilation of SPTA intensity ranges from several sources. It can be seen that output intensities have a large range, with the highest being 250,000 times the lowest. Imaging instruments dominate the lower portion of the range, whereas Doppler instruments dominate the higher portion. Within specific classes of instruments, intensity ranges vary by factors as small as 24 (phased-arrays stopped) and as large as 4800 (linear-arrays scanning).

These output intensity measurements are usually made with the use of hydrophones and radiation-force balances located in the beam in a water bath. Attenuation in water is low compared to that in tissues, so that an intensity at a comparable location within tissue would be less than that in water. Models designed to account for the tissue attenuation have been proposed.[38,43] These approaches have yielded the following, somewhat conflicting, conclusions:

1. Total attenuation to the human fetus averages approximately 11 dB at 3.5 MHz.

2. A realistic estimate of the minimum expected attenuation in early pregnancy is, in decibels, one or two times the frequency in megahertz. This seems reasonable for transvaginal imaging also (Fig. 7.20).

The United States Food and Drug Administration (FDA), in its *Guide for Measuring and Reporting Acoustic Output of Diagnostic Ultrasound Medical Devices* and *Diagnostic Ultrasound Guidance Update of 1987* for the "fetal imaging and other" category, list the following as the highest known SPTA intensities emitted from pre-1976 diagnostic ultrasound devices: 94 mW/cm² (calculated *in situ* value) and 180 mW/cm² (water value). There is a 2.8-dB difference between these two values.

To compare instrument output intensities with bioeffects knowledge, (*AIUM Statement on In Vivo Mammalian Bioeffects*), let us assume 7-dB attenuation (see Fig. 7.20). This corresponds to an intensity reduc-

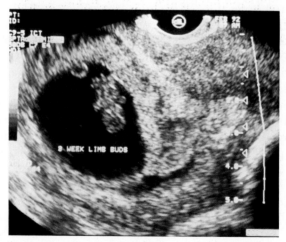

Figure 7.20. A display that includes spatial peak–temporal average (SPTA) intensity (reduced by estimated tissue attenuation) and mechanical index (MI). The tissue attenuation path in this transvaginal scan is about 2 cm and the operating frequency is 7 MHz. Assuming 0.5 dB/cm-MHz attenuation, the beam is attenuated by 7 dB by the time it arrives at the fetus.

TABLE 7.2
Upper Limits of Attenuated* Spatial Peak–Temporal Average (SPTA)
Output Intensities from Table 7.1

Type of Instrument	SPTA Output Intensity (mW/cm²)
All instruments	500
Imaging instruments	136
Scanning	88
Stopped	136
Doppler instruments	500
Continuous wave	500
Pulsed	389

* 7 dB, to account for human tissue path

tion of 80 per cent. Reducing the values in Table 7.1 by 80 per cent
yields upper limits as given in Table 7.2. Because most of the bioeffects
studies were done in small animals, such as mice and rats, the attenuation would be negligible; moreover, the values in Table 7.2 can be compared to the *AIUM Statement* value of 1 W/cm² for focused beams, as
virtually all diagnostic ultrasound uses focused beams. It can be seen
from this comparison that, on the basis of experimental animal studies,
clinical bioeffects would not be expected to occur from outputs of current and past diagnostic instrumentation.

Regulatory Activities

Manufacturers are required to submit premarket notifications to the
FDA prior to marketing a device for a specific application. The FDA
then reviews this notification to determine whether the device is substantially equivalent, with regard to safety and effectiveness, to instruments
on the market prior to the enactment of the Medical Device Amend-
ments (1976). If the device is determined to be substantially equivalent,
the manufacturer may then market it for that application. Part of the
FDA evaluation involves output data for the instrument, which are then
compared to maximum values found for pre-1976 devices. These values
are given in the *510(k) Guide for Measuring and Reporting Acoustic Output of
Diagnostic Ultrasound Medical Devices* and are presented in Table 7.3.
Some of the values have been updated since the 1985 publication of this
guide. The current values are shown in the table. Until recently, fetal
Doppler imaging was not approved by the FDA, primarily because of
efficacy considerations. However, some devices are now approved for
this application. Part of the requirements for this approval is the real-
time display of output information on the instrument. Recently, a volun-

TABLE 7.3
Spatial Peak–Temporal Average (SPTA) *In Situ* Intensity Upper
Limits Listed in the EDA *510(k) Guide for Measuring and Reporting
Acoustic Output of Diagnostic Ultrasound Medical Devices*

Physiological Application	SPTA Intensity (mW/cm²)
Cardiac	430
Peripheral vessel	720
Ophthalmic	17
Fetal imaging and other*	94

* Abdominal, intraoperative, pediatric, small organ (breast, thyroid, testes), neonatal cephalic, adult cephalic

tary output display standard was developed by a joint committee involving the AIUM, FDA, National Electrical Manufacturers Association (NEMA), and several other ultrasound-related professional societies. The goal of this activity was to develop a voluntary standard that would provide a parallel pathway to the current regulatory *510(k)* process. It would allow exemption from the upper limits given in the *510(k) Guide* in exchange for presenting output information on the display. The standard[43] includes two indexes that would be displayed: thermal and mechanical. The thermal index is defined as the transducer acoustic output power divided by the estimated power required to raise tissue temperature by 1°C. The mechanical index is equal to the peak rarefactional pressure divided by the square root of the center frequency of the pulse bandwidth. In the case of both indexes, display would not be required if the instrument were incapable of exceeding index values of 1. The standard was adopted by the AIUM in 1992. Displays, including mechanical index and SPTA intensity incorporating tissue attenuation, appeared in 1991 (see Fig. 7.20).

Epidemiology

A dozen or so epidemiologic studies have been conducted and published.[35] These indicate that epidemiologic studies and surveys in widespread clinical usage over 25 years have yielded no evidence of any adverse effect from diagnostic ultrasound. One recent study included 806 children, approximately half of whom had been exposed to diagnostic ultrasound *in utero*. The study measured Apgar scores, gestational age, head circumference, birth weight, length, congenital abnormalities, neonatal infection, and congenital infection at birth, and included conductive and nerve measurements of hearing, visual acuity and color vision, cognitive function, behavior, and complete and detailed neurologic examinations of children ages 7 to 12 years. No biologically significant differences between exposed and unexposed children were found. Another study compared the head circumference, height, and weight of 149 sibling pairs of the same sex, one of whom had been exposed to diagnostic ultrasound *in utero*. No statistically significant differences in head circumference at birth or in height and weight between birth and 6 years of age were found between ultrasound-exposed and unexposed siblings.

Although these studies have limitations and some flaws, they have not revealed a risk in clinical use of diagnostic ultrasound. The AIUM developed and approved in 1987 the following statements[37] regarding epidemiology:

1. Widespread clinical use over 25 years has not established any adverse effect arising from exposure to diagnostic ultrasound.

2. Randomized clinical studies are the most rigorous method for assessing potential adverse effects of diagnostic ultrasound. Studies using this methodology show no evidence of an effect on birthweight in humans.*

3. Other epidemiologic studies have shown no causal association of diagnostic ultrasound with any of the adverse fetal outcomes studied.*

Prudent Use

Epidemiologic studies have revealed no known risk in the use of diagnostic ultrasound. Experimental animal studies show bioeffects to be occurring at intensities higher than those expected at relevant tissue locations during ultrasound imaging and flow measurements. Thus, a comparison of instrument output data adjusted for tissue attenuation with experimental bioeffects data does not indicate any risk. However, we must be open to the possibility that unrecognized, but none-zero, risk may exist. Such risk, if it does exist, may have eluded detection up to this point because it is either subtle, delayed, or of incidence rates close to normal values. As more sensitive endpoints are studied over longer periods of time or with larger populations, such risk may be identified. On the other hand, future studies may not yield any positive effects, thus strengthening the possibility that medical ultrasound imaging is without detectable risk. In the meantime, with no known risk and with known benefit to the procedure, a conservative approach to imaging (Fig. 7.21) is justified.[36] That is, ultrasound imaging should be used when medically

---

* The acoustic exposure levels in these studies may not be representative of the full range of current fetal exposures.

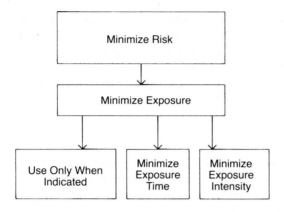

Figure 7.21. Minimize risk by minimizing exposure.

indicated with minimum exposure of the patient and fetus. Exposure is minimized by minimizing instrument output intensity and by minimizing exposure time during a study. Doppler instrument outputs can be significantly higher than those for imaging (see Table 7.1). It thus seems most likely that the greatest potential for risk in ultrasound diagnosis (although no specific risk has been identified even in this case), is in fetal Doppler studies. These combine potentially high-output intensities with stationary geometry and a fetus, which presumably is more sensitive to possible bioeffects than other subjects. Transvaginal exposure involves shorter distances to the fetus, but higher frequencies are used, resulting in comparable attenuation and fetal exposure[12] (see Fig. 7.20).

Ultrasound should be used for imaging only when medically indicated. A controversial issue relating to this is whether pregnancy constitutes a medical indication. A National Institutes of Health (NIH) consensus development panel concluded that "the data on clinical efficacy and safety do not allow a recommendation for routine screening at this time." The Royal College of Obstetricians and Gynaecologists, concentrating on the safety aspect, has stated that "the present evidence for the safety of ultrasound based on over 20 years of experience and research is sufficiently convincing for us not to recommend a change in the common practice of routine ultrasound examination between 16-18 weeks of pregnancy." The European Federation of Societies for Ultrasound in Medicine and Biology has stated that "routine clinical scanning of every woman during pregnancy is not contra-indicated by the evidence currently available from biological investigations and its performance should be left to clinical judgment."

The diagnostic methods committee of the British Institute of Radiology in 1984 created a working group to review the scientific evidence relevant to the safety of diagnostic ultrasound. The working group concluded that there was no reason to suspect that any hazard exists. The World Health Organization has stated that "the benefits of this imaging modality far outweigh any presumed risks."[44]

The AIUM[36,37] issued the following statement on clinical safety (October 1982, revised October 1983 and March 1988):

> Diagnostic ultrasound has been in use since the late 1950s. Given its known benefits and recognized efficacy for medical diagnosis, including use during human pregnancy, the American Institute of Ultrasound in Medicine herein addresses the clinical safety of such use:
>
> > No confirmed biological effects on patients or instrument operators caused by exposure at intensities typical of present diagnostic ultrasound instruments have ever been reported. Although the possibility exists that such biological effects may be identified in the future, current data indicate that the benefits to patients of the prudent use of diagnostic ultrasound outweigh the risks, if any, that may be present.

In conclusion, extensive mechanistic, *in vitro*, *in vivo*, and epidemiologic studies have revealed no known risk associated with the current ultrasound instrumentation used in medical diagnosis. However, a prudent and conservative approach to ultrasound safety is to assume that there may be unidentified risk which should be minimized in medically indicated ultrasound studies by minimizing exposure time and intensity.

It is difficult to make firm statements about the clinical safety of diagnostic ultrasound. The experimental and epidemiologic bases for risk assessment are incomplete. However, much work has been done, with no evidence of clinical harm revealed. Patients should be informed that there currently is no basis for judging that diagnostic ultrasound produces any harmful effects in patients. However, unobserved effects could be occurring. Thus, ultrasound should not be used indiscriminantly. The AIUM Clinical Safety Statement forms an excellent basis for formulating a response to patient questions and concerns. Prudence in practice is exercised by minimizing exposure time and output. Display of instrument outputs in the form of amplitudes or intensities, or the display of thermal and mechanical indexes, will greatly facilitate this approach to prudent use.

[Editorial note: Subsequent to the preparation of Sections 7.3 and 7.4, the AIUM developed and published several new statements on heating and cavitation and a new statement on mammalian biological effects. They are presented and discussed in References 45–48.]

7.5
Review

Phantoms and test objects provide means for measuring the detail resolution, distance accuracy, compensation, sensitivity, and dynamic range of diagnostic instruments. Hydrophones are used to measure the acoustic output of diagnostic instruments.

The AIUM has stated that there have been no independently confirmed, significant bioeffects reported to occur in mammalian tissues exposed to focused SPTA intensities of less than 1 W/cm. Furthermore, no risk has been identified with use of diagnostic ultrasound in humans. Because there is limited specific knowledge, a conservative approach is justified: diagnostic ultrasound should be used, with minimum exposure, when medical benefit is expected to be derived from the procedure.

The definitions for terms discussed in this chapter are listed below:

Cavitation. Production and dynamics of bubbles in sound.

Dynamic range. Ratio (in decibels) of largest power to smallest power that a system can handle, or of the largest to the smallest intensity of a group of echoes.

Hydrophone. A small transducer element mounted on the end of a narrow tube.

Phantom. Tissue-equivalent device that has some characteristics representative of tissues (e.g., scattering or attenuation properties).

Polyvinylidene fluoride. A piezoelectric film material.

PVDF. Polyvinylidene fluoride. A piezoelectric film material or a large piezoelectric membrane of small metallic electrodes for measuring acoustic output of an instrument.

Sensitivity. Ability of an imaging system to detect weak echoes.

Test object. A device without tissue-like properties that is designed to measure some characteristic of an imaging system.

EXERCISES

7.1 A tissue-equivalent _____ has an attenuation of about 0.5 dB/cm-MHz and a propagation speed of 1.54 mm/μs. A _____ _____ does not mimic tissue, but provides a means for measuring some aspect of imaging performance.

7.2 Match the parameters measured with the items used (answers may be used more than once):

a. axial resolution: _____, _____

b. lateral resolution: _____, _____

c. range accuracy: _____

d. caliper accuracy: _____

e. contrast resolution: _____

f. compensation: _____

g. sensitivity: _____

h. dynamic range: _____

i. beam profile: _____

j. section thickness: _____

1. nylon fibers
2. attenuating scattering material
3. simulated cysts
4. hyperechoic and hypoechoic simulated lesions
5. thin scattering layer

7.3 Match the parameters measured with the correlating types of observation modes (answers may be used more than once):

a. axial resolution: _____

b. lateral resolution: _____

c. range accuracy: _____

d. caliper accuracy: _____

e. compensation: _____

f. sensitivity: _____

g. dynamic range: _____, _____

1. gain settings
2. deepest scattering material imaged
3. fiber distances from the transducer or from each other on the display
4. minimum spacing of separately displayed fibers
5. lateral smearing of fibers

7.4 Test objects and phantoms are available commercially. True or false?

7.5 Test objects and phantoms can be used by the instrument operator. True or false?

7.6 A moving _____ test object is useful in checking the accuracy of Doppler spectral displays.

7.7 A _____ phantom is useful in simulating physiological _____ conditions for a Doppler instrument.

7.8 Which of the following is used for Doppler sensitivity measurements?

    a. cyst phantom
    b. profile test object
    c. string test object
    d. PIRTO
    e. none of the above

7.9 Tissue-equivalent phantoms attempt to represent some acoustic property of _____.

7.10 PIRTO is an example of a tissue-equivalent phantom. True or false?

7.11 Using a hydrophone, which of the following can be measured or calculated? (More than one correct answer.)

    a. impedance
    b. amplitude
    c. period
    d. pulse duration
    e. pulse repetition period

7.12 All hydrophones consist of a small element mounted on the end of a needle. True or false?

7.13 A needle hydrophone contains a small _____ element.

7.14 Because of its small size, a hydrophone can measure spatial details of a sound beam. True or false?

7.15 A hydrophone

    a. interacts with light
    b. produces a voltage
    c. measures intensity directly
    d. measures total energy
    e. none of the above

7.16 Match the items in column A with those in B and C (answers may be used more than once). (Note: *A* can be calculated from *B* if *C* is known.)

A:
    a. frequency: _____, _____
    b. pulse repetition frequency:_____, _____
    c. duty factor: _____, _____
    d. wavelength: _____, _____
    e. spatial pulse length:_____, _____

B:
    1. wavelength
    2. period
    3. pulse repetition period
    4. frequency
    5. energy
    6. power

f. energy: _____, _____

g. intensity: _____, _____

C:

7. number of cycles in the pulse
8. pulse duration
9. propagation speed
10. exposure time
11. beam area
12. nothing else

7.17 The piezoelectric material commonly used in hydrophones is
a. quartz
b. PZT
c. PVDF
d. PDQ
e. PVC

7.18 The important characteristic of the material used in hydrophones (Problem 7.17) is
a. impedance
b. propagation speed
c. efficiency
d. density
e. bandwidth

7.19 Heating depends most directly on
a. SATA intensity
b. SATP intensity
c. SPTP intensity
d. pressure

7.20 Conditions under which cavitation may occur are best described by
a. SATA intensity
b. SATP intensity
c. SPTP intensity
d. pressure

7.21 Bioeffects have been observed in experimental animals with intensities greater than
a. 100 mW/cm² SPTA
b. 1 W/cm² SPTA
c. 10 W/cm² SPTA
d. 1 mW/cm² SPTP
e. 10 mW/cm² SPTP

7.22 Bioeffects have been observed in experimental animals with focused intensities greater than
a. 100 mW/cm² SPTA
b. 1 W/cm² SPTA

    c. 10 W/cm² SPTA
    d. 1 mW/cm² SPTP
    e. 10 mW/cm² SPTP

7.23 Focal lesions have been observed in experimental animals with intensities greater than
    a. 100 mW/cm² SPTA
    b. 1 W/cm² SPTA
    c. 10 W/cm² SPTA
    d. 1 mW/cm² SPTP
    e. 10 mW/cm² SPTP

7.24 The available epidemiologic data are sufficient to make a final judgment on the safety of diagnostic ultrasound. True or false?

7.25 Exposure is minimized by using diagnostic ultrasound
    a. only when indicated
    b. with minimum intensity
    c. with minimum time
    d. all of the above
    e. none of the above

7.26 Which of the following is (are) currently used to indicate output on the display?
    a. per cent
    b. dB
    c. SPTA intensity
    d. Mechanical index (MI)
    e. all of the above

7.27 Which of the following affect(s) the exposure of a fetus?
    a. intensity at the transducer
    b. distance to the fetus
    c. frequency
    d. receiver gain
    e. more than one of the above
    f. all of the above

7.28 There is no possible hazard involved in the diagnostic use of ultrasound. True or false?

7.29 Ultrasound should not be used as a diagnostic tool because of the bioeffects it can produce. True or false?

7.30 No independently confirmed, significant bioeffects in mammalian tissues have been reported at intensities below
    a. 10 W/cm² SPTP
    b. 100 mW/cm² SPTA
    c. 10 mW/cm² SPTA
    d. 10 mW/cm² SATA
    e. 1 mW/cm² SATP

7.31 Is there any known risk with the current use of diagnostic ultrasound?

7.32 Are there any bioeffects that ultrasound produces in small animals under experimental conditions? Yes or no?

7.33 Which of the following are mechanisms by which ultrasound can produce bioeffects?
(More than one correct answer)
a. direction ionization
b. absorption
c. photoelectric effect
d. cavitation
e. Compton effect

7.34 Which of the following relates to heating?
a. impedance
b. sound speed
c. absorption
d. refraction
e. diffraction

7.35 Which of the following endpoints is documented well enough in the scientific literature to allow a risk assessment for diagnostic ultrasound to be based on it?
a. fetal weight
b. sister chromatid exchange
c. fetal abnormalities
d. carcinogenesis
e. none

7.36 More than one epidemiologic study has shown a statistically significant effect of ultrasound exposure on which of the following endpoints?
a. fetal activity
b. birth weight
c. fetal abnormalities
d. dyslexia
e. none

7.37 Which of the following acoustic parameters have been documented in ultrasound epidemiologic studies published thus far?
a. frequency
b. exposure time
c. intensity and pulsing conditions
d. scanning patterns
e. none

7.38 A device commonly used to measure the output of diagnostic ultrasound instruments is a(n)

    a. hydrophone
    b. optical interferometer
    c. Geiger counter
    d. photoelectric cell
    e. absorption radiometer

7.39 A typical output intensity (SPTA) for an ultrasound imaging instrument is
    a. 1540 W
    b. 13 kW/mm^2
    c. 3.5 MHz
    d. 1 mW/cm^2
    e. 2 dB/cm

7.40 Which of the following typically have the highest output intensity?
    a. fetal monitor Doppler
    b. duplex pulsed Doppler
    c. static imager
    d. mechanical real-time imager
    e. phase-array, real-time imager

7.41 As far as we know now, which of the following is the most correct and informative response to a patient's question, "Will this hurt me or my baby?"
    a. no
    b. yes
    c. I don't know.
    d. The risks are well understood but the benefits always outweigh them
    e. There is no known risk with ultrasound imaging as applied currently

7.42 To minimize whatever (unidentified) risk there may be with ultrasound imaging, which of the following should be done? (More than one correct answer)
    a. scan for family album pictures
    b. scan to determine fetal sex
    c. minimize exposure time
    d. scan for medical indication(s) only
    e. minimize exposure intensity

7.43 Which of the following controls affect instrument output intensity?
    a. dynamic range, compression
    b. transmit, output
    c. near gain, far gain
    d. overall gain
    e. slope, TGC

7.44 Which of the following are correct for a duplex pulsed Doppler instrument? (More than one correct answer)
  a. tissue anywhere in the Doppler beam is exposed to ultrasound
  b. tissue anywhere in the imaging plane is exposed to ultrasound
  c. imaging intensities are higher than for conventional real-time instruments
  d. Doppler intensities are higher than for continuous-wave fetal monitoring

7.45 The tissue of greatest concern with regard to bioeffects in an abdominal scan is the
  a. spleen
  b. pancreas
  c. liver
  d. kidney
  e. fetus

7.46 Would it be wise to substitute a duplex pulsed Doppler device for an inoperative fetal monitor for long-term (e.g., 24-hour) monitoring in labor?
  a. yes
  b. no
  c. depends on frame rate of image
  d. depends on frequency of Doppler beam
  e. depends on gate location

7.47 Which of the following is (are) likely to be exposed to ultrasound during a diagnostic study?
  a. patient
  b. sonographer
  c. sonologist
  d. observers in the room
  e. more than one of the above

CHAPTER 8

Summary

Ultrasound is sound (a wave of traveling acoustic variables: pressure, density, temperature, and particle motion) of a frequency greater than 20 kHz. It is described by frequency, period, wavelength, propagation speed, amplitude, intensity, and attenuation. Pulsed ultrasound is described by additional terms: pulse repetition frequency (PRF), pulse repetition period, pulse duration, duty factor, and spatial pulse length. Propagation speed and impedance are characteristics of the medium that are determined by density and stiffness. Attenuation increases with frequency and path length. Imaging depth decreases with increasing frequency. Several intensities are used to describe pulsed ultrasound, including spatial average–temporal average (SATA), spatial peak–temporal average (SPTA), spatial average–pulse average, spatial peak–pulse average (SPPA), spatial average–temporal peak (SATP), and spatial peak–temporal peak (SPTP). The average soft tissue propagation speed is 1.54 mm/μs, and the average attenuation coefficient is 0.5 dB/cm for each megahertz of frequency.

When, with perpendicular incidence, sound encounters boundaries between media with different impedances, part of the sound is reflected and part is transmitted. If the two media have the same impedance, there is no reflection. With oblique incidence, the sound is refracted at a boundary between media where propagation speeds are different. Incidence and reflection angles are always equal. For oblique incidence, there may be a reflection when the impedances are equal (if the propagation speeds are different), or there may not be a reflection even if the impedances are different. Scattering occurs at rough media boundaries and within heterogeneous media. The range equation is used to determine distance to reflectors. The round-trip travel time is 13 μs/cm.

Transducers convert energy from one form to another. Ultrasound transducers convert electric energy to ultrasound energy and vice versa. They operate on the piezoelectricity principle. Transducers may be operated in burst-excited mode or shock-excited mode. The preferred operating frequency depends on the element thickness. Axial resolution is equal to one half the spatial pulse length. Pulsed transducers have damping material to shorten the spatial pulse length. Transducers produce sound in the form of beams with near and far zones. Lateral resolution is equal to beam width. Beam width may be reduced by focusing. Linear, convex, and annular are types of array construction. Sequenced, phased, and vector are types of array operation. Phasing provides electronic control of focus. Detail resolution improves with increasing frequency.

Diagnostic ultrasound imaging systems are of the pulse-echo type. These use the direction, strength, and arrival time of received echoes to generate B-mode and M mode displays. Imaging systems consist of a pulser, a beam former, a transducer, a receiver, a memory, and a display. Receivers amplify, compensate, compress, demodulate, and reject echoes. Compensation equalizes differences in received echo amplitudes caused by attenuation. B and M modes use a brightness display. M mode shows reflector motion in time. The B scan shows an anatomic cross section through the scanning plane. Scan converters (memories) store gray-scale image information and permit image display on television monitors. Digital scan converters are computer memories that store echo information as numbers in memory elements. Contrast resolution improves with increasing bits per pixel. Real-time imaging is the rapid sequential display of ultrasound images resulting in a moving presentation. Such imaging requires rapid, repeatable, sequential scanning of the sound beam through the tissue. This is accomplished by mechanical real-time transducers and by electronic transducer arrays. Rectangular or sector display formats result from such scanning techniques. Temporal resolution improves with increasing frame rate.

Flow in vessels depends on pressure difference and resistance. Viscosity, vessel length, and vessel diameter contribute to resistance. Flow types include steady, pulsatile, plug, laminar (parabolic), disturbed, and turbulent. The Doppler effect is a change in frequency resulting from reflector or scatterer motion toward or away from the transducer. Doppler instruments make use of this frequency shift to yield information regarding motion and flow. Continuous-wave (CW) systems provide motion and flow information without depth information or selection capability. Pulsed Doppler systems provide depth information and the ability to select the depth at which Doppler information is generated. Spectral analysis provides information on the distribution of received frequencies resulting from the distribution of scatterer velocities (speeds and directions) encountered. In addition to audible output, imaging of vessel flow spectra is possible in Doppler systems. Combined (duplex) systems utilizing dynamic B-scan imaging and CW and pulsed Doppler are available. Color-flow systems provide displays of two-dimensional, real-time flow superimposed on gray-scale anatomic scans.

Axial resolution is determined by spatial pulse length. Lateral resolution is determined by beam width. The beam width perpendicular to the scan plane causes section-thickness artifacts. Apparent resolution close to the transducer is not directly related to tissue texture, but is a result of interference effects from a distribution of scatterers in the tissue (speckle). Reverberation produces a set of equally spaced artifactual echoes distal to the real reflector. Refraction displaces echoes laterally. In a mirror-image artifact, objects that are present on one side of a strong reflector are presented on the other side as well. Enhancement results from low-attenuation objects in the sound path. Propagation speed error and refraction can cause objects to be displayed improperly in terms of location or size, or both. Refraction can also cause edge shadowing.

Artifacts with Doppler ultrasound include aliasing, range ambiguity, color-flow image and Doppler signal mirroring, and spectral trace mirroring. Aliasing is the most common artifact. It occurs when the Doppler shift frequency exceeds one half the PRF. It can be reduced or eliminated by increasing the PRF or Doppler angle, using baseline shift, reducing the operating frequency, or using a CW instrument.

Phantoms and test objects provide means for measuring detail resolution, distance accuracy, compensation, sensitivity, and dynamic range of diagnostic instruments. Hydrophones are used to measure the acoustic output of diagnostic instruments.

There have been no independently confirmed, significant bioeffects reported in mammalian tissues exposed to focused SPTA intensities of less than 1 W/cm^2. No risk with use of diagnostic ultrasound in humans has been identified. Because there is limited specific knowledge, however, a conservative approach is appropriate—that is, diagnostic ultrasound should be performed only with minimum exposure and when medical benefit is expected to be derived from the procedure.

EXERCISES

8.1 Increasing the frequency
  a. improves the resolution
  b. increases the imaging depth
  c. increases refraction
  d. both a and b
  e. both a and c

8.2 Increasing the pulse repetition frequency
    a. improves detail resolution
    b. increases maximum depth imaged unambiguously
    c. decreases maximum depth imaged unambiguously
    d. both a and b
    e. both a and c

8.3 Increasing the intensity produced by the transducer
    a. is accomplished by increasing the pulser voltage
    b. increases the sensitivity of the system
    c. increases the possibility of bioeffects
    d. all of the above
    e. none of the above

8.4 Increasing the spatial pulse length
    a. is accomplished by transducer damping
    b. is accompanied by decreased pulse duration
    c. improves the axial resolution
    d. all of the above
    e. none of the above

8.5 Dynamic imaging is made possible by
    a. scan converters
    b. mechanically driven transducers
    c. gray-scale display
    d. arrays
    e. both b and d

8.6 Phantoms with nylon lines measure
    a. detail resolution
    b. pulse duration
    c. SATA intensity
    d. wavelength
    e. all of the above

8.7 Ultrasound bioeffects
    a. do not occur
    b. do not occur with diagnostic instruments
    c. are not confirmed below an SPTA intensity of 100 mW/cm^2
    d. both b and c
    e. none of the above

8.9 The diagnostic ultrasound frequency range is
    a. 2 to 10 mHz
    b. 2 to 10 kHz
    c. 2 to 10 MHz
    d. 3 to 15 kHz
    e. none of the above

8.10 Small transducers always produce smaller beam diameters. True or false?

8.11 No reflection occurs if media impedances are equal. True or false?

8.12 No refraction occurs if media impedances are equal. True or false?

8.13 Gray-scale display is made possible by
  a. array transducers
  b. cathode ray storage tubes
  c. scan converters
  d. both b and c
  e. all of the above

8.14 Attenuation is corrected by
  a. demodulation
  b. desegregation
  c. decompression
  d. compensation

8.15 Time is one dimension on which type of display?
  a. B mode
  b. color-flow
  c. M mode
  d. a la mode
  e. none of the above

8.16 The Doppler effect for a scatterer moving toward the transducer causes scattered sound (compared with incident sound) received by the transducer to have _____.
  a. increased intensity
  b. decreased intensity
  c. increased impedance
  d. increased frequency
  e. increased wavelength

8.17 An ultrasound instrument that could represent 64 shades of gray would require an eight-bit memory. True or false?

8.18 Continuous-wave sound is used in _____.
  a. all imaging instruments
  b. some imaging instruments
  c. all Doppler instruments
  d. some Doppler instruments
  e. none of the above

8.19 What is the transmitted intensity if the incident intensity is 1 and the impedances are 1.00 and 2.64?
  a. 0.2
  b. 0.4
  c. 0.6

    d. 0.8

    e. 1.0

8.20 A thin–scattering-layer test object measures:

    a. contrast resolution

    b. beam profile

    c. axial resolution

    d. section thickness

    e. more than one of the above

8.21 An advantage of continuous-wave Doppler instruments is that they have _____.

    a. no aliasing

    b. depth information and selectivity

    c. bidirectional information

    d. amplitude information

    e. all of the above

8.22 An advantage of pulsed Doppler instruments is that they have _____.

    a. no aliasing

    b. depth information

    c. bidirectional information

    d. amplitude information

    e. all of the above

8.23 A digital memory with one bit per pixel would have a _____ display.

    a. bidirectional

    b. biscattering

    c. bistable (black and white)

8.24 If a transducer element 19 mm in diameter is focused to produce a minimum beam diameter of 2 mm, the intensity at the focus is approximately _____ times the intensity at the transducer.

    a. 2

    b. 3

    c. 19

    d. 100

    e. 500

8.25 The largest number that can be stored in a pixel of a seven-bit digital memory is _____.

    a. 16

    b. 32

    c. 127

    d. 255

    e. 256

8.26 Digital calipers are used to calculate the distance between
_____.
a. potentiometers
b. bits
c. optical encoders
d. pixels
e. all of the above

8.27 Which of the following produce(s) a sector-scan format?
a. convex array
b. oscillating mechanical real-time transducer
c. phased array
d. vector array
e. all of the above

8.28 A digital imaging instrument divides the cross-sectional image into
_____.
a. frequencies
b. bits
c. pixels
d. binaries
e. wavelengths

8.29 A 6-bit memory with a dynamic range of 65 dB has a contrast resolution of _____ dB/shade.
a. 1
b. 6
c. 16
d. 64
e. 65

8.30 The binary number 10111 is equal to the decimal number
_____.
a. 10
b. 16
c. 20
d. 23
e. 111

8.31 The axial resolution for a two-cycle pulse of 5 MHz in tissue is
_____ mm.
a. 0.1
b. 0.2
c. 0.3
d. 0.4
e. 0.5

8.32 The best lateral resolution for an unfocused 13-mm transducer element is _____ mm.
   a. 2.5
   b. 4.5
   c. 6.5
   d. 815
   e. 13

8.33 Which is not improved by multiple transmit focus?
   a. detail resolution
   b. temporal resolution
   c. lateral resolution
   d. image detail
   e. none of the above

8.34 If the frame rate with one focus is 30 Hz, what is the likely frame rate with 3 transmit focuses?
   a. 3
   b. 10
   c. 15
   d. 20
   e. 30

8.35 If pulse repetition frequency is increased, the SPTA intensity is _____.
   a. increased
   b. unchanged
   c. decreased
   d. eliminated
   e. none of the above

8.36 If the thickness of a transducer element is decreased, the frequency is _____.
   a. increased
   b. unchanged
   c. decreased
   d. intensified
   e. none of the above

8.37 In Exercise 8.36, the near-zone length is _____.
   a. increased
   b. unchanged
   c. decreased
   d. intensified
   e. none of the above

8.38 With increased damping, which of the following is increased?
   a. bandwidth
   b. pulse duration

    c. spatial pulse length
    d. Q factor
    e. all of the above

8.39 As frequency is increased, which of the following is (are) decreased?
    a. propagation speed
    b. PRF
    c. imaging depth
    d. more than one of the above
    e. none of the above

8.40 If the pulse repetition frequency is 3 kHz and the frame rate is 30 per second, there will be _____ scan lines in the image (single focus).
    a. 3
    b. 100
    c. 300
    d. 3000
    e. 30,000

8.41 If linear preprocessing is used and the echo dynamic range is 40 dB, a 20-dB echo will be assigned the number _____ in a six-bit memory.
    a. 0
    b. 16
    c. 32
    d. 48
    e. 64

8.42 If linear postprocessing is used, a stored 48 in a six-bit memory will produce _____ per cent brightness on the display.
    a. 0
    b. 15
    c. 50
    d. 75
    e. 100

8.43 A five-bit memory can store which of the following decimal numbers?
    a. 64
    b. 32
    c. 31
    d. 55
    e. more than one of the above

8.44 Television monitors produce _____ frames per second.
    a. 10
    b. 24

c. 30

d. 60

e. none of the above

8.45 Duplex Doppler instruments include _____.

a. pulsed Doppler

b. continuous-wave Doppler

c. color-flow imaging

d. gray-scale imaging

e. more than one of the above

8.46 If the Doppler shifts from normal arteries and from stenotic carotid arteries are 4 kHz and 10 kHz, respectively, for which will a pulse repetition frequency of 7 kHz be a problem?

a. normal

b. stenotic

c. both

d. neither

8.47 The problem in Exercise 8.46 is

a. refraction

b. resolution

c. range ambiguity

d. aliasing

e. mirror

8.48 Compensation (swept gain) makes up for the fact that echoes from deeper reflectors arrive at the transducer later. True or false?

8.49 Which of the following affects contrast resolution the most?

a. number of pixels

b. number of bits per pixel

c. pulse duration

d. frequency

e. focusing

8.50 Which of the following requires a phased array as a receiving transducer?

a. dynamic range

b. dynamic imaging

c. dynamic focusing

d. dynamic personality

e. none of the above

8.51 *Across:*

1. Referring to sound

2. Abbreviation for cosine

3. Not perpendicular to a boundary

4. Occurs at boundaries with perpendicular incidence

5. Material through which sound is passing

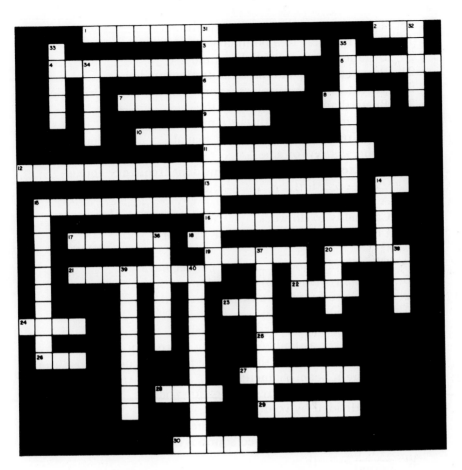

6. Pulsed Doppler requires _____ the receiver
7. The duty _____ is sound-on fraction
8. Beam diameter decreases in the _____ zone
9. Intensity is power divided by _____
10. Reflector motion produces a Doppler _____
11. Sound of a frequency of 20 kHz or higher
12. Parallel to sound direction
13. Maximum variation of an acoustic variable
14. Abbreviation for continuous wave
15. Attenuation _____ is expressed in decibels per centimeter
16. Power divided by area
17. $\dfrac{1}{\text{frequency}}$

18. The range equation yields the distance _____ a reflector
19. Perpendicular to a boundary
20. Distance moved divided by time
21. Propagation speed depends on density and _____
22. _____ scale displays several values of spot brightness
23. Beam diameter increases in the _____ zone
24. Force multipled by distance moved
25. Axial resolution depends on spatial _____ length
26. Abbreviation for sine
27. Reflected frequency minus incident frequency equals _____ shift
28. A traveling variation
29. Capability to do work
30. Complete variation of a wave variable

Down:

14. One hertz is one _____ per second
15. The abbreviation CW stands for _____ wave
20. A line produced on a display is called a _____ line
31. (A message for you)
32. Traveling wave of acoustic variables
33. Transducer assembly containing more than one element
34. _____ length is the distance from a focused transducer to minimum beam diameter
35. Density multiplied by propagation speed
36. Mass divided by volume
37. Another name for a hydrophone
38. Fraction of time a pulsed sound is on is the _____ factor
39. $\dfrac{1}{\text{period}}$
40. Ability of an imaging system to detect weak reflections

8.52 *Across:**

1. The ratio of the largest to the smallest power that a system can handle is called the _____ range.
2. At a distance of one near-zone length from a disk transducer, beam diameter is approximately equal to disk diameter divided by _____.
3. Passing only echoes that arrive at a certain time after the transducer has produced a pulse is called _____.
4. Several frames per second is called _____ time imaging.

---

* From Kremkau, F.W.: Crossword puzzle. Med. Ultrasound, *4*:38, 1980. Reprinted by permission of John Wiley & Sons, Inc.

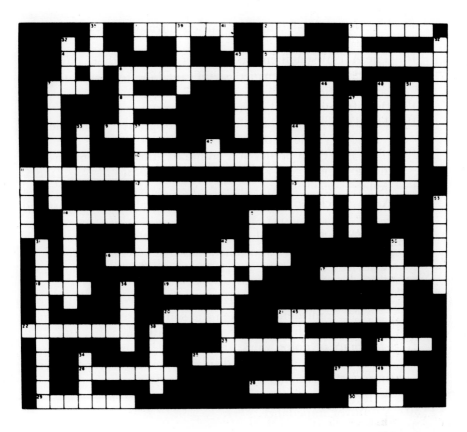

5. The process by which small voltages are increased to larger ones.
6. The speed with which a wave moves through a medium is called _____ speed.
7. The region of a sound beam where the beam diameter increases with distance from the transducer is called the _____ zone.
8. Another word for a reflection.
9. Acoustic means having to do with _____.
10. If propagation speeds of two media are equal, incidence angle equals _____ angle.
11. A device that stores a gray-scale image and allows it to be displayed on a television monitor is called a scan _____.
12. Conversion of sound to heat.
13. Power divided by area.
14. An echo-free region on a display is called _____.

15. The fraction of time that pulsed ultrasound is on is called
    _____ factor.
16. The AIUM statement on bioeffects says that there have been
    no _____ confirmed significant bioeffects at intensities
    below 100 mW/cm².
17. Density multiplied by sound propagation speed.
18. The display of several values of spot brightness is possible on a
    _____ scale display.
19. If no reflection occurs at a boundary, this always means that
    media impedances are equal in the case of _____ inci-
    dence.
20. A few cycles of ultrasound may be called an ultrasound
    _____.
21. Maximum variation of an acoustic variable or voltage.
22. Reverberations are also called _____ reflections.
23. A device that converts energy from one form to another.
24. Prefix meaning 1000.
25. Abbreviation for megahertz.
26. _____ incidence is when the sound direction is not per-
    pendicular to the boundary of the medium.
27. Capability of doing work.
28. Number of complete scans displayed per unit of time in a real-
    time system is called the _____ rate.
29. Perpendicular to the direction of sound travel.
30. A unit for impedance.

Down:
1. Abbreviation for decibel.
2. Sound _____ through a medium improves as attenuation
   decreases.
3. Ratio of output to input electric power for an amplifier.
6. A Greek prefix meaning pressure.
7. Number of cycles per second.
11. One hertz is one _____ per second.
14. An _____ array is made up of ring-shaped elements.
15. Imaging _____ decreases with increasing frequency.
31. Along the direction of sound travel (axial).
32. Focusing produces decreased beam _____.
33. A sound _____ is a traveling variation of acoustic vari-
    ables.
34. Most two-dimensional imaging is done with B _____ dis-
    plays.
35. To sweep a sound beam to produce an image.

36. Rate at which work is done; rate at which energy is trans-
    ferred.
37. Sound having a frequency of greater than 20 kHz.
38. To concentrate the sound beam into a smaller area.
39. A transducer _____ is an assembly containing more than
    one transducer element.
40. Abbreviation for millimeter.
41. Abbreviation for continuous wave.
42. Frequency unit.
43. A _____ array is made up of rectangular elements in a
    line.
44. Propagation speed increases with decreasing _____.
45. Material through which a wave travels.
46. Decrease of amplitude and intensity as a wave travels through
    a medium.
47. Length of space over which a cycle occurs.
48. Change of sound direction on passing from one medium to
    another.
49. A cathode _____ tube is a common display device.
50. Diffusion or redirection of sound in several directions.
51. Speed, with direction of motion specified.
52. Perpendicular _____ occurs when sound direction is per-
    pendicular to the boundary of the medium.
53. The _____ effect is a frequency change of a reflected
    sound wave secondary to reflector motion.

8.53 Identify the physical/ultrasound parameters for which the following units of measure are appropriate.*

Across:
1. joule
2. microsecond
3. rayl
4. joule
5. decibel
6. kelvin
7. millimeter
8. gram
9. milliliter
10. hertz

Down:
5. radian

---

* From Kremkau, F.W.: Ultrapuzzles. Reflections 6:85, 1980. Reprinted by permission
of the American Institute of Ultrasound in Medicine.

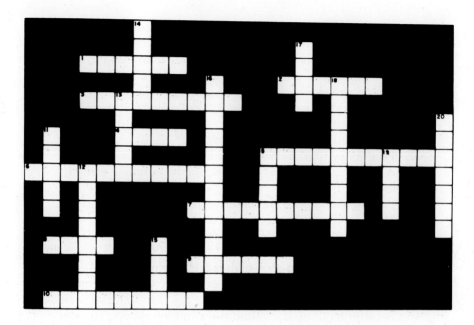

11. meter/second
12. newton/meter
13. watt
14. newton
15. decibel
16. meter/second^2
17. centimeter^2
18. watt/centimeter^2
19. second
20. gram/milliliter

8.54 For the following review, determine the appropriate word to fill in the blank. Then, in the figure, begin at the upper left and draw a line to one letter at a time in any direction (horizontal, vertical, or diagonal) to spell out the word for each blank. All letters are used in a continuous line. Do not cross over your line. Use each letter only once. The words should be found in the same order as they are needed for the blanks.

Ultrasound is a _____ of traveling _____ variables. Pulsed ultrasound is commonly used in ultrasound imaging. Pulses contain a range of _____. Soft tissue _____ _____ is 1.54 mm/μs and the _____ coefficient is 0.5 dB/cm for each _____ of frequency. _____ occurs at rough boundaries

START

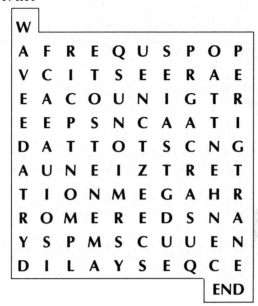

and within heterogeneous media. _____ convert electric energy to ultrasound energy and vice versa. Imaging systems consist of a pulser, transducer, receiver, _____, and _____. Real-time instruments display a rapid _____ of static pictures (frames).

8.55 Propagation speed increases with increasing
   a. stiffness
   b. density
   c. absorption
   d. attenuation
   e. both a and b

8.56 Reflections are produced by changes in
   a. stiffness
   b. density
   c. absorption
   d. attenuation
   e. both a and b

8.57 If no reflection occurs at a boundary, this always means that media impedances are equal in the case of
   a. perpendicular incidence
   b. oblique incidence

    c. refraction
    d. both a and b
    e. both b and c
8.58 If the propagation speeds in two media are unequal, the incidence angle equals the
    a. reflection angle
    b. transmission angle
    c. Doppler angle
    d. both a and b
    e. both b and c
8.59 At a distance of one near-zone length from a disk transducer, the beam diameter is equal to the disk diameter divided by
    a. one
    b. two
    c. three
    d. four
    e. one fourth
8.60 Velocity is _____.
    a. speed
    b. direction
    c. acceleration
    d. a and b
    e. all of the above
8.61 Decibels are _____ ratio units.
    a. amplitude
    b. power
    c. neper
    d. more than one of the above
    e. all of the above
8.62 Which of the following are real-time displays? (More than one correct answer)
    a. B mode
    b. B scan
    c. M mode
    d. Doppler
    e. color flow
8.63 A television monitor scans _____ fields per second.
    a. 10
    b. 30
    c. 60
    d. 512
    e. 525

8.64 A television monitor field is _____ a frame.
 a. $\frac{1}{10}$
 b. $\frac{1}{4}$
 c. $\frac{1}{2}$
 d. $\frac{3}{4}$
 e. more than one of the above

8.65 Frame rate is _____ by dynamic focus.
 a. increased
 b. decreased
 c. strengthened
 d. unaffected
 e. doubled

8.66 Which of the following produce(s) a sector scan format?
 a. convex array
 b. oscillating mechanical transducer
 c. phased array
 d. linear array
 e. more than one of the above

8.67 Which of the following produce(s) a rectangular scan format?
 a. convex array
 b. oscillating mechanical transducer
 c. phased array
 d. linear array
 e. more than one of the above

8.68 Gray-scale displays present brightness corresponding to echo
 a. frequency
 b. amplitude
 c. bandwidth
 d. impedance
 e. more than one of the above

8.69 If approximately 100 different gray levels can be distinguished by a human observer, how many bits per pixel would be a good choice for an ultrasound memory?
 a. 4
 b. 6
 c. 8
 d. 10
 e. 12

8.70 Which of the following memories will have sufficient contrast resolution to distinguish adjacent 25-dB and 26-dB echoes within a dynamic range of 0 to 40 dB, assuming straight line preprocessing and postprocessing characteristics?

   a. 5 bit
   b. 6 bit
   c. 7 bit
   d. b and c
   e. all of the above

8.71 A digital scan converter stores _____ corresponding to echo amplitudes.
   a. numbers
   b. electrical charges
   c. lines
   d. frames
   e. none of the above

8.72 The intensity of returning echoes changes with the angle in Doppler flow measurements. True or false?

8.73 The intensity of returning echoes changes with the flow speed in Doppler ultrasound. True or false?

8.74 Figure 8.1 describes which type of resolution?
   a. axial
   b. lateral
   c. contrast
   d. detail
   e. a and d

8.75 In which part of Figure 8.1 (*a* or *b*) are the two reflectors resolved?

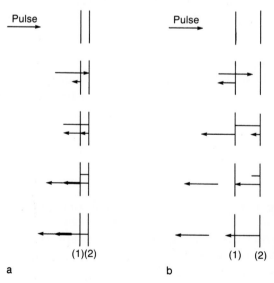

a   b

Figure 8.1. (From Kremkau, F.W.: Basic principles and biological effects of ultrasound. *In* Resnick, M.I., and Sanders, R.C. [eds.]: Ultrasound in Urology. © 1979, The Williams & Wilkins Co., Baltimore. Reprinted with permission.)

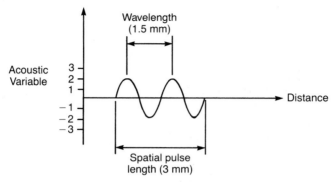

a

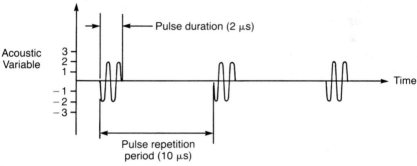

b

Figure 8.2. (From Kremkau, F.W.: Basic principles and biological effects of ultrasound. *In* Resnick, M.I., and Sanders, R.C. [eds.]: Ultrasound in Urology. © 1979, The Williams & Wilkins Co., Baltimore. Reprinted with permission.)

8.76 In Figure 8.2, give the following:
   a. number of cycles in a pulse
   b. amplitude
   c. wavelength
   d. spatial pulse length
   e. pulse repetition period
   f. pulse repetition frequency
   g. pulse duration
   h. period
   i. frequency
   j. duty factor
   k. propagation speed
8.77 In Figure 8.3, if the frequency is 4 MHz, the attenuation from the source to the tissue boundary is _____ dB. If the intensity

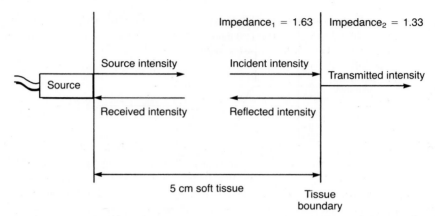

Figure 8.3. (From Kremkau, F.W.: Basic principles and biological effects of ultrasound. *In* Resnick, M.I., and Sanders, R.C. [eds.]: Ultrasound in Urology. © 1979, The Williams & Wilkins Co., Baltimore. Reprinted with permission.)

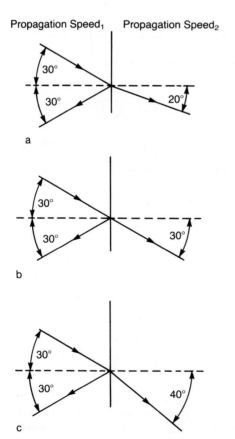

Figure 8.4. (From Kremkau, F.W.: Basic principles and biological effects of ultra- sound. *In* Resnick, M.I., and Sanders, R.C. [eds.]: Ultrasound in Urology. © 1979, The Williams & Wilkins Co., Balti- more. Reprinted with permission.)

emitted by the source (transducer) is 10 mW/cm, the intensity arriving at the boundary (incident intensity) is _____ mW/cm. The intensity reflection coefficient at the boundary is _____. The reflected intensity is _____ mW/cm and the received intensity at the source is _____ mW/cm.

8.78 In which part of Figure 8.4 (*a*, *b*, or *c*) is speed 2 greater than speed 1? Is speed 2 less than speed 1? Is speed 2 equal to speed 1? Is there no refraction?

8.79 Figure 8.5 shows that a higher frequency yields a (longer, shorter) near-zone length and that a larger transducer produces a (longer, shorter) near-zone length. By curving them, which of these transducers (*a*, *b*, *c*, or *d*) can be focused at 25 cm? at 15 cm? at 4 cm?

8.80 In Figure 8.6, the wave type is (continuous-wave, pulsed). If the lower portion of the figure represents 4 μs later than the upper portion, the propagation speed is _____ mm/μs, the wavelength for a frequency of 1 MHz is _____ mm, and the spatial pulse length is _____ mm.

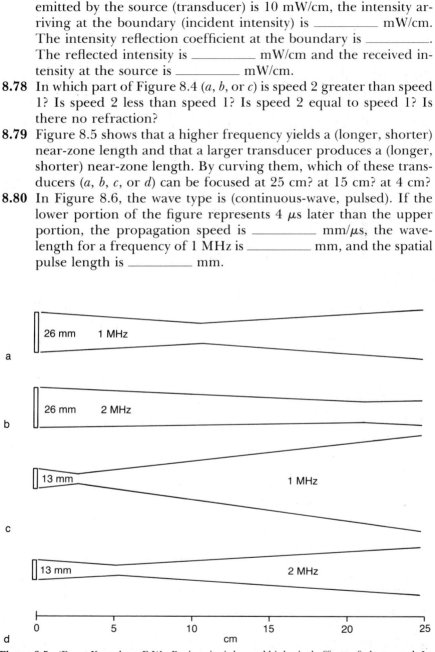

Figure 8.5. (From Kremkau, F.W.: Basic principles and biological effects of ultrasound. *In* Resnick, M.I., and Sanders, R.C. [eds.]: Ultrasound in Urology. © 1979, The Williams & Wilkins Co., Baltimore. Reprinted with permission.)

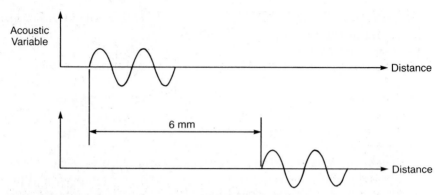

Figure 8.6. (From Kremkau, F.W.: Basic principles and biological effects of ultrasound. *In* Resnick, M.I., and Sanders, R.C. [eds.]: Ultrasound in Urology. © 1979, The Williams & Wilkins Co., Baltimore. Reprinted with permission.)

8.81 In Figure 8.7, the frequency is _____ MHz, the period is _____ μs, the amplitude is _____ units, the wave type is (continuous-wave, pulsed), and for soft tissue, the wavelength is _____ mm.

8.82 In Figure 8.8, which of the following have occurred?
   a. reflection
   b. refraction
   c. transmission
   d. a and b
   e. a and c

8.83 In Figure 8.9, as the pulse travels to the right, the amplitude decreases. This is called _____. If the amplitude at the right is one half the amplitude at the left, the attenuation is _____ dB.

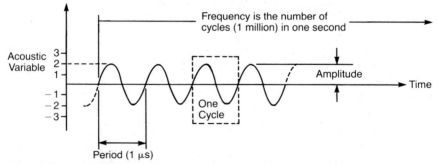

Figure 8.7. (From Kremkau, F.W.: Basic principles and biological effects of ultrasound. *In* Resnick, M.I., and Sanders, R.C. [eds.]: Ultrasound in Urology. © 1979, The Williams & Wilkins Co., Baltimore. Reprinted with permission.)

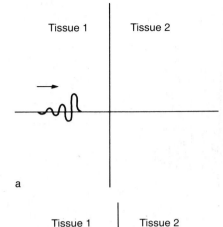

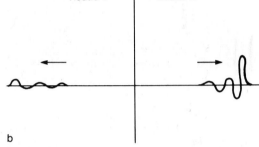

Figure 8.8. (From Kremkau, F.W.: Ultrasound instrumentation: Physical principles. *In* Callen, P.W. [ed.]: Ultrasonography in Obstetrics and Gynecology. Philadelphia, W.B. Saunders Co., 1982. Reprinted with permission.)

If the distance from left to right is 3 cm, the attenuation coefficient is _____ dB/cm. If the travel were in soft tissue, the frequency of the pulse would be approximately _____ MHz.

8.84 In Figure 8.10, which is the higher-frequency pulse (both in same medium)?

a. a
b. b
c. neither

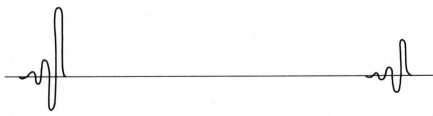

Figure 8.9. (From Kremkau, F.W.: Ultrasound instrumentation: Physical principles. *In* Callen, P.W. [ed.]: Ultrasonography in Obstetrics and Gynecology. Philadelphia, W.B. Saunders Co., 1982. Reprinted with permission.)

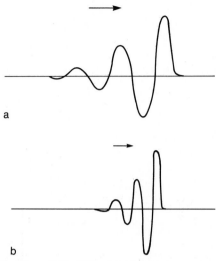

Figure 8.10. (From Kremkau, F.W.: Ultrasound instrumentation: Physical principles. *In* Callen, P.W. [ed.]: Ultrasonography in Obstetrics and Gynecology. Philadelphia, W.B. Saunders Co., 1982. Reprinted with permission.)

8.85 In Figure 8.10, which pulse travels faster?
  a. a
  b. b
  c. neither

8.86 In Figure 8.10, which pulse travels farther (i.e., experiences less attenuation)?
  a. a
  b. b
  c. neither

8.87 In Figure 8.10, which pulse has better axial resolution?
  a. a
  b. b
  c. neither

8.88 In Figure 8.10, which pulse has the greater amplitude?
  a. a
  b. b
  c. neither

8.89 As frequency increases, which of the following (more than one) decrease?
  a. period
  b. wavelength
  c. propagation speed

   d. amplitude
   e. intensity
   f. attenuation coefficient
   g. penetration
   h. reflection coefficient
   i. transmission coefficient
   j. refraction
   k. pulse duration
   l. spatial pulse length
   m. pulse repetition frequency
   n. pulse repetition period
   o. duty factor
   p. near-zone length
   q. imaging depth
   r. axial resolution
   s. impedance

8.90 In Figure 2.19, what is the approximate amount of attenuation (dB) that can be tolerated by the instrument before imaging ceases (at the imaging depth)?
   a. 60
   b. 50
   c. 40
   d. 30
   e. 10

8.91 The approximate frequencies (MHz) for attenuations in soft tissue shown in Figure 2.16(*a* through *c*) are:
   a. 3.5, 7.5, 7.5
   b. 2, 4, 6
   c. 6, 4, 25
   d. 6, 2, 20
   e. 3, 1, 10

8.92 For a (flat) disk transducer element that is 13 mm in diameter, the lateral resolution at two times the near-zone length is:
   a. 6.5
   b. 13
   c. 19.5
   d. 26
   e. none of the above

8.93 As period increases, _____ increases.
   a. pulse duration
   b. frequency
   c. pulse repetition period

    d. amplitude

    e. intensity

8.94 As duty factor increases, _____ increases.

    a. SPPA intensity

    b. SAPA intensity

    c. SATA intensity

    d. frequency

    e. amplitude

8.95 As PRF increases, _____ increases.

    a. penetration

    b. SPPA intensity

    c. amplitude

    d. pulse duration

    e. frame rate

8.96 Which produces a sector display that comes to a point at the top?

    a. linear array

    b. convex array

    c. phased array

    d. annular array

    e. vector array

8.97 A typical dynamic range for ultrasound instruments is:

    a. 1540 m/s

    b. 2–10 MHz

    c. 3 dB

    d. 50 dB

    e. 0.5 dB/cm

8.98 To maintain a comparable width focus as it moves deeper, _____ must be increased.

    a. frequency

    b. aperture

    c. delays

    d. amplitude

    e. apodization

8.99 Find the words to complete the blanks below that are hidden in the puzzle (horizontally, vertically, or diagonally; forward or backward).

A _____ is a traveling variation in some quantity, such as pressure. _____ is the number of cycles of variation in a second. The spatial length of a cycle is called _____. _____ is the maximum variation from the normal value. Related to this is _____, which is power divided by area. A _____ is a few cycles of ultrasound. The weakening of a wave as it travels is called _____. It is composed of _____ (conversion of sound to

I	P	M	O	E	T	S	A	R	T	N	O	C	K	F	F	B	B	Z
Z	P	D	R	E	C	E	I	V	E	R	T	A	V	R	T	K	S	X
I	N	A	Z	A	I	L	G	C	U	F	K	E	P	H	L	A	V	
N	J	M	E	Q	R	D	N	E	U	H	C	Q	M	Q	U	Q	Y	Q
G	L	P	X	N	X	R	C	O	T	L	U	I	M	E	M	L	K	M
U	Q	L	A	M	O	H	A	G	S	E	X	J	K	A	M	R	S	X
R	U	I	X	T	O	H	N	Y	N	O	D	B	T	W	E	O	F	E
H	E	T	R	E	T	E	P	C	W	O	J	E	C	A	A	B	R	R
L	J	U	S	S	L	E	Y	O	A	I	I	R	T	P	L	V	Y	Y
M	G	D	I	E	L	T	N	F	R	V	B	T	Q	A	L	I	E	W
C	T	E	V	N	L	M	R	U	R	D	I	Z	P	H	I	S	T	L
D	Y	A	D	G	T	V	P	A	A	I	Y	T	P	R	G	L	A	Z
B	W	A	R	R	J	E	E	G	N	T	Z	H	A	J	O	N	M	T
E	Z	S	N	S	D	F	N	J	I	S	I	E	L	T	V	S	W	D
M	I	Q	B	B	P	D	T	S	X	N	D	O	J	Q	I	H	B	E
N	C	N	X	G	K	G	X	R	I	R	W	U	N	Y	Y	O	N	A
V	U	L	E	S	W	G	X	E	C	T	N	K	C	N	P	Z	N	E
X	R	T	E	M	P	O	R	A	L	J	Y	L	F	E	O	P	H	B
W	B	U	D	I	B	B	U	G	U	Q	F	T	J	B	R	P	R	X

heat) and _____; which represent anatomic structures on the display. A _____ converts voltage impulses or bursts to pressure pulses. An _____ transducer contains many piezoelectric elements. The ultrasound emitted by a scanhead propagates through a region of space called a _____. Pulse length and width determine _____ resolution. The _____ amplifies echoes, compensates for attenuation, and converts echoes from radio frequency to video form. A digital scan converter is a computer _____. The number of bits per pixel determines _____ resolution. The display is a _____. The number of frames displayed per second relates to _____ resolution. A _____ is used to detect and quantify transducer acoustic output. Heating and _____ are two mechanisms relevant to ultrasound bioeffects and safety.

Glossary

The terms defined here are also listed at the beginning and defined at the end of the chapter in which they are discussed.

A mode. Mode of operation in which the display records a spot deflection for each echo delivered from the receiver (no longer used).

Absorption. Conversion of sound to heat.

Acoustic. Having to do with sound.

Acoustic propagation properties. Characteristics of a medium that affect the propagation of sound through it.

Acoustic variables. Pressure, density, temperature, and particle motion; things that change with location and time in a sound wave.

Aliasing. Improper Doppler shift information from a pulsed Doppler or color flow instrument when true Doppler shift exceeds one half the pulse repetition frequency.

Amplification. The process of increasing small voltages to larger ones.

Amplifier. A device that accomplishes amplification.

Amplitude. Maximum variation of an acoustic variable or voltage.

Analog. Related to a procedure or system in which data are represented by continuously variable physical quantities (e.g., electric voltage).

Analog-to-digital converter (ADC). A device that converts voltage amplitude to a (digital) number.

Anechoic. Echo-free.

Annular. Ring-shaped.

Annular array. Array made up of ring-shaped elements arranged concentrically.

Aperture. Transducer width.

Apodization. Reduction of grating lobes by driving elements nonuniformly.

Array. Transducer array.

Attenuation. Decrease in amplitude and intensity as a wave travels through a medium.

Attenuation coefficient. Attenuation per centimeter of wave travel.

Autocorrelation. A rapid technique, used in color-flow instruments, for obtaining mean Doppler shift frequency.

Axial. In the direction of the transducer axis (sound-travel direction).

Axial resolution. Minimum reflector separation along the sound path that is required to produce separate echoes.

B mode. Mode of operation in which the display records a spot brightening for each echo pulse delivered from the receiver.

B scan. A brightness image that represents a cross section of an object through the scanning plane.

Backscatter. Sound scattered back in the direction from which it originally came.

Bandwidth. Range of frequencies contained in an ultrasound pulse; range of frequencies within which a material, device, or system can operate.

Beam. Region containing continuous-wave sound; region through which a sound pulse propagates.

Beam area. Cross-sectional area of a sound beam.

Beam former. The part of an instrument that accomplishes electronic beam scanning, apodization, steering, focusing, and aperture with arrays.

Bidirectional. Indicating Doppler instruments that are capable of distinguishing between positive and negative Doppler shifts (forward and reverse flow).

Bistable. Having two possible states (e.g., on or off; white or black).

Bistable display. Display in which all recorded spots have the same brightness.

Bit. Binary digit.

Burst. A cycle or two of voltage variation.

Burst-excited mode. Operative mode in which the transducer is driven by a burst from the pulser.

Cathode ray tube. A display device that produces an image by scanning an electron beam over a phosphor-coated screen.

Cavitation. Production and behavior of bubbles in sound.

Channel. An independent electronic path consisting of a separate transducer element and electronics (amplifier, delay, etc.).

Color-flow display. The presentation of two-dimensional, real-time Doppler or time shift information superimposed on a real-time, grayscale anatomic cross-sectional image. Flow directions toward and away from the transducer (i.e., positive and negative Doppler or time shifts) are presented as different colors on the display.

Comet tail. A series of closely spaced reverberation echoes.

Compensation. Equalization of received echo amplitude differences caused by attenuation.

Composite. Combination of a piezoelectric ceramic and a nonpiezoelectric polymer.

Compressibility. Ability of a material to be reduced to a smaller volume under external pressure.

Compression. Reduction in differences between small and large amplitudes; region of high density and pressure in a compressional wave.

Constructive interference. Combination of positive or negative pressures.

Continuous mode. Continuous-wave mode.

Continuous wave. A wave in which cycles repeat indefinitely; not pulsed.

Continuous-wave mode. Mode of operation in which continuous-wave sound is used.

Contrast resolution. Ability of a gray-scale display to distinguish between echoes of slightly different amplitude or intensity.

Convex array. Linear array with a curved (bowed out) shape.

cos. Abbreviation for cosine.

Cosine. The cosine of angle A in Figure 5.4 is the length of side b divided by the length of side c.

Coupling medium. Gel used to provide a good sound path between the transducer and the skin.

CRT. Cathode ray tube.

Crystal. Element.

Curie point. Temperature at which an element material loses its piezo-electric properties.

CW. Abbreviation for continuous wave.

Cycle. Complete variation of an acoustic variable.

Damping. Material placed behind the rear face of a transducer element to reduce pulse duration; also, the process of pulse duration reduction.

dB. Abbreviation for decibel.

Dead zone. Region close to the transducer in which imaging cannot be performed.

Decibel. Unit of power or intensity ratio; the number of decibels is 10 times the logarithm (to the base 10) of the power or intensity ratio.

Demodulation. Converting voltage pulses from RF to video form.

Density. Mass divided by volume.

Destructive interference. Combination of positive and negative pressures.

Detail resolution. Ability to image fine detail and to distinguish closely spaced reflectors. (See axial and lateral resolution.)

DGC. Depth gain compensation meaning, simply, compensation.

Digital. Related to a procedure or system in which data are represented by discrete units (numerical digits).

Digital scan converter. Computer memory that stores echo information.

Digital-to-analog converter (DAC). A device that converts a (digital) number to a proportional voltage amplitude.

Disk. Thin, flat, circular object.

Displacement. Distance that an object has moved.

Disturbed flow. Flow that cannot be described by straight, parallel streamlines.

Doppler angle. The angle between the sound beam and the flow direction.

Doppler effect. Frequency change of a reflected sound wave as a result of reflector motion relative to the transducer.

Doppler shift. Reflected frequency minus incident frequency.

Duplex. Combination of B-mode imaging and pulsed-wave Doppler.

Duty factor. Fraction of time that pulsed ultrasound is on.

Dynamic aperture. Aperture that increases with increasing focal length (to maintain constant focal width).

Dynamic focusing. Continuously variable receiving focus that follows the changing position of the transmitted pulse.

Dynamic imaging. Rapid-frame-sequence imaging; real-time imaging.

Dynamic range. Ratio (in decibels) of the largest power to the smallest power that a system can handle, or of the largest to the smallest intensity of a group of echoes.

Echo. Reflection.

Electric current. The rate of flow of electrons in an electric conductor.

Electric pulse. A brief excursion of electric voltage from its normal value impulse, usually zero.

Electric resistance. The characteristic of electric components that limits the electric current for a given voltage.

Electric resistor. A device that limits the electric current for a given voltage.

Electric voltage. Electric potential or potential difference expressed in volts.

Electricity. A form of energy associated with the displacement or flow of electrons.

Element. A small piece of piezoelectric material in a transducer assembly.

Energy. Capability of doing work.

Enhancement. Increase in echo amplitude from reflectors that lie behind a weakly attenuating structure.

External focus. A focus produced by a lens attached to a transducer element.

f number. Focal length divided by aperture.

Far zone. The region of a sound beam in which the beam diameter increases as the distance from the transducer increases; also called far field.

Fast Fourier transform. Rapid digital implementation of Fourier transform.

FFT. Fast Fourier transform.

Fluid. A material that flows and conforms to the shape of its container; a gas or liquid.

Focal length. Distance from a focused transducer to the center of a focal region or to the location of the spatial peak intensity.

Focal region. Region of minimum beam diameter and area.

Focal zone. Focal region.

Focus. The concentration of a sound beam into a smaller beam area than would exist otherwise.

Force. That which changes the state of rest or motion of an object.

Fourier transform. A mathematical technique for obtaining a Doppler frequency spectrum.

Fractional bandwidth. Bandwidth divided by operating frequency.

Frame. A single display image produced by one complete scan of the sound beam.

Frame rate. Number of frames displayed per unit of time.

Fraunhofer zone. Far zone.

Freeze frame. Constant display of the last frame entered into memory.

Frequency. Number of cycles per second.

Frequency spectrum. The range of frequencies present. In a Doppler instrument, the range of Doppler shift frequencies present in the returning echoes.

Fresnel zone. Near zone.

Gain. Ratio of output to input electrical power.

Generator gate. The electronic portion of a pulsed Doppler system that converts the continuous voltage of the voltage generator to a pulsed voltage.

Grating lobes. Additional minor beams of sound traveling out in directions different from the primary beam. These result from the multielement structure of transducer arrays.

Gray scale. Range of brightnesses between white and black.

Gray-scale display. Display in which several values of pixel brightness may be displayed.

Heat. Energy resulting from thermal molecular motion.

Hertz. Unit of frequency, one cycle per second; unit of pulse repetition frequency, one pulse per second; frame rate unit, one frame per second.

Hydrophone. A small transducer element mounted on the end of a narrow tube. Piezoelectric membrane with small metallic electrodes.

Hz. Abbreviation for hertz.

Impedance. Density multiplied by sound propagation speed.

Impulse. A brief excursion of electric voltage from its normal value, usually zero.

Incidence angle. Angle between incident sound direction and a line perpendicular to the boundary of the medium.

Intensity. Power divided by area.

Intensity reflection coefficient. Reflected intensity divided by incident intensity.

Intensity transmission coefficient. Transmitted intensity divided by incident intensity.

Interference. Combination of positive and/or negative pressures.

Internal focus. A focus produced by a curved transducer element.

kHz. Abbreviation for kilohertz.

Kilohertz. One thousand hertz.

Laminar flow. Flow in which fluid layers slide over each other to produce a parabolic flow speed profile.

Lateral. Perpendicular to the direction of sound travel.

Lateral resolution. Minimum reflector separation perpendicular to the sound path that is required to produce separate echoes.

Lead zirconate titonate. A ceramic piezoelectric material.

Lens. A curved material that focuses a sound beam.

Linear. Adjectival form of line.

Linear array. Array made up of rectangular elements in a line.

Linear phased array. Linear array operated by applying voltage pulses to all elements, but with small time differences to direct ultrasound pulses out in various directions.

Linear sequenced array. Linear array operated by applying voltage pulses to groups of elements sequentially.

log. Abbreviation for logarithm.

Logarithm. The logarithm (to the base of 10) of a number is equal to the number of tens that must be multiplied together to result in that number.

Longitudinal wave. Wave in which the particle motion is parallel to the direction of wave travel (compressional wave).

M mode. Mode of operation in which the display presents a spot brightening for each pulse delivered from the receiver, producing a two-dimensional recording of reflector position (motion) versus time.

Mass. Measure of an object's resistance to acceleration.

Matching layer. Material placed in front of the front face of a transducer element to reduce the reflection at the transducer surface.

Mechanical transducer. A transducer that contains moving parts and scans the sound beam with a motor drive.

Medium. Material through which a wave travels.

Megahertz. One million hertz.

MHz. Abbreviation for megahertz.

Mirror image. An artifactual image appearing on the opposite side of a strong reflector from the real structure.

Multipath. Paths to and from a reflector that are not the same.

Multiple reflection. Several reflections produced by a pulse encountering a pair of reflectors. Reverberation.

Near zone. The region of a sound beam in which the beam diameter decreases as the distance from the transducer increases; also called near field.

Noise. Thermally generated, random variations in a voltage signal.

Nyquist limit. The Doppler-shift frequency above which aliasing occurs; one half the pulse repetition frequency.

Oblique incidence. Sound direction that is not perpendicular to a medium's boundary.

Operating frequency. Preferred (maximum efficiency) frequency of operation of a transducer.

Parabolic flow. Laminar flow.

Particle. Small portion of a medium.

Particle motion. Displacement, speed, velocity, and acceleration of a particle.

Penetration. Imaging depth.

Period. Time per cycle.

Perpendicular. Geometrically related by 90 degrees.

Perpendicular incidence. Sound direction that is perpendicular to a medium's boundary.

Phantom. A tissue-equivalent material that has some characteristics representative of tissues (e.g., scattering or attenuation properties).

Phased array. An array that steers and focuses the beam electronically (with short time delays).

Phased linear array. A linear sequenced array that adds phasing to element group firing to focus or steer the ultrasound pulses.

Piezoelectricity. Conversion of pressure to electric voltage.

Pixel. Picture element; the unit into which imaging information is divided for storage and display in a digital instrument.

Plug flow. Flow with all fluid portions traveling with nearly the same flow speed and direction.

Polyvinylidene fluoride (PVDF). A piezoelectric thin film material.

Postprocessing. Signal processing done after memory.

Preprocessing. Signal processing (gain, time gain compensation, etc.) done before memory.

Power. Rate at which work is done; rate at which energy is transferred.

Pressure. Force divided by area.

PRF. Pulse repetition frequency.

Probe. Transducer assembly.

Propagation. Progression or travel.

Propagation speed. Speed with which a wave moves through a medium.

Pulsatile flow. Flow that accelerates and decelerates with each cardiac cycle.

Pulse. A brief excursion of a quantity from its normal value; a few cycles.

Pulse duration. The time from the beginning to the end of a pulse.

Pulse-echo diagnostic ultrasound. Ultrasound imaging in which pulses are reflected and used to produce a display.

Pulse repetition frequency. Number of pulses per second; sometimes called pulse repetition rate.

Pulse repetition period. The time from the beginning of one pulse to the beginning of the next.

Pulsed mode. Mode of operation in which pulsed ultrasound is used.

Pulsed ultrasound. Ultrasound produced in pulse form by applying electric pulses to the transducer.

PVDF. Polyvinylidene fluoride.

PW. Pulsed wave.

PZT. Lead zirconate titanate.

Q factor. Quality factor.

Quality factor. Operating frequency divided by bandwidth.

Range ambiguity. Improper placement of late echoes (from a previous pulse) received after the next pulse is emitted.

Range equation. Relationship between round-trip pulse travel time, propagation speed, and distance to a reflector.

Rarefaction. Region of low density and pressure in a compressional wave.

Rayl. Unit of impedance.

Real-time. Imaging with a rapid-frame-sequence display.

Real-time display. A display that continuously images moving structures or a changing scan plane.

Receiver gate. A device that allows only echoes from a selected depth (arrival time) to pass.

Rectification. Conversion from an alternating (reversing) to a direct (one-way) form of voltage.

Reflection. Portion of sound returned from a boundary of a medium.

Reflection angle. Angle between reflected sound direction and a line perpendicular to the boundary of a medium.

Reflector. Medium boundary that produces a reflection; reflecting surface.

Refraction. Change of sound direction upon passing from one medium to another.

Rejection. Elimination of small-amplitude voltage pulses.

Resolution. The ability to separate in space, time, or strength (detail, temporal, and contrast resolutions, respectively).

Resonance frequency. Operating frequency.

Reverberation. Multiple reflection.

Radio frequency. Voltages representing echoes in cyclic form.

RF. Radio frequency

Sample volume. Region of tissue from which pulsed Doppler echoes are accepted.

Scan converter. A device that stores imaging information in one scanning format and reads it out for display in another.

Scanhead. Transducer assembly.

Scan line. A line produced on a display that represents the echoes from a pulse.

Scanning. The sweeping of a sound beam to produce an image.

Scatterer. An object that scatters sound because of its small size or its surface roughness.

Scattering. Diffusion or redirection of sound in several directions upon encountering a particle suspension or a rough surface.

Section thickness. Thickness of the scanned tissue volume perpendicular to the scan plane.

Sector. A geometric figure bounded by two radii and the arc of a circle included between them.

Sensitivity. Ability of an imaging system to detect weak echoes.

Shadowing. Reduction in echo amplitude from reflectors that lie behind a strongly reflecting or attenuating structure.

Shock-excited mode. Mode of operation in which the transducer is driven by an impulse from the pulser.

Side lobes. Minor beams of sound traveling out from a single-element transducer in a direction different from that of the primary beam.

Sound. Traveling wave of acoustic variables.

Sound beam. The region of a medium that contains virtually all of the sound produced by a transducer.

Spatial pulse length. Length of space over which a pulse occurs.

Speckle. The granular appearance of images caused by the interference of echoes from the distribution of scatterers in tissue.

Spectral analysis. Use of fast Fourier transform to determine Doppler-shift frequency range several times each second.

Spectral broadening. The widening of the Doppler-shift spectrum; i.e., an increase in the range of Doppler shift frequencies present as a result of a broader range of flow velocities encountered by the sound beam. This occurs with normal flow in small vessels and with turbulent flow in any vessel.

Specular reflection. Reflection from a large, flat, smooth boundary.

Speed. Displacement divided by the time over which displacement occurs.

Speed error. A propagation speed that is different from the assumed value (1.54 mm/μs).

Stiffness. Property of a medium; applied pressure divided by the fractional volume change produced by the pressure.

Strength. Nonspecific term referring to amplitude or intensity.

Temperature. Condition of a body that determines transfer of heat to or from other bodies.

Temporal resolution. Ability to distinguish closely spaced events in time; improves with increased frame rate.

Test object. A device without tissue-like properties that is designed to measure some characteristic of an imaging system.

TGC. Time gain compensation.

Time gain compensation. Compensation.

Transducer. Device that converts energy from one form to another.

Transducer array. Transducer assembly containing many transducer elements.

Transducer assembly. Transducer elements with damping and matching materials assembled in a case.

Transducer element. Piece of piezoelectric material in a transducer assembly.

Transmission angle. Angle between the transmitted sound direction and a line perpendicular to the boundary of a medium.

Turbulence. Random, chaotic, multidirectional flow of a fluid.

Turbulent flow. See turbulence.

Ultrasound. Sound having a frequency greater than 20 kHz.

Ultrasound transducer. Device that converts electric energy to ultrasound energy and vice versa.

Variable focusing. Transmit focus with various focal lengths.

Variance. Spread around a mean value.

Vector array. Linear sequenced array that emits pulses from different starting points and (by phasing) in different directions.

Velocity. Speed, with direction of motion specified.

Video. Demodulated amplitude voltages representing echoes.

Viscosity. Resistance of a fluid to flow.

Voltage pulse. Brief excursion of voltage from its normal value.

Wave. Traveling variation of wave variables.

Wave variables. Things that are functions of space and time in a wave.

Wavelength. Length of space over which a cycle occurs.

Work. Force multiplied by displacement.

ANSWERS TO EXERCISES

Chapter 1

1.1 pulses, ultrasound, echoes, image
1.2 pulse, echo
1.3 strength
1.4 parallel
1.5 origin (starting point)
1.6 rectangular
1.7 slice, pie
1.8 pulse, echo, location, strength, location, brightness

Chapter 2

2.1.1 wave variables
2.1.2 acoustic variables
2.1.3 20,000
2.1.4 pressure, density, temperature, particle motion
2.1.5 c, d, e
2.1.6 a, e
2.1.7 cycles
2.1.8 hertz, Hz
2.1.9 time
2.1.10 frequency
2.1.11 space
2.1.12 wave
2.1.13 propagation speed, frequency
2.1.14 density, stiffness
2.1.15 e
2.1.16 1540, 1.54

2.1.17 e
2.1.18 a, c, b
2.1.19 0.22
2.1.20 decreases
2.1.21 10
2.1.22 higher
2.1.23 d (fastest in solids)
2.1.24 b
2.1.25 higher
2.1.26 mechanical longitudinal
2.1.27 doubled
2.1.28 1
2.1.29 unchanged (determined by the medium)
2.1.30 energy, information
2.1.31 e
2.1.32 false
2.1.33 true
2.1.34 1,540,000 (propagation speed is 1540 m/s)
2.1.35 true
2.1.36 true
2.1.37 density, propagation speed
2.1.38 a. 0.1 μs, 10 MHz; b. 0.25 μs, 4 MHz
2.1.39 1.54
2.1.40 0.38
  2.2.1 continuous wave
  2.2.2 pulses
  2.2.3 pulses
  2.2.4 pulses
  2.2.5 period
  2.2.6 decreases
  2.2.7 time
  2.2.8 length, space
  2.2.9 duty factor
2.2.10 period
2.2.11 wavelength
2.2.12 1 (100 per cent)
2.2.13 6
2.2.14 2
2.2.15 1.3 (period is 0.33 μs; soft tissue is irrelevant)
2.2.16 1
2.2.17 0.0013 (0.13 per cent)
2.2.18 d
2.2.19 e (answer is 50,000)

2.2.20 c
2.2.21 less than
 2.3.1 variation
 2.3.2 power, area
 2.3.3 W/cm^2 or mW/cm^2
 2.3.4 amplitude
 2.3.5 doubled
 2.3.6 halved
 2.3.7 unchanged
 2.3.8 quadrupled
 2.3.9 5
2.3.10 100
2.3.11 temporal, average
2.3.12 b
2.3.13 100
2.3.14 2
2.3.15 3, 4
2.3.16 amplitude, intensity
2.3.17 absorption, reflection, scattering
2.3.18 centimeter
2.3.19 dB, dB/cm
2.3.20 0.5
2.3.21 1.5 dB/cm
2.3.22 increases
2.3.23 doubled, doubled, quadrupled
2.3.24 unchanged
2.3.25 sound, heat
2.3.26 no (absorption is one part of attenuation)
2.3.27 higher
2.3.28 50, 50, 80
2.3.29 5
2.3.30 2.5
2.3.31 frequency
2.3.32 decreases
2.3.33 0.32 (intensity ratio is 0.16)
2.3.34 0.00000002
2.3.35 c ($0.5 \times 7.5 \times 0.8 = 3$ dB)
2.3.36 a. 1; b. -1; c. 2; d. -3
2.3.37 6 dB (intensity ratio is 0.25)
2.3.38 20, 4
2.3.39 1.9
 2.4.1 impedances
 2.4.2 impedances, intensity

2.4.3 impedances
2.4.4 0.0008, 1.9992
2.4.5 0.0002, 1.9998
2.4.6 0.0008, 1.9992
2.4.7 0.01, 1 (incident intensity not needed)
2.4.8 0.99, 99
2.4.9 20 (intensity ratio of 0.01; use Table 2.3)
2.4.10 0.01
2.4.11 0 (impedances are equal)
2.4.12 5, 0 (total reflection)
2.4.13 true, for perpendicular incidence
2.4.14 false, in general (true only if propagation speeds are also equal)
2.4.15 false, in general (true only if densities are also equal)
2.4.16 false
2.4.17 0.9990
2.4.18 air, reflection
2.4.19 0.01
2.4.20 0.43
2.4.21 d
2.4.22 direction, propagation speed
2.4.23 larger than, equal to
2.4.24 smaller than, equal to
2.4.25 equal to, equal to
2.4.26 30, 21
2.4.27 30, 30
2.4.28 30, 39
2.4.29 0.04 (incidence angle and intensity are not needed; the propaga-
       tion speeds are equal, so that the calculation is the same as with
       perpendicular incidence)
2.4.30 0.2 (no refraction; calculate as with perpendicular incidence)
2.4.31 perpendicular incidence, media propagation speeds are equal
2.4.32 media propagation speeds are equal (no refraction)
2.4.33 density, propagation speed
2.4.34 32
2.4.35 1.7
2.4.36 scattering
2.4.37 true
2.4.38 false
2.4.39 a
2.4.40 true
2.4.41 c
2.4.42 pulses, echoes, display
2.4.43 propagation speed, time

2.4.44 4
2.4.45 7
2.4.46 7.7
2.4.47 1
2.4.48 3 cm
2.4.49 10
2.4.50 65 μs
 2.5.1 a
 2.5.2 e
 2.5.3 a. 4; b. 1; c. 3; d. 5; e. 2
 2.5.4 a. 1; b. 2; c. 3
 2.5.5 a. 3; b. 4, c. 1; d. 2; e. 6; f. 5
 2.5.6 a. 3; b. 4; c. 1; d. 2; e. 1; f. 10; g. 11; h. 5; i. 8; j. 7; k. 6; l. 9
 2.5.7 a. 1; b. 2, 3; c. 3; d. 1; e. 2
 2.5.8 a. 1.54; b. 0.77; c. 3.1; d. 0.5; e. 2; f. 1; g. 0.002; h. 500; i. 1; j. 3.0;
        k. 3; l. 0.5; m. 0.5; n. 0.25; o. 250; p. 125; q. 1,630,000
 2.5.9 c
2.5.10 a
2.5.11 increased
2.5.12 100 μs, 50 μs, 0.5, 10 kHz, 17 μs, 59 kHz
2.5.13 propagation speeds, equal
2.5.14 d
2.5.15 e
2.5.16 d
2.5.17 0.04
2.5.18 impedances
2.5.19 densities or impedances, propagation speeds
2.5.20 18
2.5.21 23
2.5.22 false
2.5.23 80 (9-dB increase)

Chapter 3

3.1.1 energy
3.1.2 electric, ultrasound
3.1.3 piezoelectricity
3.1.4 disks
3.1.5 thickness
3.1.6 element, assembly
3.1.7 element, assembly
3.1.8 pulses, frequency

3.1.9 pulses, thickness
3.1.10 decreases
3.1.11 cycles, axial resolution, bandwidth, quality (Q) factor
3.1.12 efficiency, sensitivity
3.1.13 one, three
3.1.14 0.2
3.1.15 e
3.1.16 reflection
3.1.17 air
3.1.18 e (unitless)
3.1.19 false
3.1.20 frequencies
3.1.21 c
3.1.22 a. 3; b. 0.33 (33 per cent); c. 2.5; d. 3.5; e. 3
3.1.23 rectangles
3.1.24 probes, scanheads
3.1.25 resonance frequency
3.1.26 composites
3.1.27 burst excitation
3.1.28 no (because these frequencies are outside the 2.5-MHz band-width [3.75–6.25 MHz])
3.2.1 4
3.2.2 near, far
3.2.3 near-zone
3.2.4 frequency or wavelength, diameter, distance
3.2.5 transducer diameter, frequency
3.2.6 wavelength
3.2.7 one half
3.2.8 two
3.2.9 decreases
3.2.10 increases
3.2.11 increases
3.2.12 c
3.2.13 30
3.2.14 3, 6, 9
3.2.15 longer
3.2.16 shorter
3.2.17 false
3.2.18 c
3.2.19 quadruples
3.2.20 doubles
3.2.21 doubled

3.2.22 e (all of the above)
3.2.23 false
3.2.24 focal length
3.2.25 c
3.2.26 b (wavelength is 0.3 mm; f number is 2)
3.2.27 a. 3; b. 2; c. 2; d. 1; e. 1
 3.3.1 element
 3.3.2 linear, convex, annular
 3.3.3 sequencing
 3.3.4 a. 1; b. 2, 3; c. 2, 3; d. 3, 1, 2; e. 1, 3; f. 1; g. 3; h. 1, 2, 3
 3.3.5 one
 3.3.6 two
 3.3.7 motor drive
 3.3.8 a. 1; b. 2; c. 2
 3.3.9 b
3.3.10 a
3.3.11 c
3.3.12 a, c, f
3.3.13 b, d, e
3.3.14 c
3.3.15 the same, different
3.3.16 different
3.3.17 convex, vector
 3.4.1 sound travel or scan line, echoes
 3.4.2 spatial pulse length
 3.4.3 true
 3.4.4 1.5
 3.4.5 1
 3.4.6 0.77, 0.15
 3.4.7 halved
 3.4.8 doubled
 3.4.9 false
3.4.10 false
3.4.11 2
3.4.12 10 (less than 10 MHz in many applications)
3.4.13 wavelength, spatial pulse length
3.4.14 attenuation
3.4.15 separation, echoes
3.4.16 beam width
3.4.17 c, d, f
3.4.18 true
3.4.19 true

3.4.20 false, in general (only true near the transducer)
3.4.21 b, c, e, f
 3.5.1 a. 4; b. 3; c. 2; d. 1
 3.5.2 a, d
 3.5.3 a. 10; b. 0.31; c. 14; d. 6.5; e. 13; f. 14
 3.5.4 c
 3.5.5 one half, near-zone
 3.5.6 focal
 3.5.7 6.5 (frequency not needed)
 3.5.8 0.7 (size not needed)
 3.5.9 true
3.5.10 false
3.5.11 focal
3.5.12 true
3.5.13 false
3.5.14 a. 1, 2, 3; b. 2; c. 2; d. 1
3.5.15 a
3.5.16 e
3.5.17 a
3.5.18 b, c, d
3.5.19 true
3.5.20 resolution, penetration
3.5.21 2, 10
3.5.22 0.5, 1.5
3.5.23 3 mm, 2 mm
3.5.24 4 cm
3.5.25 2 or 3 mm
3.5.26 a. 4; b. 1; c. 4; d. 3; e. 5; f. 4; g. 2

Chapter 4

4.1.1 pulse or burst
4.1.2 amplitude, intensity
4.1.3 a (an echo reception time of 130 μs is required)
4.2.1 amplification, compensation, compression, demodulation, rejection
4.2.2 a. 2; b. 5; c. 3; d. 1; e. 4
4.2.3 10, 100, 20
4.2.4 1
4.2.5 10
4.2.6 b, e
4.2.7 depth, distance

4.2.8 times
4.2.9 dynamic, eyes
4.2.10 2.0
4.2.11 RF, video
4.2.12 false
4.2.13 a
4.2.14 zero, linearly, higher, weaker
4.2.15 30
4.2.16 50, 75, 87.5
4.2.17 20
4.2.18 10
4.2.19 40
4.2.20 32
4.2.21 45, 32,000
4.2.22 −2, 2, 0.63
4.3.1 a. 6; b. 9; c. 10; d. 13; e. 14
4.3.2 a (43/32)
4.3.3 c (45/64)
4.3.4 a. 5; b. 3; c. 2; d. 6; e. 1; f. 4
4.3.5 e
4.3.6 a. 4; b. 5; c. 6; d. 7; e. 8
4.3.7 50,000
4.3.8 c
4.3.9 e
4.3.10 a
4.3.11 two
4.3.12 bit
4.3.13 two
4.3.14 a. 3; b. 7; c. 8; d. 5; e. 4; f. 2; g. 1; h. 6
4.3.15 25
4.3.16 1101
4.3.17 a. 5; b. 10; c. 3; d. 1; e. 9; f. 2; g. 8; h. 7; i. 4; j. 6
4.3.18 a. 1 (0); b. 1 (1); c. 3 (101); d. 4 (1010); e. 5 (11001); f. 5 (11110);
    g. 6 (111111); h. 7 (1000000); i. 7 (1001011); j. 7 (1100100)
4.3.19 a. 3 (111); b. 4 (1111); c. 2 (11); d. 9 (111111111); e. 10
    (1111111111); f. 6 (111111); g. 8 (11111111); h. 1 (1); i. 7
    (1111111); j. 5 (11111)
4.3.20 a. 1 (0, 1); b. 2 (00, 01, 10, 11); c. 3 (000, 001, 010, 011, 100, 101,
    110, 111); d. 4; e. 4; f. 5; g. 5; h. 6; i. 7; j. 7
4.4.1 B, M (brightness and motion)
4.4.2 a. 1, 2, 4; b. 2, 3, 5
4.4.3 cathode ray
4.4.4 deflection

4.4.5 electromagnetic
4.4.6 M
4.4.7 scanning
4.4.8 gray-scale, B-mode
4.4.9 scan converter
4.4.10 c
4.4.11 d
4.4.12 33
4.4.13 63
4.4.14 a. 1; b. 2; c. 2; d. 2; e. 2; f. 2
4.4.15 40
4.4.16 1200
4.4.17 true (10 × 1 × 100 × 30 = 30,000 [<77,000])
4.4.18 c
4.5.1 pulser, beam former, transducer, receiver, memory, display
4.5.2 a. 4; b. 1; c. 2; d. 5; e. 3
4.5.3 a. 2; b. 2; c. 2, 3; d. 3; e. 1; f. 1; g. 2; h. 1, 2; i. 2, 3; j. 2, 3; k. 1, 2; l. 1, 2; m. 2, 3; n. 2, 3; o. 1, 2; p. 1, 2
4.5.4 a
4.5.5 b
4.5.6 d
4.5.7 c
4.5.8 d
4.5.9 c
4.5.10 b
4.5.11 b
4.5.12 d
4.5.13 2, 60
4.5.14 b
4.5.15 echoes
4.5.16 pulse-echo
4.5.17 brightness
4.5.18 strength, direction, time
4.5.19 b
4.5.20 display, voltages
4.5.21 receiver
4.5.22 pulser
4.5.23 receiver
4.5.24 a
4.5.25 f
4.5.26 transducer
4.5.27 e
4.5.28 c

4.5.29 d
4.5.30 c
4.5.31 b
4.5.32 a
4.5.33 false
4.5.34 M
4.5.35 B
4.5.36 mechanical, electronic
4.5.37 frame
4.5.38 pulsed
4.5.39 lines, frame
4.5.40 frame rate
4.5.41 increase
4.5.42 improved, decreases, increased
4.5.43 $512 \times 512 = 262{,}144$
4.5.44 b; a, c
4.5.45 $1000/20 = 50$ lines per frame (one scan line for each pulse)

Chapter 5

5.1.1 b
5.1.2 difference
5.1.3 a
5.1.4 pressure, resistance
5.1.5 a
5.1.6 decreases
5.1.7 vessels
5.1.8 d
5.1.9 b
5.1.10 e
5.1.11 e
5.1.12 disturbed
5.1.13 turbulent
5.1.14 stenosis
5.1.15 d
5.1.16 a
5.1.17 d, g
5.1.18 a, b, f
5.1.19 c, d, e, f, g
5.2.1 frequency or wavelength, motion
5.2.2 higher
5.2.3 lower

5.2.4 equal to
5.2.5 motion
5.2.6 0.02, 1.02
5.2.7 0.026
5.2.8 -0.026
5.2.9 reflected or echo, incident or operating
5.2.10 cosine
5.2.11 0.01, 1.01 (the Doppler shift is cut in half)
5.2.12 0, 1.00 (no Doppler shift at 90 degrees)
5.2.13 110
5.2.14 0.8
5.2.15 0
5.2.16 20
5.2.17 presence, direction, speed, character
5.3.1 false
5.3.2 direction, bidirectional
5.3.3 false
5.3.4 voltage generator, source transducer, receiving transducer, receiver, loudspeaker, memory, display
5.3.5 fast Fourier transform
5.3.6 Doppler shift, time
5.3.7 gray, color
5.3.8 flow velocities
5.3.9 true
5.3.10 gates, transducer elements
5.3.11 continuous, burst
5.3.12 depths, arrival times
5.3.13 false
5.3.14 true
5.4.1 flow, anatomy
5.4.2 e
5.4.3 time
5.4.4 autocorrelation, mean
5.4.5 d
5.4.6 false
5.4.7 b
5.4.8 c
5.4.9 false
5.4.10 false
5.5.1 Doppler shift
5.5.2 false
5.5.3 two
5.5.4 frequencies

5.5.5 false
5.5.6 motion, cosine
5.5.7 gate
5.5.8 display
5.5.9 gate, voltage generator
5.5.10 depth
5.5.11 fast Fourier
5.5.12 false
5.5.13 true
5.5.14 2.6
5.5.15 b
5.5.16 Doppler, flow
5.5.17 frequency
5.5.18 d

Chapter 6

6.1 5.1
6.2 77
6.3 c
6.4 false
6.5 a
6.6 e (a, b, d)
6.7 false. This is the display of the interference pattern (speckle) of scattered sound from the distribution of scatterers in the tissue.
6.8 section-thickness
6.9 c, d, e, f
6.10 true
6.11 6.4b
6.12 a. 1; b. 2, 3; c. 3; d. 4, 5; e. 4, 5; f. 2, 4
6.13 separation
6.14 weaker
6.15 b
6.16 d
6.17 true
6.18 b
6.19 b
6.20 b
6.21 c
6.22 refraction (double image)
6.23 e
6.24 e (c and d)

6.25 e
6.26 a
6.27 true
6.28 continuous-wave
6.29 red, blue, blue, red

Chapter 7

7.1 phantom, test object
7.2 a. 1, 3; b. 1, 3; c. 1; d. 1; e. 4; f. 2; g. 2; h. 2; i. 5; j. 5
7.3 a. 4; b. 5; c. 3; d. 3; e. 1; f. 2; g. 1, 2
7.4 true
7.5 true
7.6 string
7.7 flow, flow
7.8 e
7.9 tissues
7.10 false
7.11 b, c, d, e
7.12 false
7.13 transducer or piezoelectric
7.14 true
7.15 b
7.16 a. 2, 12; b. 3, 12; c. 3, 8; d. 4 or 2, 9; e. 1, 7; f. 6, 10; g. 6, 11
7.17 c
7.18 e
7.19 a
7.20 d
7.21 a
7.22 b
7.23 c
7.24 false
7.25 d
7.26 e
7.27 e (a, b, c)
7.28 false
7.29 false
7.30 b
7.31 no
7.32 yes
7.33 b and d
7.34 c

7.35 e
7.36 e
7.37 e
7.38 a
7.39 d
7.40 b
7.41 e
7.42 c, d, e
7.43 b
7.44 a, b, d
7.45 e (pregnancy possibility in fertile female)
7.46 b
7.47 a

Chapter 8

8.1 a
8.2 c
8.3 d
8.4 e
8.5 e
8.6 a
8.7 a
8.8 c
8.9 c (ophthalmic and intravascular are higher)
8.10 false (only true near the transducer)
8.11 false (only true for perpendicular incidence or oblique incidence
      when densities and propagation speeds of the media are equal)
8.12 false (see comment for 8.11)
8.13 c
8.14 d
8.15 c
8.16 d
8.17 false (6 bits)
8.18 d
8.19 d
8.20 e (b and d)
8.21 a
8.22 b
8.23 c
8.24 d (areas are 284 and 3 mm^2)
8.25 c

8.26 d
8.27 e
8.28 c
8.29 a
8.30 d
8.31 c
8.32 c
8.33 b
8.34 b
8.35 a
8.36 a
8.37 a
8.38 a
8.39 c
8.40 b
8.41 c
8.42 d
8.43 c
8.44 c
8.45 e (a and d)
8.46 c
8.47 d
8.48 false
8.49 b
8.50 c
8.51 See p. 357
8.52 See p. 358
8.53 See p. 359
8.54 See p. 359
8.55 a
8.56 e
8.57 a
8.58 a
8.59 b
8.60 d
8.61 b
8.62 a, b, c, d, e
8.63 c
8.64 c
8.65 d
8.66 e (a, b, c)
8.67 d
8.68 b

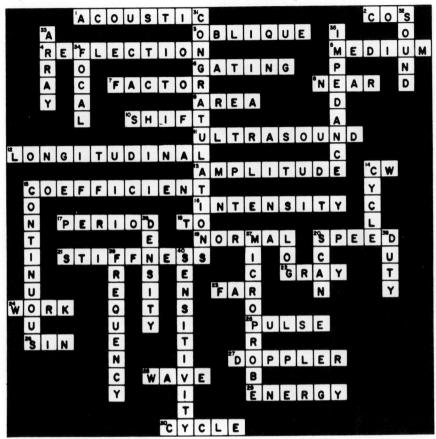

Exercise 8.51

8.69 c

8.70 d

8.71 a

8.72 false

8.73 false

8.74 e

8.75 b

8.76 a. 2; b. 2; c. 1.5 mm; d. 3 mm; e. 10 μs; f. 100 kHz; g. 2 μs; h. 1 μs; i. 1 MHz; j. 0.2; k. 1.5 mm/μs

8.77 10, 1, 0.01, 0.01, 0.001

8.78 c, a, b, b

8.79 longer; longer; none; b; a, b, and d

8.80 pulsed, 1.5, 1.5, 3

8.81 1, 1, 2, continuous-wave, 1.54

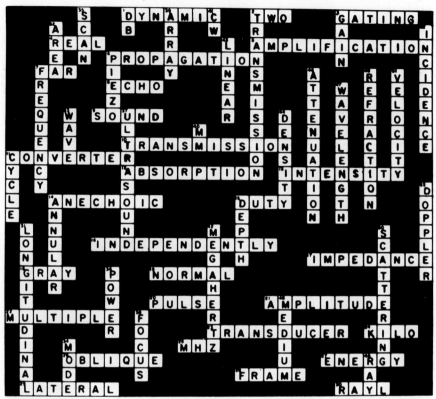

Exercise 8.52

8.82 e
8.83 attenuation, 6, 2, 4
8.84 b
8.85 c
8.86 a
8.87 b
8.88 c
8.89 a, b, g, k, l, o, q, r (improved)
8.90 c
8.91 d
8.92 b
8.93 a
8.94 c
8.95 e

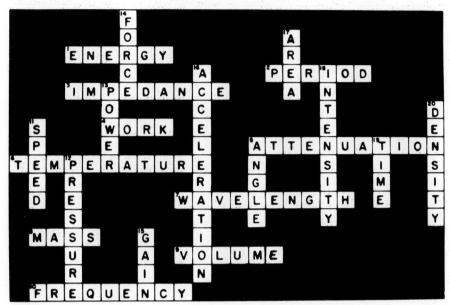

Exercise 8.53

START

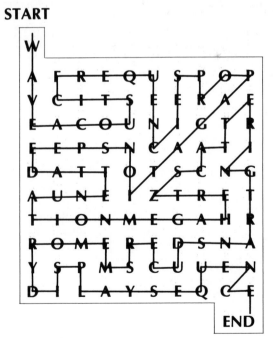

END

Exercise 8.54

8.96 c
8.97 d
8.98 b
8.99

```
. . . . . T S A R T N O C . . F . . .
. . . R E C E I V E R . . . R . . . .
. . A . A . . . . . . . E P . . . .
. . M E . R . . E . H . Q M . U . . .
. . P . N . R C . T . U . M E . L . .
. . L A . O H A G . E . . . A M . S .
. . I . T O H N Y N . D . . W E O . E
. . T . E T E P C . O . E . . A B R .
. . U S . L E Y O A . I . T . . V . Y
. . D I E . T N . R V . T . A . . E .
. . E V N . . R U . D I . P . I . . .
. . A . . T . . A A . Y T . R L . . .
. W . . . . E . . N T . H A . O . . .
. . . . . . N . . S I . . T . S . . .
. . . . . . T S . . D O . . I . B .
. . . . . . . R I . . U N . . O . A
. . . . . . . . C T . . C . . . N .
. . T E M P O R A L . Y . . E . . . .
. . . . . . . . . . . . . . R . . .
```

APPENDIX A
SYMBOLS, ABBREVIATIONS, AND EQUATIONS

The following symbols and abbreviations are used in the equations in this appendix and those in Chapters 2 through 5.

a	attenuation
a_c	attenuation coefficient
A	area
A_B	beam area
BW	bandwidth
c	sound propagation speed
c_m	transducer element material propagation speed
d	distance to reflector
D_B	beam diameter
D_T	transducer diameter
DF	duty factor
f	frequency
f_D	Doppler shift
f_o	operating frequency
f_e	echo frequency
FR	frame rate
I	intensity, current
I_i	incident intensity
I_r	reflected intensity
I_{SA}	spatial average intensity
I_{SP}	spatial peak intensity
I_{TA}	temporal average intensity
I_{PA}	pulse average intensity
IRC	intensity reflection coefficient
ITC	intensity transmission coefficient
L	path length
LPF	lines per frame
n	number of cycles in a pulse
NF	number of focuses

NZL	near-zone length
P	power, penetration
PD	pulse duration
PRF	pulse repetition frequency
PRP	pulse repetition period
Q	quality factor
R	resistance
R_A	axial resolution
R_L	lateral resolution
SPL	spatial pulse length
t	time, pulse round-trip time
T	period
v	reflector speed
w	transducer thickness
z	impedance
λ	wavelength
ρ	density
θ	Doppler angle
θ_i	incidence angle
θ_r	reflection angle
θ_t	transmission angle

For convenient reference, 35 equations relevant to material in this book are compiled here. One asterisk over the equals symbol indicates that the equation is specifically for soft tissues. Two asterisks over the equals symbol indicate that the equation is specifically for perpendicular incidence. The 12 most fundamental and important equations (that appear in the text) are indicated with arrows ($\leftarrow$).

Chapter 2

$$\text{period } (\mu s) = \frac{1}{\text{frequency (MHz)}} \qquad T = \frac{1}{f}$$

$$\text{wavelength (mm)} = \frac{\text{propagation speed (mm/}\mu s)}{\text{frequency (MHz)}} \qquad \lambda = \frac{c}{f} \qquad \leftarrow$$

$$\text{wavelength (mm)} \overset{*}{=} \frac{1.54}{\text{frequency (MHz)}} \qquad \lambda \overset{*}{=} \frac{1.54}{f}$$

$$\underset{\text{(rayl)}}{\text{impedance}} = \underset{\text{(kg/m}^3)}{\text{density}} \times \underset{\text{speed (m/s)}}{\text{propagation}} \qquad z = \rho c \qquad \leftarrow$$

$$\frac{\text{pulse repetition}}{\text{period (ms)}} = \frac{1}{\text{pulse repetition frequency (kHz)}} \qquad PRP = \frac{1}{PRF}$$

$$\frac{\text{pulse}}{\text{duration } (\mu s)} = \frac{\text{number of cycles}}{\text{in the pulse}} \times \text{period } (\mu s) \qquad PD = nT$$

$$\frac{\text{pulse}}{\text{duration } (\mu s)} = \frac{\text{number of cycles in the pulse}}{\text{frequency (MHz)}} \qquad PD = \frac{n}{f}$$

$$\frac{\text{duty}}{\text{factor}} = \frac{\text{pulse duration } (\mu s)}{\text{pulse repetition period (ms)} \times 1000} \qquad DF = \frac{PD}{PRP \times 1000} \qquad \leftarrow$$

$$\frac{\text{duty}}{\text{factor}} = \frac{\text{pulse duration } (\mu s) \times \dfrac{\text{pulse repetition}}{\text{frequency (kHz)}}}{1000} \qquad DF = \frac{PD \times PRF}{1000}$$

$$\frac{\text{spatial pulse}}{\text{length (mm)}} = \frac{\text{number of cycles in the pulse}}{\times \text{wavelength (mm)}} \qquad SPL = n\lambda$$

$$\frac{\text{spatial pulse}}{\text{length (mm)}} = \frac{\begin{array}{c}\text{number of cycles in the pulse}\\ \times \text{ propagation speed (mm/}\mu s)\end{array}}{\text{frequency (MHz)}} \qquad SPL = \frac{nc}{f}$$

$$\frac{\text{spatial pulse}}{\text{length (mm)}} \overset{*}{=} \frac{\begin{array}{c}\text{number of cycles}\\ \text{in the pulse} \times 1.54\end{array}}{\text{frequency (MHz)}} \qquad SPL \overset{*}{=} \frac{n \times 1.54}{f}$$

$$\text{intensity (W/cm}^2) = \frac{\text{power (W)}}{\text{area (cm}^2)} \qquad I = \frac{P}{A} \qquad \leftarrow$$

$$\frac{\text{temporal average}}{\text{intensity (W/cm}^2)} = \frac{\text{duty factor} \times \text{pulse}}{\text{average intensity (W/cm}^2)} \qquad I_{TA} = DF \times I_{PA}$$

$$\text{attenuation (dB)} = \frac{\text{attenuation coefficient (dB/cm)}}{\times \text{ path length (cm)}} \qquad a = a_o L$$

$$\text{attenuation (dB)} \overset{*}{=} \tfrac{1}{2} \times \frac{\text{frequency (MHz)} \times}{\text{path length (cm)}} \qquad a \overset{*}{=} \tfrac{1}{2}fL \qquad \leftarrow$$

$$\begin{array}{l}\text{intensity reflection}\\ \text{coefficient}\end{array} = \dfrac{\text{reflected intensity (W/cm}^2)}{\text{incident intensity (W/cm}^2)} \qquad \text{IRC} = \dfrac{I_r}{I_i}$$

$$\overset{**}{=} \left[\dfrac{\begin{array}{l}\text{medium two impedance}\\ -\ \text{medium one impedance}\end{array}}{\begin{array}{l}\text{medium two impedance}\\ +\ \text{medium one impedance}\end{array}} \right]^2 \quad \overset{**}{=} \left[\dfrac{z_2 - z_1}{z_2 + z_1} \right]^2 \qquad \leftarrow$$

$$\begin{array}{l}\text{intensity transmission}\\ \text{coefficient}\end{array} = \dfrac{\text{transmitted intensity (W/cm}^2)}{\text{incident intensity (W/cm}^2)} \qquad \text{ITC} = \dfrac{I_t}{I_i}$$

$$\overset{**}{=} 1 - \text{intensity reflection coefficient} \qquad \overset{**}{=} 1 - \text{IRC} \qquad \leftarrow$$

$$\text{reflection angle (°)} = \text{incidence angle (°)} \qquad \theta_r = \theta_i$$

$$\begin{array}{l}\text{transmission}\\ \text{angle (°)}\end{array} = \begin{array}{l}\text{incidence}\\ \text{angle (°)}\end{array} \times \left[\dfrac{\begin{array}{c}\text{medium two}\\ \text{propagation speed (mm/}\mu\text{s)}\end{array}}{\begin{array}{c}\text{medium one}\\ \text{propagation speed (mm/}\mu\text{s)}\end{array}} \right] \quad \theta_t = \theta_i \left[\dfrac{c_2}{c_1} \right]$$

$$\begin{array}{l}\text{distance to}\\ \text{reflector (mm)}\end{array} = \begin{array}{l}\frac{1}{2}[\text{propagation speed (mm/}\mu\text{s)}\\ \times\ \text{pulse round-trip time (}\mu\text{s)}]\end{array} \qquad d = \tfrac{1}{2}\,ct \qquad \leftarrow$$

$$\begin{array}{l}\text{distance to}\\ \text{reflector (mm)}\end{array} \overset{*}{=} 0.77 \times \text{pulse round-trip time (}\mu\text{s)} \qquad d \overset{*}{=} 0.77t$$

Chapter 3

$$\text{operating frequency (MHz)} = \dfrac{\begin{array}{c}\text{element}\\ \text{propagation speed (mm/}\mu\text{s)}\end{array}}{2 \times \text{thickness (mm)}} \qquad f_o = \dfrac{c_m}{2w}$$

$$\text{quality factor} = \dfrac{\text{operating frequency (MHz)}}{\text{bandwidth (MHz)}} \qquad Q = \dfrac{f_o}{BW}$$

$$\text{near-zone length (mm)} = \dfrac{[\text{transducer diameter (mm)}]^2}{4 \times \text{wavelength (mm)}} \qquad \text{NZL} = \dfrac{D_T^2}{4\lambda}$$

$$\text{near-zone length (mm)} \overset{*}{=} \frac{[\text{transducer diameter (mm)}]^2 \times \text{frequency (MHz)}}{6} \qquad \text{NZL} \overset{*}{=} \frac{D_T^2 f}{6}$$

$$\text{beam area (cm}^2) = 0.8 \times [\text{beam diameter (cm)}^2] \qquad A_B = 0.8\, D_B^2$$

$$\text{axial resolution} = \frac{\text{spatial pulse length (mm)}}{2} \qquad R_A = \frac{SPL}{2} \qquad \leftarrow$$

$$\text{axial resolution} \overset{*}{=} \frac{0.77 \times \text{number of cycles in the pulse}}{\text{frequency (MHz)}} \qquad R_A \overset{*}{=} \frac{0.77n}{f}$$

$$\text{lateral resolution (mm)} = \text{beam diameter (mm)} \qquad R_L = D_B$$

Chapter 4

$$\text{pulse repetition frequency (Hz)} = \frac{\text{number of focuses} \times \text{lines}}{\text{per frame} \times \text{frame rate}} \qquad PRF = NF \times LPF \times FR$$

$$\text{maximum unambiguous imaging depth (cm)} = \frac{77}{\text{pulse repetition frequency (kHz)}} \qquad d_m = \frac{77}{PRF}$$

$$\text{penetration (cm)} \times \text{number of focuses} \times \text{lines per frame} \times \text{frame rate} \leq 77{,}000 \qquad \leftarrow$$

$$P \times NF \times LPF \times FR \leq 77{,}000$$

Chapter 5

$$\text{Doppler shift (MHz)} = \text{echo frequency (MHz)} - \text{operating frequency (MHz)}$$

$$= \frac{2 \times \text{operating frequency (MHz)} \times \text{reflector speed (m/s)} \times \cos\theta}{\text{propagation speed (m/s)}} \qquad \leftarrow$$

$$f_D = f_e - f_o = \frac{2\, f_o\, v \cos\theta}{c}$$

$$\text{reflector speed} = \frac{\text{propagation speed} \times \text{Doppler shift}}{2 \times \text{operating frequency} \times \cos\theta} \qquad \leftarrow$$

$$v \text{ (cm/s)} = \frac{77 \, f_D \text{ (kHz)}}{f_o \text{ (MHz)} \cos\theta}$$

APPENDIX B
COMPREHENSIVE EXAMINATION

For each question, choose the best answer. This examination should take less than two hours to complete (averaging less than 1 minute per question). The correct answers are found at the end of the appendix.

1. Which of the following frequencies is within the ultrasound range?
   a. 15 Hz
   b. 15 kHz
   c. 15 MHz
   d. 17,000 Hz
   e. 17 km
2. The average propagation speed in soft tissues is
   a. 1.54 mm/μs
   b. 0.501 m/s
   c. 1540 dB/cm
   d. 37.0 km/min
   e. 2 to 10 MHz
3. Pulse duration is the _____ for a pulse to occur.
   a. space
   b. time
   c. delay
   d. pressure
   e. reciprocal
4. Spatial pulse length equals the number of cycles in the pulse times
   a. period
   b. impedance
   c. beam width
   d. resolution
   e. wavelength
5. If pulse duration is 1 μs and pulse repetition period is 100 μs, duty factor is

367

a. 1 per cent
b. 10 per cent
c. 50 per cent
d. 90 per cent
e. 100 per cent

6. Which of the following depends significantly on frequency in soft tissues?
   a. propagation speed
   b. density
   c. stiffness
   d. attenuation
   e. impedance

7. The attenuation of 5-MHz ultrasound in 4 cm of soft tissue is
   a. 5 dB/cm
   b. 10 dB
   c. 2.5 MHz/cm
   d. 2 cm
   e. 5 dB/MHz

8. If the maximum value of an acoustic variable in a sound wave is 10 units and the normal (no sound) value is 7 units, the amplitude is _____ units.
   a. 1
   b. 3
   c. 7
   d. 10
   e. 17

9. Impedance equals propagation speed multiplied by
   a. density
   b. stiffness
   c. frequency
   d. attenuation
   e. path length

10. Which of the following cannot be determined from the others?
    a. frequency
    b. amplitude
    c. intensity
    d. power
    e. beam area

11. For perpendicular incidence, in medium one, density = 1 and propagation speed = 3; in medium two, density = 1.5 and propagation speed = 2. What is the intensity reflection coefficient?
    a. 0
    b. 1

c. 2

d. 3

e. 4

12. For perpendicular incidence, if the intensity transmission coefficient is 96 per cent, what is the intensity reflection coefficient?

a. 2 per cent

b. 4 per cent

c. 6 per cent

d. 8 per cent

e. 10 per cent

13. The quantitative presentation of frequencies contained in echoes is called

a. preamplification

b. digitizing

c. optical encoding

d. spectral analysis

e. all of the above

14. For oblique incidence and medium-two speed that is equal to twice medium-one speed, the transmission angle will be about _____ times the incidence angle.

a. ½

b. 17

c. 2

d. 4

e. 5

15. The range equation describes the relationship of

a. reflector distance, propagation time, and sound speed

b. distance, propagation time, and reflection coefficient

c. number of cows and sheep on a ranch

d. propagation time, sound speed, and transducer frequency

e. dynamic range and system sensitivity

16. Axial resolution in a system equals

a. four times the spatial pulse length

b. ratio of reflector size to transducer frequency

c. maximum reflector separation expected to be displayed

d. minimum reflector separation expected to be displayed

e. spatial pulse length

17. The Doppler frequency shift is caused by

a. relative motion between the transducer and the reflector

b. patient shivering in a cool room

c. a high transducer frequency and real-time scanner

d. small reflectors in the transducer beam

e. changing transducer thickness

18. A small (relative to the transducer wavelength) reflector is said to
_____ an incident sound beam.
   a. focus
   b. speculate
   c. scatter
   d. shatter
   e. amplify

19. In soft tissue, two boundaries that generate reflections are separated in axial distance (depth) by 1 mm. With a two-cycle pulse of ultrasound, the minimum frequency that will axially resolve these boundaries is
   a. 1.0 MHz
   b. 2.0 MHz
   c. 3.0 MHz
   d. 4.0 MHz
   e. 5.0 MHz

20. The frequency of an ultrasound transducer is determined primarily by which of the following:
   a. element diameter
   b. element thickness
   c. speed of sound in tissue
   d. voltage applied
   e. all of the above

21. The fundamental operating principle of medical ultrasound transducers is
   a. Snell's law
   b. Doppler's law
   c. magnetostrictive effect
   d. piezoelectric effect
   e. impedance effect

22. Transducers operating properly in pulse-echo imaging systems have a quality factor of approximately
   a. 1–3
   b. 7–10
   c. 25–50
   d. 100
   e. 500

23. The axial resolution of a transducer is determined primarily by the
   a. spatial pulse length
   b. the near-field limit
   c. the transducer diameter
   d. the acoustic impedance of tissue
   e. density

24. The lateral resolution of a transducer is determined primarily by the
    a. spatial pulse length
    b. damping
    c. the transducer diameter
    d. the acoustic impedance of tissue
    e. applied voltage
25. Which of the following quantities varies most with distance from the transducer face?
    a. axial resolution
    b. lateral resolution
    c. frequency
    d. wavelength
    e. period
26. The near-zone length for a 13-mm diameter, unfocused, 5-MHz, circular transducer is greater than that for which of the following 5-MHz transducers with diameters as listed?
    a. 19 mm
    b. 15 mm
    c. 9 mm
    d. depends on impedance
    e. none of the above
27. If the near-zone length of an unfocused transducer that is 13 mm in diameter extends (in soft tissue) 6 cm from the transducer face, at which of the following distances from the face can the lateral resolution be improved by focusing the sound from this transducer?
    a. 13 cm
    b. 8 cm
    c. 3 cm
    d. 9 cm
    e. none of the above
28. The lateral resolution of an ultrasound system depends upon
    a. the transducer diameter
    b. the transducer frequency
    c. the speed of sound in soft tissue
    d. memory and display
    e. all of the above
29. Which of the following is a characteristic of a medium through which sound is propagating?
    a. impedance
    b. intensity
    c. amplitude

    d. frequency
    e. period
30. Which of the following cannot be determined from the others?
    a. frequency
    b. period
    c. amplitude
    d. wavelength
    e. propagation speed
31. For perpendicular incidence, if the impedances of the two media are the same, there will be no
    a. inflation
    b. reflection
    c. refraction
    d. calibration
    e. b and c
32. What is the transmitted intensity if the incident intensity is 1 and the impedances are 1.00 and 2.64?
    a. 0.2
    b. 0.4
    c. 0.6
    d. 0.8
    e. 1.0
33. Increasing frequency
    a. improves resolution
    b. increases imaging depth
    c. increases refraction
    d. a and b
    e. a and c
34. Increasing intensity produced by the transducer
    a. is accomplished by increasing pulser voltage
    b. increases sensitivity of the system
    c. increases the possibility of biologic effects
    d. all of the above
    e. none of the above
35. Ultrasound bioeffects
    a. do not occur
    b. do not occur with diagnostic instruments
    c. are not confirmed below 100 mW/cm^2 SPTA
    d. b and c
    e. none of the above
36. Diagnostic ultrasound frequency range is:
    a. 2 to 10 mHz
    b. 2 to 10 kHz

c. 2 to 10 MHz
d. 3 to 15 kHz
e. none of the above

37. If propagation speeds of two media are equal, incidence angle equals
   a. reflection angle
   b. transmission angle
   c. Doppler angle
   d. a and b
   e. b and c

38. If no reflection occurs at a boundary, it always means that media impedances are equal in the case of
   a. perpendicular incidence
   b. oblique incidence
   c. refraction
   d. a and b
   e. b and c

39. Increasing spatial pulse length
   a. accompanies increased transducer damping
   b. is accompanied by decreased pulse duration
   c. improves axial resolution
   d. all of the above
   e. none of the above

40. Place the media in order of increasing sound propagation speed.
   a. gas, solid, liquid
   b. solid, liquid, gas
   c. gas, liquid, solid
   d. liquid, solid, gas
   e. solid, gas, liquid

41. What is the wavelength of 1-MHz ultrasound in tissue with a propagation speed of 1540 m/s?
   a. 1×10^6 m
   b. 1.54 mm
   c. 1540 m
   d. 1.54 cm
   e. 0.77 cm

42. What is the spatial pulse length for two cycles of ultrasound having a wavelength of 2 mm?
   a. 4 cm
   b. 4 mm
   c. 7 mm
   d. 1.5 mm
   e. 3 mm

43. Increased damping produces
a. increased bandwidth
b. decreased Q factor
c. decreased efficiency
d. all of the above
e. none of the above

44. The Doppler effect is a change in
a. intensity
b. wavelength
c. frequency
d. all of the above
e. b and c

45. What determines the lower and upper limits of the frequency range that is useful in diagnostic ultrasound?
a. resolution and imaging depth
b. intensity and resolution
c. intensity and propagation speed
d. scattering and impedance
e. impedance and wavelength

46. If no refraction occurs as an oblique sound beam passes through the boundary between two materials, what is unchanged as the boundary is crossed?
a. impedance
b. propagation speed
c. intensity
d. sound direction
e. b and d

47. If the spatial average intensity in a beam is 1 W/cm^2 and the transducer is 5 cm^2 in area, what is the total acoustic power?
a. 1 W
b. 2 W
c. 3 W
d. 4 W
e. 5 W

48. How does the propagation speed in bone compare to that in soft tissue?
a. lower
b. the same
c. higher
d. cannot say unless soft tissue is specified
e. b and c

49. Attenuation along a sound path is a decrease in
   a. frequency
   b. amplitude
   c. intensity
   d. b and c
   e. impedance

50. Reverberation causes us to think there are reflectors that are too great in
   a. impedance
   b. attenuation
   c. brightness
   d. size
   e. number

51. Doppler shift is zero when the angle between the sound direction and the movement (flow) direction is _____ degrees.
   a. 30
   b. 60
   c. 90
   d. 45
   e. none of the above

52. A focused transducer that is 13 mm in diameter has a lateral resolution at the focus of better than (i.e., smaller than)
   a. 26 mm
   b. 13 mm
   c. 6.5 mm
   d. depends on frequency
   e. none of the above

53. An important factor in the selection of a transducer for a specific application is the ultrasonic attenuation of tissue. Owing to this attenuation, a 7.5-MHz transducer should generally be used for
   a. imaging deep structures
   b. imaging superficial structures
   c. imaging both deep and shallow structures
   d. imaging adult intracranial structures
   e. all of the above

54. A real-time scan
   a. consists of many frames produced per second
   b. depends on how short a time the sonographer takes to make a scan
   c. is made only between 8 a.m. and 5 p.m.

  d. gives a gray-scale image, where the other scans give only an M-mode display
  e. none of the above

55. Which of the following is determined by the pulser in an instrument?
  a. amplitude
  b. pulse repetition frequency
  c. length of time required for a pulse to reach a specific reflector and return to the instrument
  d. more than one of the above
  e. none of the above

56. The standard United States television scanning format has _____ lines per frame and _____ frames per second.
  a. 625, 25
  b. 512, 512
  c. 512, 640
  d. 525, 30
  e. 625, 30

57. In an ultrasound imaging instrument, a cathode ray tube is used as a
  a. pulser
  b. receiver
  c. memory
  d. display
  e. scan convector

58. If the power at the output of an amplifier is 1000 times the power at the input, the gain is
  a. 60 dB
  b. 30 dB
  c. 1000 dB
  d. 1000 volts
  e. none of the above

59. The dynamic range of an ultrasound system is defined as
  a. the speed with which ultrasound examination can be performed
  b. the range over which the transducer can be manipulated
  c. the ratio of the maximum to the minimum intensity that can be displayed
  d. the range of pulser voltages applied to the transducer
  e. none of the above

60. The display will generally have a _____ dynamic range than other portions of the ultrasound instrument.
  a. larger
  b. smaller

61. The compensation (swept gain) control serves to
   a. compensate for machine instability in the warm-up time
   b. compensate for attenuation
   c. compensate for transducer aging and the ambient light in the examining room
   d. decrease patient examination time
   e. none of the above
62. A digital scan converter is a
   a. compressor
   b. receiver
   c. display
   d. computer memory
   e. none of the above
63. The number 30 in binary is
   a. 0110
   b. 1110
   c. 1001
   d. 1111
   e. none of the above
64. An ultrasound instrument that could represent 64 shades of gray would require an 8-bit memory.
   a. true
   b. false
65. Mechanical real-time devices may be designed such that
   a. a transducer is "rocked" at the skin surface
   b. a transducer is not moved at all
   c. a transducer is rocked and the beam passed through a liquid path
   d. a and c
   e. all of the above
66. Phased array systems involve the sequential switching of a small group of elements along the array.
   a. true
   b. false
67. Duplex Doppler presents:
   a. anatomic (structural) information
   b. physiologic (flow) information
   c. impedance data
   d. more than one of the above
   e. all of the above
68. Doppler shift frequencies are usually in a relatively narrow range above 20 kHz.
   a. true
   b. false

69. Enhancement is caused by a
   a. strongly reflecting structure
   b. weakly attenuating structure
   c. strongly attenuating structure
   d. frequency error
   e. propagation speed error

70. For a two-cycle pulse of 5 MHz in soft tissue, the axial resolution is
   a. 0.1 mm
   b. 0.3 mm
   c. 0.5 mm
   d. 0.7 mm
   e. 0.9 mm

71. Postprocessing is the process of assigning numbers to be placed in memory.
   a. true
   b. false

72. The minimum displayed axial dimension of a reflector is approximately equal to _____.
   a. beam diameter
   b. ½ × beam diameter
   c. 2 × beam diameter
   d. spatial pulse length
   e. ½ × spatial pulse length
   f. 2 × spatial pulse length

73. The minimum displayed lateral dimension of a reflector is approximately equal to _____.
   a. beam diameter
   b. ½ × beam diameter
   c. 2 × beam diameter
   d. spatial pulse length
   e. ½ × pulse length
   f. 2 × spatial pulse length

74. In a digital instrument, echo intensity is represented in memory by
   a. positive charge distribution
   b. a number
   c. electron density of the scan converter writing beam
   d. a and c
   e. all of the above

75. M-mode recordings have _____ dimension(s).
   a. two spatial
   b. one spatial and one temporal

c. one Doppler and one temporal
d. one Doppler and one spatial
e. b and c
76. In a mechanical sector scanner (assuming constant lines per frame) the higher the frame rate, the greater the unambiguously displayed depth.
   a. true
   b. could be true, depending on the sector angle chosen
   c. false
   d. depends on whether or not it is an annular array
   e. depends on impedance
77. Another name for rejection is
   a. threshold
   b. depth gain compensation
   c. swept gain
   d. compression
   e. demodulation
78. The binary number 01001 is _____ in decimal.
   a. 1
   b. 3
   c. 5
   d. 7
   e. 9
79. Reflectors may be added to the display because of
   a. reverberation
   b. propagation speed error
   c. enhancement
   d. oblique reflection
   e. Doppler shift
80. If the propagation speed in a soft-tissue path is 1.60 mm/μs, a diagnostic instrument assumes a propagation speed too _____ and will show reflectors too _____ the transducer.
   a. high, close to
   b. high, far from
   c. low, close to
   d. low, far from
   e. none of the above
81. The reflector information that can be obtained from an M-mode display includes
   a. distance and motion pattern
   b. transducer frequency, reflection coefficient, and distance
   c. acoustic impedance, attenuation, and motion pattern

d. all of the above
e. none of the above

82. Increasing the gain generally produces the same effect as
   a. decreasing the attenuation
   b. increasing the compression
   c. increasing the rectification
   d. both b and c
   e. all of the above

83. A gray-scale display shows
   a. gray color on a white background
   b. reflections with one brightness level
   c. a white color on a gray background
   d. a range of reflection amplitudes or intensities
   e. none of the above

84. Electric pulses from the pulser are applied to the
   a. pulser
   b. transducer
   c. receiver
   d. display
   e. memory

85. Rectification and smoothing (filtering) are parts of
   a. amplipression
   b. rejection
   c. a and b
   d. compression
   e. demodulation

86. Which of the following is performed in a receiver?
   a. amplification
   b. compensation
   c. compression
   d. demodulation
   e. all of the above

87. Continuous-wave sound is used in
   a. all ultrasound imaging instruments
   b. only bistable instruments
   c. all Doppler instruments
   d. some Doppler instruments
   e. some Fourier instruments

88. If the gain of an amplifier is reduced by 3 dB and input power is unchanged, the output power of the amplifier is _____ what it was before.
   a. equal to
   b. twice

    c. one half

    d. greater than

    e. none of the above

89. Increasing the pulse repetition frequency

    a. improves detail resolution

    b. increases maximum depth imaged unambiguously

    c. decreases maximum depth imaged unambiguously

    d. both a and b

    e. both a and c

90. If gain was 30 dB and output power is reduced by one half, the new gain is _____ dB.

    a. 15

    b. 60

    c. 33

    d. 27

    e. none of the above

91. If four shades of gray are shown on a display, each twice the brightness of the preceding one, the brightest shade is _____ times the brightness of the dimmest shade.

    a. 2

    b. 4

    c. 8

    d. 16

    e. 32

92. The dynamic range displayed in Problem 91 is _____ dB.

    a. 100

    b. 9

    c. 5

    d. 2

    e. 0

93. Phantoms with nylon lines measure

    a. resolution

    b. pulse duration

    c. SATA intensity

    d. wavelength

    e. all of the above

94. The following measure acoustic output:

    a. hydrophone

    b. optical encoder

    c. 100-mm test object

    d. all of the above

    e. none of the above

95. Real-time imaging is made possible by
a. scan converters
b. mechanically driven transducers
c. gray-scale display
d. arrays
e. both b and d

96. Gain and attenuation are usually expressed in
a. dB
b. dB/cm
c. cm
d. cm/dB
e. none of the above

97. Gray-scale display is made possible by
a. array transducers
b. cathode ray storage tubes
c. scan converters
d. b and c
e. all of the above

98. An advantage of continuous-wave Doppler over pulsed Doppler is
a. depth information
b. bidirectional
c. no aliasing
d. b and c
e. all of the above

99. With which of the following is time on one axis?
a. B mode
b. B scan
c. M mode
d. a la mode
e. none of the above

100. In Doppler color-flow instruments, color represents
a. sign (+ or −) of Doppler shift
b. flow direction
c. magnitude of the Doppler shift
d. amplitude of the Doppler shift
e. more than one of the above

101. Attenuation is corrected by
a. demodulation
b. desegregation
c. decompression
d. compensation
e. decompensation

102. What must be known to calculate distance to a reflector?
  a. attenuation, speed, density
  b. attenuation, impedance
  c. attenuation, absorption
  d. travel time, speed
  e. density, speed

103. Which of the following improve(s) sound transmission from the transducer element into the tissue?
  a. matching layer
  b. Doppler effect
  c. damping material
  d. coupling medium
  e. a and d

104. Lateral resolution is improved by
  a. damping
  b. pulsing
  c. focusing
  d. reflecting
  e. absorbing

105. Voltage pulses occur at the output of the
  a. pulser
  b. transducer
  c. receiver
  d. display
  e. a, b, and c

106. The Doppler effect for a scatterer moving toward the sound source causes the scattered sound (compared to the incident sound) received by the transducer to have
  a. increased intensity
  b. decreased intensity
  c. increased impedance
  d. increased frequency
  e. decreased impedance

107. Axial resolution is improved by
  a. damping
  b. pulsing
  c. focusing
  d. reflecting
  e. absorbing

108. Which of the following is (are) dynamic (real-time)?
  a. Doppler
  b. B scan

   c. M mode

   d. all of the above

   e. none of the above

109. Duplex Doppler instruments include _____.

   a. pulsed Doppler

   b. continuous-wave Doppler

   c. B-scan imaging

   d. dynamic imaging

   e. more than one of the above

110. If the Doppler shifts from normal and stenotic carotid arteries are 4 kHz and 10 kHz, respectively, for which will there be a problem with a pulse repetition frequency of 7 kHz?

   a. normal

   b. stenotic

   c. both

   d. neither

111. The receiver in a Doppler system compares the _____ of the voltage generator and the voltage from the receiving transducer.

   a. wavelength

   b. intensity

   c. impedance

   d. frequency

   e. all of the above

112. A digital imaging instrument divides the cross-sectional image into _____.

   a. frequencies

   b. bits

   c. pixels

   d. binaries

   e. wavelengths

113. Which of the following produce(s) a sector-scan format?

   a. rotating mechanical real-time transducer

   b. oscillating mechanical real-time transducer

   c. phased array

   d. oscillating mirror

   e. all of the above

114. The piezoelectric effect describes how _____ is converted into _____ by a _____.

   a. electricity, an image, display

   b. incident sound, reflected sound, boundary

   c. ultrasound, electricity, transducer

   d. ultrasound, heat, tissue

   e. none of the above

115. Propagation speed in soft tissues
   a. is directly proportional to frequency
   b. is inversely proportional to frequency
   c. is directly proportional to intensity
   d. is inversely proportional to intensity
   e. none of the above

116. The frequencies used in diagnostic ultrasound imaging
   a. are much lower than those used in Doppler measurements
   b. determine imaging depth in tissue
   c. determine imaging resolution
   d. all of the above
   e. b and c

117. As frequency is increased
   a. wavelength increases
   b. a three-cycle ultrasound pulse decreases in length
   c. imaging depth decreases
   d. propagation speed decreases
   e. b and c

118. In the Doppler equation

$$f_D = \frac{2 \, fv \cos \theta}{c - v \cos \theta}$$

which can normally be ignored?
   a. $v \cos \theta$ in the denominator
   b. $v \cos \theta$ in the numerator
   c. f
   d. f_D
   e. b and c

119. For which of the following is the reflected frequency less than the incident frequency?
   a. advancing flow
   b. receding flow
   c. perpendicular flow
   d. laminar flow
   e. all of the above

120. Focusing
   a. improves lateral resolution
   b. improves axial resolution
   c. increases beam width in the focal region
   d. shortens pulse length
   e. increases duty factor

Comprehensive Examination Answers

Following each answer is the section number in which the subject is discussed. Some answers also have explanatory comments.

   1. c. 2.1. Ultrasound is sound having a frequency greater than 20 kHz (0.02 MHz). Answer e is not expressed in frequency units.
   2. a. 2.1. Propagation speeds in soft tissues are in the range of about 1.4 to 1.6 mm/μs. Answers c and e are not expressed in speed units.
   3. b. 2.2.
   4. e. 2.2. The wavelength is the length of each cycle in a pulse.
   5. a. 2.2. Duty factor is pulse duration divided by pulse repetition period.
   6. d. 2.3. Propagation speed and impedance increase only slightly with frequency.
   7. b. 2.3. The attenuation coefficient of 5-MHz ultrasound is approximately 2.5 dB/cm. The attenuation coefficient multiplied by the path length yields the attenuation in dB. Only answer b is given in attenuation (dB) units.
   8. b. 2.3. Amplitude is the maximum amount that an acoustic variable varies from the normal value. In this case, 10 minus 7 units.
   9. a. 2.1. This is the characteristic impedance.
  10. a. 2.3. Amplitude, intensity, power, and beam area are all related to each other. If two of these are known, the others can be found. Frequency is independent of these. All four of them can be known and yet frequency can remain undetermined.
  11. a. 2.4. Impedance 1 equals 3, which equals impedance 2; thus, there is no reflection.
  12. b. 2.4. If 96 per cent of the intensity is transmitted, 4 per cent was reflected because what is not reflected is transmitted (i.e., the two must add up to 100 per cent).
  13. d. 3.1 and 6.3. Spectral comes from "spectrum," referring to color spectrum. A prism is an optical spectrum analyzer that breaks down white light into its component colors.
  14. c. 2.4. If the second speed is twice the first speed, then the transmission angle is twice the incidence angle.
  15. a. 2.4. Reflector distance equals ½ × speed × time.
  16. d. 3.4. If reflectors are separated by less than the axial resolution, they are not separated on the display.
  17. a. 5.2.
  18. c. 2.4. Scattering occurs with rough surfaces and with hetero-

geneous media (made up of small particles relative to the wavelength). Large flat smooth surfaces produce specular reflections.

19. b. 3.4. Axial resolution is equal to one half the spatial pulse length. Spatial pulse length is equal to the number of cycles in the pulse multiplied by wavelength. Wavelength is equal to propagation speed divided by frequency. For 1 MHz, wavelength is 1.54 mm, spatial pulse length is 2×1.54, and axial resolution is 1.54 mm, so that two reflectors separated by 1 mm would not be resolved. For 2 MHz, the resolution is 0.77 and the reflectors will be resolved.

20. b. 3.1. The operating frequency of a transducer is such that its thickness is equal to one half the wavelength in the transducer element material.

21. d. 3.1. Transducer elements expand and contract when a voltage is applied, and, conversely, when returning echoes apply pressure to the element, a voltage is generated.

22. a. 3.1. For highly damped transducers, the quality factor (Q) is approximately equal to the number of cycles in the pulse.

23. a. 3.4. Axial resolution is equal to one half the spatial pulse length.

24. c. 3.4. Lateral resolution is equal to beam width. Near-zone length is dependent on transducer diameter and, thus, so is the lateral resolution at any given distance from the transducer.

25. b. 3.4. Beam width changes with distance from transducer and, thus, so does lateral resolution.

26. c. 3.2. Near-zone length increases with transducer diameter so that the only transducer that would have a shorter near-zone length would be a transducer of smaller diameter.

27. c. 3.2. Focusing can only be accomplished in the near zone of a beam.

28. e. 3.4. Answers a, b, and c all affect the beam. Resolution of the system is also affected by the electronics of the instrument.

29. a. 2.1. All the others are characteristics of the sound.

30. c. 2.1. Frequency, period, wavelength, and propagation speed are all related to each other. However, all four of these can be known and yet the amplitude can remain undetermined.

31. e. 2.4. For perpendicular incidence, there is no refraction. For equal impedances, there is no reflection.

32. d. 2.4.

$$\text{IRC} = \left[\frac{2.64 - 1.00}{2.64 + 1.00}\right]^2 = \left[\frac{1.64}{3.64}\right]^2 = (0.45)^2 = 0.2$$

For an intensity reflection coefficient of 0.2 and an incident intensity of one, the reflected intensity is 0.2 and the transmitted intensity is 0.8.

33. a. 3.4, 2.3, and 2.4. Imaging depth decreases with increasing frequency and frequency has no effect on refraction.

34. d. 4.1 and 7.3.

35. c. 7.3. This is the AIUM statement on *in vivo* mammalian bioeffects.

36. c. 3.4. Frequencies lower than this range do not provide the needed resolution, whereas frequencies greater than this range do not allow for adequate imaging depth for medical purposes.

37. d. 2.4. Incidence angle always equals reflection angle and, for equal propagation speeds, it equals transmission angle as well.

38. a. 2.4. For oblique incidence, it is possible to have no reflection, even if media impedances are unequal.

39. e. 2.2, 3.1, and 3.4. Increased transducer damping decreases the spatial pulse length. Increasing spatial pulse length is accompanied by increased pulse duration and degraded axial resolution.

40. c. 2.1

41. b. 2.1. Wavelength is equal to propagation speed divided by frequency.

42. b. 2.2. Spatial pulse length is equal to wavelength multiplied by the number of cycles in the pulse.

43. d. 3.1.

44. e. 5.2. If frequency changes, wavelength changes also.

45. a. 3.4. See answer to Problem 36.

46. e. 2.4. No refraction means that there is no change in sound direction. This is a result of no change in propagation speed (equal propagation speeds on both sides of the boundary).

47. e. 2.3. If there is 1 W in each square centimeter of area, then there are 5 W in 5 cm² of area.

48. c. 2.1. Speeds in solids are higher than in liquids. Soft tissue behaves acoustically as a liquid (it is mostly water).

49. d. 2.3

50. e. 6.1. Reverberation adds additional reflectors on the display deeper than the true ones.

51. c. 5.2.

52. c. 3.2. An unfocused 13-mm transducer has a beam width of 6.5 mm at the near-zone length. Focusing would reduce the lateral resolution below this value (i.e., improve it).

53. b. 2.3. A 7.5-MHz transducer can image to a depth of only a few centimeters in tissue.

54. a. 3.3 and 4.4. The other answers make little sense.

55. d. 4.2 (a and b).

56. d. 4.4.

57. d. 4.4.

58. b. 4.2. For each 10 dB, there is a factor of 10 increase in power.

59. c. 4.2.

60. b. 4.2.

61. b. 4.2.

62. d. 4.3.

63. e. 4.3. Decimal numbers greater than 15 require at least five bits in a binary number. The number 30 in binary is 11110.

64. b. 4.3. 64 shades require a 6-bit memory.

65. e. 3.3. In the answer b, the beam can be reflected off an oscillating acoustic mirror (reflector).

66. b. 3.3. This is a description of a linear switched or sequenced array, rather than a phased array.

67. d. 5.3. Answers a and b are both correct. Anatomic data are provided by the real-time B scan and physiologic data are provided by the pulsed Doppler portion of the instrument.

68. b. 5.2. Physiologic Doppler shift frequencies are usually in the audible frequency range.

69. b. 6.2.

70. b. 3.4.

$$AR = \tfrac{1}{2}SPL = \tfrac{1}{2}n \times \frac{c}{f} = \tfrac{1}{2}(2)\frac{1.54}{5} = 0.3$$

71. b. 4.3. Postprocessing is the assignment of display brightness to numbers coming out of memory.

72. e. 3.4.

73. a. 3.4.

74. b. 4.3.

75. b. 4.4. In M mode, echo depth is displayed as a function of time.

76. c. 6.1. For constant lines per frame, a constant number of pulses must be emitted per frame, and the higher the frame rate, the greater the pulse repetition frequency. Therefore unambiguously displayed depth would decrease (less time for echoes to return before the next pulse is emitted).

77. a. 4.2.

78. e. 4.3. One plus eight equals nine.

79. a. 6.1.

80. c. 2.4. The instrument assumes a speed of 1.54 mm/μs. Echoes will arrive sooner because of their higher propagation speed and will be placed in closer proximity than they should be.

81. a. 4.4.

82. a. 2.3 and 4.2. Increasing gain and decreasing attenuation each increase echo intensity.

83. d. 4.3 and 4.4.

84. b. 3.1 and 4.1.

85. e. 4.2.

86. e. 4.2.

87. d. 5.3. All imaging instruments and some Doppler instruments use pulsed ultrasound.

88. c. 4.2. A reduction of 3 dB is a 50 per cent reduction.

89. c. 3.4, 4.4. Pulse repetition frequency has no effect on detail resolution.

90. d. 4.2. See answer to Problem 88.

91. c. 4.3 and 4.4.

92. b. 4.2. A factor of 8 is three doublings (i.e., 3 + 3 + 3 dB).

93. a. 7.1.

94. a. 7.2.

95. e. 3.3.

96. a. 2.3 and 4.2.

97. c. 4.3.

98. c. 5.3.

99. c. 4.4.

100. e. 5.4 (a, b, and c).

101. d. 4.2.

102. d. 2.4. The range equation relates these three quantities.

103. e. 3.1. The matching layer improves sound transmission by reducing the reflection at the transducer–skin boundary. A coupling medium improves sound transmission by removing the air layer between the transducer and the skin.

104. c. 3.2.

105. e. 3.1, 4.1, and 4.2.

106. d. 5.2.

107. a. 3.4.

108. d. 4.4, 5.3, 5.4. All of these modes are updated many times each second.

109. e. 5.3. They include pulsed Doppler and dynamic (B-scan) imaging.

110. c. 6.3. Both Doppler shifts exceed one half the pulse repetition frequency. The problem is aliasing.

111. d. 5.3.

112. c. 4.3.

113. e. 3.3.

114. c. 3.1.

115. e. 2.1. Propagation speed is independent of frequency and intensity.
116. e. 2.3 and 3.4.
117. e. 2.2 and 2.3.
118. a. 5.2. Physiologic flow speeds are small compared to the speed of sound in tissues.
119. b. 5.2.
120. a. 3.2 and 3.4.

References

1. Kremkau, F.W.: Doppler Ultrasound: Principles and Instruments. Philadelphia, W.B. Saunders Co., 1990.

2. McDicken, W.N.: Diagnostic Ultrasonics: Principles and Use of Instruments, 3rd ed. New York, Churchill Livingstone, 1991.

3. Hykes, D.L., Hedrick, W.R., and Starchman, D.E.: Ultrasound Physics and Instrumentation, 2nd ed. St. Louis, Mosby–Year Book, 1991.

4. Fish, P.: Physics and Instrumentation of Diagnostic Medical Ultrasound. New York, John Wiley & Sons, 1990.

5. Hill, C.R.: Physical Principles of Medical Ultrasonics. Chichester, England, Ellis Horwood, 1986.

6. Hussey, M.: Basic Physics and Technology of Medical Diagnostic Ultrasound. New York, Elsevier, 1985.

7. Powis, R.L., and Powis, W.J.: A Thinker's Guide to Ultrasonic Imaging. Baltimore, Urban & Schwarzenberg, 1984.

8. Evans, D.H., McDicken, W.N., Skidmore, R., and Woodcock, J,P.: Doppler Ultrasound: Physics, Instrumentation, and Clinical Applications. New York, John Wiley & Sons, 1989.

9. Powis, R.L., and Schwartz, R.A.: Practical Doppler Ultrasound for the Clinician. Baltimore, Williams and Wilkins, 1991.

10. Smith, H.J., and Zagzebski, J.A.: Basic Doppler Physics. Madison, WI, Medical Physics Publishing, 1991.

11. Duck, F.A.: Physical properties of tissue. *In* Acoustic Properties of Tissue at Ultrasonic Frequencies. New York, Academic Press, 1990.

12. Nelson, L.H., and Kremkau, F.W.: Introduction to transvaginal imaging. Obstet. Gynecol. Clin. North Am. *18:*683–692, 1991.

13. Zemanek, J.: Beam behavior within the nearfield of a vibrating piston. J. Acoust. Soc. Am. *49:*181–191, 1971.

14. Kremkau, F.W.: Clinical benefit of higher acoustic output levels. Ultrasound Med. Biol. *15* (Suppl. 1): 69–70, 1989.

15. Pizer, S.M., and Zimmerman, J.B.: Color display in ultrasonography. Ultrasound Med. Biol. *9:*331–345, 1983.

16. Thickman, D.I., Ziskin, M.C., and Goldenberg, N.J.: Effect of display format on detectability. J. Ultrasound Med. *2:*117–121, 1983.

17. Kremkau, F.W.: Doppler principles. Semin. Roentgenol. *27:*6–16, 1992.

18. Kremkau, F.W.: Principles of color flow imaging. J. Vascular Technol. *15:*104–111, 1991.

19. Kremkau, F.W.: Principles and instrumentation. *In* Merritt, C.R.B.: Doppler Color Imaging. New York, Churchill Livingstone, 1992.

20. Kremkau, F.W.: Principles and pitfalls of real-time color-flow imaging. *In* Bernstein, E.F.: Vascular Diagnosis, 4th ed. St. Louis, Mosby–Year Book, 1993.

21. Tegeler, C.H., Kremkau, F.W., and Hitchings, L.P.: Color velocity imaging: Introduction to a new ultrasound technology. J. Neuroimaging *1:*85–90, 1991.

22. Kremkau, F.W., and Taylor, K.J.W.: Artifacts in ultrasound imaging. J. Ultrasound Med. *5:*227–237, 1986.

23. Sanders, R.C.: Atlas of Ultrasonographic Artifacts and Variants, 2nd ed. St. Louis, Mosby–Year Book, 1992.

24. Goldstein, A.: Quality Assurance in Diagnostic Ultrasound. Bethesda, MD, American Institute of Ultrasound in Medicine, 1980.

25. Banjavic, R.A.: Design and maintenance of a quality assurance program for diagnostic ultrasound equipment. Semin. Ultrasound, *4:*10–26, 1983.

26. AIUM Standards Committee: Standard Methods for Measuring Performance of Pulse-Echo Ultrasound Imaging Equipment. Rockville, MD, American Institute of Ultrasound in Medicine, 1991.

27. Ziskin, M.C., and Lewin, P.A. (ed.): Ultrasonic Exposimetry. Boca Raton, CRC Press, 1993.

28. Kremkau, F.W. (ed.): IEEE Guide for Medical Ultrasound Field Parameter Measurements. New York, Institute of Electrical and Electronics Engineers, 1990.

29. Preston, R.C.: Output Measurement for Medical Ultrasound. New York, Springer-Verlag, 1991.

30. Acoustic Output Task Group: Acoustic Output Measurement and Labeling Standard for Diagnostic Ultrasound Equipment. Rockville, MD, American Institute of Ultrasound in Medicine, 1992.

31. Macdonald, M.C., and Madsen, E.L.: Method for determining the SATA and SAPA intensities for real-time ultrasonographic scanning modes. J. Ultrasound Med. *11:*11–23, 1992.

32. AIUM Manufacturers' Commendation Panel: Acoustical Data for Diagnostic Ultrasound Equipment. Rockville, MD, American Institute of Ultrasound in Medicine, 1984, 1991.

33. Ide, M., Zagzebski, J.A., and Duck, F.A.: Acoustic output of diagnostic equipment. Ultrasound Med. Biol. *15* (Suppl. 1): 47–65, 1989.

34. Duck, F.A., and Martin, K.: Trends in diagnostic ultrasound exposure. Phys. Med. Biol. *36:*1423–1432, 1991.

35. Kremkau, F.W.: Biologic effects and safety. *In* Rumack, C.M., Wilson, S.R., and Charboneau, J.W. (eds.): Diagnostic Ultrasound. St. Louis, Mosby–Year Book, 1991, pp. 19–29.

36. Bioeffects Committee: Safety Considerations for Diagnostic Ultrasound. Rockville, MD, American Institute of Ultrasound in Medicine, 1991.

37. American Institute of Ultrasound in Medicine: Bioeffects Considerations for the Safety of Diagnostic Ultrasound. J. Ultrasound Med., 7 (Suppl. S1–S38): 1988.

38. National Council on Radiation Protection and Measurements: Biological Effects of Ultrasound: Mechanisms and Clinical Applications. Bethesda, MD, National Council on Radiation Protection, 1983.

39. National Council on Radiation Protection and Measurements: Exposure Criteria for Medical Diagnostic Ultrasound: I. Criteria Based on Thermal Mechanisms. Bethesda, MD, National Council on Radiation Protection, 1992.

40. Nyborg, W.L., and Ziskin, M.C.: Biological Effects of Ultrasound. New York, Churchill Livingstone, 1985.

41. Repacholi, M.H., Grandolfo, M., and Rindi, A.: Ultrasound: Medical Applications, Biological Effects, and Hazard Potential. New York, Plenum Press, 1987.

42. Suslick, K.S.: Ultrasound: Its Chemical, Physical, and Biological Effects. New York, VCH Publishers, 1988.

43. Output Display Standard Joint Task Group: Standard for Real-Time Display of Thermal and Mechanical Acoustic Output Indices on Diagnostic Ultrasound Equipment. Rockville, MD, American Institute of Ultrasound in Medicine, 1992.

44. World Health Organization: Environmental Health Criteria 22: Ultrasound. Geneva, Switzerland, World Health Organization, 1982.

45. AIUM: Bioeffects and Safety of Diagnostic Ultrasound. Rockville, MD, American Institute of Ultrasound in Medicine, 1993.

46. Kremkau, F.W.: Bioeffects and safety I. Heat. J. Diagnostic Med. Sonography 9: in press.

47. Kremkau, F.W.: Bioeffects and safety II. Cavitation. J. Diagnostic Med. Sonography 9: in press.

48. Kremkau, F.W.: Bioeffects and safety III. Output Indices and Bioeffects Statement. J Diagnostic Med. Sonography 9: in press.

INDEX

Note: page numbers in *italics* refer to illustrations; those followed by t indicate tables.